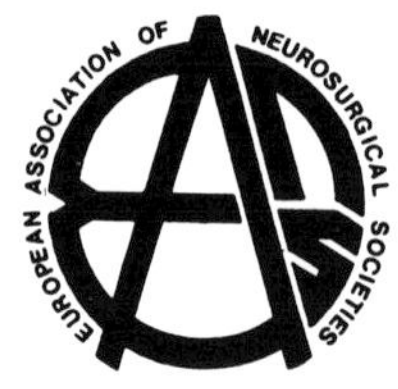

Sponsored by the
European Association of Neurosurgical Societies

Advances
and Technical Standards
in Neurosurgery

Vol. 23

Edited by
F. Cohadon, Bordeaux (Editor-in-Chief),
V. V. Dolenc, Ljubljana, J. Lobo Antunes, Lisbon,
H. Nornes, Oslo, J. D. Pickard, Cambridge,
H.-J. Reulen, Munich, A. J. Strong, London,
N. de Tribolet, Lausanne, C. A. F. Tulleken, Utrecht

SpringerWienNewYork

With 89 partly coloured Figures

© 1997 Springer-Verlag/Wien
Printed in Austria

Library of Congress Catalogue Card Number 74-10499

Printing: A. Holzhausens Nfg., A-1070 Wien
Graphic design: Ecke Bonk

Printed on acid-free and chlorine-free bleached paper

ISSN 0095-4829

ISBN 3-211-82827-3 Springer-Verlag Wien New York

Valedictory Note

At the time of his retirement from active practice in 1995, *Professor Lindsay Symon* stepped down as Editor-in-Chief of "Advances and Technical Standards in Neurosurgery". I would like to express, in the name of all the members of the Editorial Board, our appreciation and gratitude to him for his distinguished service to our Publication over the last ten years. Under his direction "Advances and Technical Standards" has maintained and reinforced its position as a major source of references in Neurosurgery throughout Europe and beyond, amply fulfilling the aims of its founders in 1974.

During his period of office it was the priviledge of the Board to meet every first Saturday of December at the National Hospital, Queen Square; the intellectual vigor and integrity, and the spirit of leadership of *Lindsay Symon* has made each one of these meetings a feast of shared knowledge and friendship. The work of the Editorial Board continues in Bordeaux in the same tradition, dedicated to academic excellence, professional reliability and, not the least, European friendship.

François Cohadon
Editor-in-Chief

Preface

As an addition to the European postgraduate training system for young neurosurgeons we began to publish in 1974 this series of Advances and Technical Standards in Neurosurgery which was later sponsored by the European Association of Neurosurgical Societies.

This series was first discussed in 1972 at a combined meeting of the Italian and German Neurosurgical Societies in Taormina, the founding fathers of the series being Jean Brihaye, Bernard Pertuiset, Fritz Loew and Hugo Krayenbühl. Thus were established the principles of European co-operation which have been born from the European spirit, flourished in the European Association, and have throughout been associated with this series.

The fact that the English language is well on the way to becoming the international medium at European scientific conferences is a great asset in terms of mutual understanding. Therefore we have decided to publish all contributions in English, regardless of the native language of the authors.

All contributions are submitted to the entire editorial board before publication of any volume.

Our series is not intended to compete with the publications of original scientific papers in other neurosurgical journals. Our intention is, rather, to present fields of neurosurgery and related areas in which important recent advances have been made. The contributions are written by specialists in the given fields and constitute the first part of each volume.

In the second part of each volume, we publish detailed descriptions of standard operative procedures, furnished by experienced clinicians; in these articles the authors describe the techniques they employ and explain the advantages, difficulties and risks involved in the various procedures. This part is intended primarily to assist young neurosurgeons in their postgraduate training. However, we are convinced that it will also be useful to experienced, fully trained neurosurgeons.

The descriptions of standard operative procedures are a novel feature of our series. We intend that this section should make available the findings of European neurosurgeons, published perhaps in less familiar languages, to neurosurgeons beyond the boundaries of the authors' countries and of Europe. We will however from time to time bring to the notice of our European colleagues, operative procedures from colleagues in the United

States and Japan, who have developed techniques which may now be regarded as standard. Our aim throughout is to promote contacts among neurosurgeons in Europe and throughout the world neurosurgical community in general.

We hope therefore that surgeons not only in Europe, but throughout the world will profit by this series of Advances and Technical Standards in Neurosurgery.

The Editors

Contents

A. Advances

A Critical Review of the Current Status and Possible Developments in Brain Transplantation. By S. REHNCRONA, Department of Neurosurgery, University Hospital of Lund, Lund (Sweden)

The Normal and Pathological Physiology of Brain Water. By K. G. Go, Department of Neurosurgery, University of Groningen, Groningen (The Netherlands)

B. Technical Standards

Transfacial Approaches to the Skull Base. By D. UTTLEY, Department of Neurosurgery, Atkinson Morley's Hospital, Wimbledon, London (U.K.)

Presigmoid Approaches to Skull Base Lesions. By M. T. Lawton,[1] C. P. Daspit,[2] and R. F. Spetzler[1], Division of [1]Neurological Surgery and [2]Neuro-Otology, Barrow Neurological Institute, St. Joseph's Hospital and Medical Center, Phoenix, AZ (U.S.A.)

Anterior Approaches to Non-Traumatic Lesions of the Thoracic Spine. By A. Monteiro Trindade and J. Lobo Antunes, Hospital Santa Maria, Lisbon (Portugal)

The Far Lateral Approach to Lumbar Disc Herniations. By F. PORCHET, H. FANKHAUSER, and N. DE TRIBOLET, Department of Neurosurgery, University of Lausanne (Switzerland)

List of Contributors

Daspit, C. P., MD, Division of Neuro-Otology, Barrow Neurological Institute, St. Joseph's Hospital and Medical Center, Phoenix, AZ, U.S.A.

Fankhauser, H., MD, Service de Neurochirurgie, Centre Hospitalier, Universitaire Vaudois, CH-1011 Lausanne, Switzerland.

Go, K. G., MD, PD, Department of Neurosurgery, University of Groningen, Oostersingel 59, Postbus 30.001, NL-9700 RB Groningen, The Netherlands.

Lawton, M. T., MD, c/o Neuroscience Publ. Office, Barrow Neurological Institute, 350 West Thomas Road, Phoenix, AZ 85013-496, U.S.A.

Lobo Antunes, J., MD, PhD, Hospital de Santa Maria, Universidade de Lisboa, Faculdade de Medicino-Neurocirurgia, Av. Prof. Egas Moniz, P-1699 Lisboa, Portugal.

Monteiro Trindade, A., MD, Hospital de Santa Maria, Universidade de Lisboa, Faculdade de Medicino-Neurocirurgia, Av. Prof. Egas Moniz, P-1699 Lisboa, Portugal.

Porchet, F., MD, Service de Neurochirurgie, Centre Hospitalier, Universitaire Vaudois, CH-1011 Lausanne, Switzerland.

Rehncrona, S., MD, PhD, Department of Neurosurgery, University Hospital, S-22185 Lund, Sweden.

Spetzler, R. F., MD, c/o Neuroscience Publ. Office, Barrow Neurological Institute, 350 West Thomas Road, Phoenix, AZ 85013-496, U.S.A.

de Tribolet, N., MD, Service de Neurochirurgie, Centre Hospitalier, Universitaire Vaudois, CH-1011 Lausanne, Switzerland.

Uttley, D., MD, Department of Neurosurgery, Atkinson Morley's Hospital, Wimbledon, London SW20 0NE, U.K.

A. Advances

A Critical Review of the Current Status and Possible Developments in Brain Transplantation

S. REHNCRONA

Department of Neurosurgery, University Hospital of Lund, Lund (Sweden)

With 4 Figures

Contents

Introduction

Currently much interest is focussed on the possibilities for treatment of neurodegenerative disorders by transplantation of specific transmitter releasing cells to the central nervous system. The term "neurodegenerative" is used to describe disorders characterized by cell loss in the central nervous system and includes Parkinson's disease, Huntington's disease, Alzheimer's disease and amyotrophic lateral sclerosis. They all have in common that their exact etiology and pathogenesis is unknown and that they curtail both the quality and quantity of life. They often slowly progress to a state of severe incapacitation of the sufferer with neurological symptoms related to which specific cell type(s) and neurotransmitter systems are affected. Since no therapy can be offered against the basic etiologies, the treatment, if any, is directed towards symptomatic relief (for comprehensive reviews the reader is referred to Calne 1994). The exciting progress made by biomedical science during the last two decades in understanding the basic mechanisms of growth, behaviour and function of neural transplants in the mammalian central nervous system has opened the possibility for a different and, at least in theory, curative therapeutic strategy aiming at repairing the brain (Dunnett and Björklund 1994). The concept may include possibilities for either a partial or even total recovery of function by replacement of lost cell populations to restore specific neurotransmitter systems, neural circuits or to remyelinate fibers in demyelination disorders.

The clinical application of such a strategy must fulfil certain basic requirements. First, it must rely upon solid data from cell biology and experimental research using relevant animal models that mimic the human disease as closely as possible. Second, neural grafting presumes the loss of a known specific cell population and not a widespread cell death in the central nervous system. Third, other therapies must either be lacking or ineffective. Fourth, there should be a reasonable chance that the graft remains unaffected by the disease process itself. Fifth, there must be the means to validate graft survival and function. These criteria are best fulfilled in Parkinson's disease, and most of the experimental as well as virtually all current clinical data pertain to this disease. Therefore, the present review will focus on the current experience of neural tissue grafting in Parkinson's disease, and will use this experience as a model for discussing similar therapeutic strategies in other disorders.

Grafting in Parkinson's Disease

Parkinson's disease is a disorder of movement, the cardinal symptoms being akinesia, rigidity, postural and gait abnormalities as well as tremor. The most conspicuous pathophysiological change underlying the disease is a loss of neurons in the substantia nigra, pars compacta, with degeneration of the mesostriatal pathway, leading to a depletion of dopamine releasing terminals mainly in the striatum and other forebrain regions. Clinical manifestation of the disease occurs first when about 50–70% of the nigral dopamine projections to striatum are lost (e.g. Fearnley and Lees 1994). Pharmacological treatment with the dopamine precursor L-dopa was introduced in the 1960s and caused a dramatic improvement of motor function in most cases. The L-dopa treatment was later combined with decarboxylase inhibitors and directly acting dopamine receptor agonists. However, in time it became evident that even if primarily effective the good response of medication is often only temporary. Thus, after approximately 5–10 years of medical treatment the course of the disease may reach a complication phase, characterized by severe fluctuations in motor performance with "on-off" phenomena and more or less severe pharmacological side-effects.

The classical neurosurgical treatment is to restore the balance between hyperactive central pathways and those with low activity either by selectively placed surgical lesions or, as recently introduced, by deep brain stimulation. Fifty years ago this treatment even included lesions of the head of the caudate nucleus and transsections of pallidofugal pathways while, thalamotomy and pallidotomy still have immediate importance (Meyers 1942, Browder 1948, Narabayashi *et al.* 1956, Cooper and Bravo 1958, Svennilson *et al.* 1960, Laitinen *et al.* 1992). Most recently, promising results have been achieved with thalamic and subthalamic electrical stimulation techniques using permanently implanted deep brain electrodes (BenAbid *et al.* 1991, 1993, Blond *et al.* 1992). The current clinical experience with brain tissue grafting is too limited to allow any comparisons with these methods.

Experimental Background

In 1976, experiments demonstrated survival of fetal monoaminergic neurons transplanted into the rat brain (Björklund *et al.* 1976). Three years later it was reported that striatal implants of embryonic dopamine rich allografts from the ventral mesencephalon not only survived but could reverse the symptoms in rat models of Parkinson's disease (Björklund and Stenevi 1979, Perlow *et al.* 1979). Using the same experimental model, based upon 6-OH-dopamine lesions of the mesostriatal tract in the rat, it was shown that the graft reinnervated the host brain with formation of synaptic contacts (Freund *et al.* 1985, Mahalik *et al.* 1985, Clarke *et al.* 1988b) and that the reduction in symptoms correlated to a spontaneous release of dopamine from the grafted cells (Zetterström *et al.* 1986, Strecker *et al.* 1987). Xenografts from the embryonic human ventral mesencephalon transplanted to the adult rat striatum were shown to develop, integrate and exert functional effects (Brundin *et al.* 1988, Clarke *et al.* 1988a). These results provided the necessary experimental evidence to justify human trials. Furthermore, the observations made in rats were soon reproduced in non-human primate models using either 1-methyl-4-phenyl-1,2,3,6-tetrahydropyridine (MPTP) or 6-OH-dopamine to induce striatal dopamine depletion mimicking human parkinsonism (Bakay *et al.* 1985, 1987, Dunnett and Annett 1991).

At the beginning of the 1980s the adrenal medulla was introduced as an alternative source of catecholamine-producing graft (Olson *et al.* 1980, Freed *et al.* 1981). A series of experiments both in rodents and in non-human primate models characterized the effects of chromaffin tissue grafts in striatum-denervated animals (Strömberg *et al.* 1984, 1985, Freed *et al.* 1986, Morihisa *et al.* 1987), indicating a therapeutic potential for auto-transplantation of adrenal chromaffin tissue.

Graft-Host Brain Interactions

The rationale behind clinical brain tissue/cell grafting was originally to replace dead neurons with new ones to recreate a physiologically well integrated system. A graft to the brain may, however, exert clinical effects by several mechanisms working either alone or together:

1. Trophic effects. Grafts may stimulate reinnervation by inducing sprouting from remaining non-degenerated neuronal sources in the host brain. Such a mechanism may be mediated by nerve growth factors produced either by the graft or by the host brain in response to the graft or to the surgical trauma. This possibility presumes a certain amount of remaining undisturbed host neurons and fibers to sprout from. Due to progression of cell degeneration, such a mechanism may be assumed to be only temporary.

2. Micropump-, paracrine or endocrine mechanisms. The transplanted cells may function like small localized pharmacological factories producing the specific neurotransmitter(s), that the brain is devoid of. By release and diffusion (paracrine mechanism) of the transmitter, they might affect postsynaptic receptors in the same way as medical treatment with receptor agonists. The principal difference from pharmacological treatment is that the production of transmitter occurs in the close vicinity of the receptor sites, with the possibility for a more localized receptor interaction and fewer side effects from generalized receptor interactions. An endocrine mechanism, i.e. transportation of the transmitter by the local circulation from the transplant site to receptor sites in the vicinity, implies remaining defects in the blood-brain barrier. To have clinical value these possibilities should include ways of controlling the amount of transmitter released.

3. Semi-integrated cellgrafts. Ectopically placed grafts that reinnervate host neurons by synaptic efferent connections. They may receive an afferent input, but from other sources than the normal. Nigral cell grafts in the striatum is an example of this type.

4. Totally integrated cellgrafts. The grafted cells extend axons as well as dendritic processes with both efferent and afferent synaptic connections with host brain cells allowing normal transmission as well as a normal regulatory input. Since this mechanism affords the most physiological way of restoration, it seems to be the most attractive. However, in Parkinson's disease for example complete physiologic integation would imply grafting to the substantia nigra. Considering the anatomical localization such a procedure may increase the surgical risk, and the distance for axonal growth to reach the effector cells needing reinnervation may be too long.

Rationale for the First Clincal Experiments

The first human experiments with grafting to the brain were stimulated by the findings that dopaminergic fetal cell grafts survived, were integrated and could improve symptoms in animals with experimentally induced parkinsonism. Since none of the human neurodegenerative disorders occurs in animals, the specific aims of the first human trials were to establish if results from animal experiments could be reproduced in brains affected with the human disease. First, however, the use of human fetal material for brain tissue grafting into the brain required thorough ethical consideration. Second, the risk of immunological rejection of cerebral fetal grafts had to be assessed. Since none of these questions are pertinent to autologous transplantation, the first clinical trials were conducted using chromaffin cell grafts from the patients' own adrenal medulla (Backlund *et al.* 1985, Lindvall *et al.* 1987).

Ethical Considerations

In the case of adrenal autotransplantation only the patient himself is involved. The ethical question, therefore, is simple and sets the scientific value of the trial and the potential beneficial effect for the individual patient against the possible risks and side effects of the procedure. This question is not different from other clinical trials of new treatment strategies.

The use of human embryos as the source of brain cell grafts introduces other ethical aspects and questions since it, as with other organ donations, involves other persons. It is of the utmost importance to emphasize that the question of using the fetal material for clinical (or basic scientific) purposes only has relevancy and can be raised first after the final decision only on the abortion has been taken. The use of fetal material should never, ever in any way influence the decision on abortion *per se*. Most importantly, abortions should under no circumstances be regarded as a means to procure material for transplantation purposes. Donation of fetal tissue after abortions, therefore, does not differ as a matter of principle from other organ donations from dead donors, and does not relate to the abortion any more than heart-, liver- or kidney donations relate to the accident or intracranial hemorrhage that caused the death of the donor. In Sweden we follow the ethical guidelines as formulated in 1986 by the Swedish Society for Medicine stating: 1. Material must only be taken from dead fetuses; 2. The women undergoing abortion must give their informed consent; 3. The transplantation must not in any way influence how, why, when or where the abortion is undertaken; 4. There must be no connection between donor and recipient; 5. The hospital staff must be fully informed.*

The main purposes of these guidelines are to guarantee women their right of decision and that the abortion procedure is completely unrelated to the transplantation surgery.

Other ethical aspects concern the potential consequences for the recipient of fetal brain tissue. The risk of transferring an infectious disease is similar to other organ transplantations and can be avoided by similar precautions, including preoperative serological tests and sterility during tissue preparation.

Quite naturally brain cell grafting also brings up the question of transfer of personality characteristics. Considering the fact that only small populations of less or undifferentiated embryonic cell types without any developed cell to cell communicating systems are transplanted, this risk can be assumed to be nonexsistent. An alteration of the recipient's personality can, however, not be excluded since a clinical effect of the transplant on the sufferer's disease may also include an effect on mental changes. If so, the effect must be regarded as one of the goals of the treatment and not a complicating side effect.

Preparation of Tissue Grafts

Fetal Tissue

Numerous animal studies have addressed the question of the optimal fetal donor age. This may vary between different species and depends on which cell type is to be grafted, and is influenced also by the maturity of the recipient and whether the graft is prepared as a dissociated cell suspension

---

*After July 1st 1996 transplantation of human fetal tissues is specifically regulated in the Swedish Transplantation Law (SFS 1995: 831).

or in small solid tissue pieces (Freeman *et al.* 1995). The limits of donor age seem to differ between dissociated tissue/cell suspension grafts and solid tissue grafts. In suspension grafts the optimal time period coincides with the time period when mesencephalic dopamine neurons have developed but before they start to extend axons to form the nigrostriatal tract. When small tissue pieces are used for grafting the upper time limit can be somewhat extended. The optimal human fetal donor age has been established by xenotransplantation to the rat and occurs between the 6th to 8th postconceptional (8th to 10th postmenstrual) weeks, while the upper limit for solid transplants can be extended by 1–2 weeks (Brundin *et al.* 1988, Freeman *et al.* 1995).

After suction abortion the fetus is dissected under completely sterile conditions to harvest a piece (1.5–2.0 mm^3) of the ventral mesencephalon corresponding to the substantia nigra and containing dopamine neurons Different methods have then been used to prepare the graft either as dissociated cell suspensions after trypsination (Lindvall *et al.* 1989, Widner *et al.* 1992, Henderson *et al.* 1991) or as solid fragments of the ventral mesencephalon (Madrazo *et al.* 1990, Molina *et al.* 1991, López-Lozano 1991, Spencer *et al.* 1992).

Autologous Adrenal Medulla

Standard surgical techniques have been used to resect one of the adrenal glands via either an extraperitoneal (Backlund *et al.* 1985, Allen *et al.* 1989, Apuzzo *et al.* 1990, Goetz *et al.* 1991) or an intraabdominal approach (Goetz *et al.* 1991, Kelly *et al.* 1989, López-Lozano *et al.* 1991). The medullary tissue is carefully separated from the adrenal cortex and divided into small fragments, kept cold and humid, until acutely transplanted into the patient's brain.

Surgical Techniques

Both stereotactic and open microneurosurgical techniques have been used to graft either adrenal medullary chromaffin tissue or fetal nervous dopaminergic tissue to the brain.

Stereotactic Techniques

The most widely used neurosurgical techniques for transplantation of human fetal tissue are stereotactically directed, and guided either by intraoperative CT- or MR-imaging to calculate coordinates for transplantation sites in the caudate and putamen (Lindvall *et al.* 1989, Freed *et al.* 1990, Spencer *et al.* 1992, Widner *et al.* 1992, Peschanski *et al.* 1994). It has also been used for autotransplantation of adrenal medullary tissue (Backlund *et al.* 1985, Lindvall *et al.* 1987, Jiao *et al.* 1989, Apuzzo *et al.* 1990, Fazzini *et al.* 1991). This technique allows the exact placement of one or multiple grafts in the different regions of interest including those that are inaccessible to open surgical approaches. The surgery involves only minor trauma and can be performed under local anesthesia, combined with sedatives if needed, but also under general anesthesia if motivated by the patient's condition or wish.

At the University Hospital in Lund, we have used the Leksell stereotactic system (Elekta AB, Stockholm, Sweden) and used CT for imaging of the striatum and planning for 3–7 transplantation sites unilaterally, the actual yield (from 3 to 7 abortions) of fetal material being taken into consideration (Fig. 1). CT-scans (2 or 3 mm thick) are produced closely parallel with the intercommissural line, i.e. the line between the anterior (AC) and posterior (PC) commissures. Both the caudate nucleus and putamen are generally easy to delineate, but safety is increased by relating their margins to AC and PC and by comparisons with preoperatively obtained MR-images. Two scans, 6–10 mm apart, are used for calculating pairs of target points, which are chosen so as to cover a maximum volume of the nuclei with reinnervating grafts. From the obtained stereotactic coordinates for target points in the two different planes, calculations of the lines between pairs of target points establish the direction and spherical angles of each trajectory. With small adjustments of the angles for the penetrating transplantation cannula all targets in the striatum can be reached through one single burrhole and a 2–3 mm dural incision. The brain is penetrated with a specifically designed (Rehncrona) transplantation instrument consisting of an outer guiding cannula with an blunt obturator, 22 mm shorter than an inner cannula (outer diameter 1.0 mm) containing the tissue suspension to be grafted (Fig. 1). Our first two patients were transplanted using an instrument with an outer diameter of 2.5 min, but after the second patient the original instrument was modified and the diameter reduced to 1.0 mm (Lindvall *et al.* 1989, 1992).

After advancing the instrument to the target the graft suspension (total volume 20–22.5 μL) is slowly injected in 2.5 μL aliquots during stepwise retraction of the cannula until the calculated length of each transplantation site (8–14 mm) is reached. A micrometer device is used for retraction between each deposit and, finally, the instrument is withdrawn from the brain after a 10 min. waiting period. The instrument is then reloaded with graft suspension by means of an indwelling tightly fitted piston and the procedure repeated for each transplantation site(s). Using this technique the author has now performed 22 transplantation operations (14 patients; 9 bilateral, 5 unilateral) with a total of 116 brain trajectories, without hemorrhages or any other surgical complication or side effect. In Fig. 2,

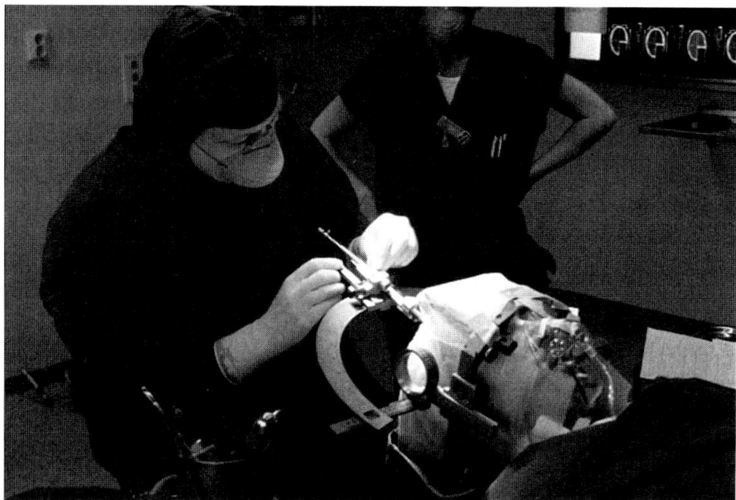

Fig. 1. Stereotactic fetal brain cell transplantation, using the Leksell G-frame (Elekta AB, Stockholm, Sweden) and the Rehncrona transplantation instrument, in a patient with idiopathic Parkinson's disease. Local anesthesia. (The Department of Neurosurgery, University Hospital, Lund, Sweden)

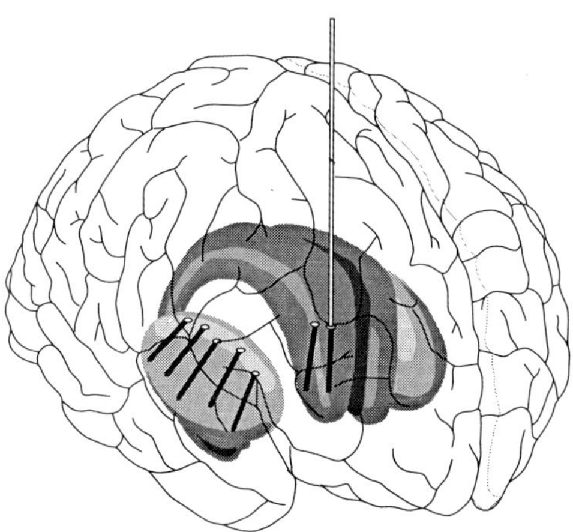

Fig. 2. Schematic illustration of the placements of human fetal brain grafts (5 transplantation sites in the right putamen and 2 in the caudate nucleus)

unilateral trajectories are schematically illustrated for five transplantation sites in the putamen and two in the caudate nucleus.

The methods for deposition of the graft material have varied among different surgeons and centres, including a spot injection of fetal mesencephalic cells suspended in 1–2 ml medium from one donor into one target point in the caudate (Hitchcock *et al.* 1991, Henderson *et al.* 1991). Others have used slow infusions of 30 μL/target in 10 transplantation sites during simultaneous withdrawal of the infusion needle (Freed *et al.* 1990).

Open Microneurosurgery

This technique was originally described by Madrazo (1987) and has mainly been used to place autografts of adrenal medulla in the caudate nucleus (Goetz *et al.* 1989, 1990, Kelly *et al.* 1989, Allen *et al.* 1989, López-Lozano *et al.* 1991, Fazzini *et al.* 1991) but also for fetal grafts (Madrazo *et al.* 1990, Molina *et al.* 1991). Through a routine frontal craniotomy the lateral ventricle is approached by transcortical dissection. The ventricular border of the head of the caudate is identified using an operating microscope and the transplant is placed subependymally after cavitation of the nucleus. The ependymal border is then closed in such a way that the grafted tissue remains embedded in the caudate parenchyma but keeps in contact with the ventricular fluid. Open microneurosurgery was also used in one case to autotransplant adrenal tissue to the right putamen via a frontotemporal bone flap and a transinsular approach (Takeuchi *et al.* 1990). General anesthesia was used in all cases of open surgical approaches and, recognising the quite extensive surgical trauma, unilateral grafting to the nondominant side has been preferred.

Human Clinical Trials

Since the first clinical trials were conducted using adrenal chromaffin tissue, data from autologous tissue grafting (Tables 1, 2, and 3) will be discussed before discussing current published results of fetal tissue transplantation (Tables 4 and 5).

Autologous Transplantation of Adrenal Medulla

The first clinical experiments with transplantation of adrenal medullary tissue in four patients with Parkinson's disease were done at the Karolinska Institute, Stockholm, and the University Hospital of Lund, Sweden in 1982 and 1985 respectively (Backlund *et al.* 1985, Lindvall *et al.* 1987). A CT-guided stereotactic technique was used to place the grafts either in the head of the caudate or in the putamen. The reason for changing transplantation site was the observation of a more severe depletion of striatal dopamine content in the putamen than in the caudate nucleus in patients with Parkinson's disease (Nyberg *et al.* 1983). Surgery was uneventful, but only minor and transient effects on the symptoms were observed. However, the preliminary results stimulated Madrazo, Mexico City, to perform medullary autotransplantation using the open microneurosurgical technique as summarized above. His first reported and very dramatic results released a kind of "tomatoketchup bottle" cascade of worldwide restrained desires to transplant into the central nervous system. It can be roughly estimated that about 600 autologous adrenal transplantations were performed in the period 1987–1992.

Tables 1 (open surgery) and 2 (stereotactical technique) summarize the main data from different centres including about 150 published cases. The exact number is uncertain since several registries are involved and some of the patients may feature in different reports. Clinical results have been evaluated using a variety of different scales including local scoring systems, the Hoehn and Yahr and Schwab-England scales, Unified Parkinson's Disease Rating Scale (UPDRS), Columbia University Rating Scale (CURS), Northwestern University Disability Scale (NWUDS) as well as different tests of psychomotor performance. The follow up periods are between 3 and 38 months. The best results using the open technique were reported by Madrazo *et al.* (1990), who found good or excellent improvements in about 50% of their (surviving) patients. Similar results were reported by López-Lozano *et al.* (1991), but both series have high mortality rates (12–15%) with 5 and 3 surgery related deaths respectively. These results conflict with the majority of other investigators who found only modest and often only temporary improvements in some of their patients (Table 1).

The morbidity rate is high in all series, including psychiatric side effects with prolonged coma, somnolence, psychosis, hallucinations, confusion, delusions, hypomania and depression as well as direct complications related to the neuro- and abdominal surgical approaches with intracerebral abscess, intracerebral hemorrhage, cerebral infarction, subdural hygromas, intercostal artery bleeding, subphrenic abscess, pancreatitis, volvulus and pneumonia.

The complication rates are by far the highest in the series with open surgery, but psychiatric side effects (transient paranoia, hallucinations, vivid dreams and depression) have also been reported after the stereotactic procedure (e.g. Backlund *et al.* 1985, Pezzoli *et al.* 1990, Apuzzo *et al.* 1990, Fazzini *et al.* 1991). The mental disturbances probably relate partly to a release of different catecholamines from the adrenal graft and partly to the frontal lobe surgical trauma. Thus, these side effects were in general considerably less after stereotactic surgery (Table 2) and similar symptoms have been noticed after fetal mesencephalic transplantations using the open surgical technique (Madrazo *et al.* 1990, Molina *et al.* 1991) but not after stereotactic fetal transplantations. Failure to find changes in lumbar spinal catecholamines after stereotactic adrenal medullary grafting (Apuzzo *et al.* 1990) does not disagree since only one patient out of 10 in that particular series experienced transient psychotic symptoms shortly after surgery. Furthermore, the symptoms in this patient seemed related

Table 1. *Adrenal Medullary Autografting Using Open Neurosurgical Procedures*

Center Authors	No. pat follow up/total	Follow up months	Transpl. site	Deaths, surgery related/ not related	Adverse effects (no.)	Clinical improvement
Mexico City, Mexico Univ. Nacional Autónoma de Mexico, Madrazo *et al.* 1987, Madrazo *et al.* 1990	2/2	3–10	Caudate n. unilat.	0	none	marked 2/2
	34/42	12–38	Caudate n. unilat.	5/5	Prolonged stupor (7), subdural hygroma (2), subphrenic absscess (2), pancreatitis (2), psychosis (2), hallucinations (11), confusion (2), aspiration (11), pneumonia (13)	good–exellent 15–20/34 moderate global group improvement in survivors
Chicago, USA Rush-Presbyterian- St. Lukes Med. Center Penn *et al.* 1988 Goetz *et al.* 1990	5/5 7/7	5 12	Caudate n. unilat.	0	Somnolence (4), depression (1), hallucinations and delusions (6) Hypomania (5), pneumonia (3)	modest in global function 6/7 modest in motor function 7/7
Rochester, USA, Mayo Clinic Kelly *et al.* 1989	7/8	6	Caudate n. unilat.	0	Somnolence (1), depression (3), confusion, hallucinations (3)	moderate in 1/7
Nashville, USA Vanderbilt Univ. Allen *et al.* 1989	17/18	6–12	Caudate n. unilat.	0/1	Intercostal artery bleeding (1), cerebral abscess (1), confusion, delusions and paranoia (4)	moderate in 4/17

Center Authors	No. pat follow up/total	Follow up months	Transpl. site	Deaths, surgery related/ not related	Adverse effects (no.)	Clinical improvement
Houston, USA Baylor College and Methodist Hospital Jankovic *et al.* 1989	3/3	8–12	Caudate n. unilat.	0/1	Prolonged somnolence, hallucinations (1)	modest in 2/3
Kyoto, Japan Utano National Hospital Takeuchi *et al.* 1990	1/1	12	Putamen unilat.	0	none	moderate transient 1/1
Madrid, Spain Clinica Puerta de Hierro Lopéz-Lozano *et al.* 1991	17/20	7	Caudate n. unilat.	3/3	Psych. disorders (13), pneumonia (3), cerebral infarction (1), interacerebr. hematom. (1)	moderate in 8–16/17
Lopéz-Lozano *et al.* 1992	3/3	5	Caudate n. and periferal nerve	0	Psych. disorders (2)	moderate
Multicenter study Goetz *et al.* 1989 Olanow *et al.* 1990	18/19	6 and 18	Caudate n. unilat.	1/1	Vegetative (1), cerebrovasc. acc. (2), pneumonia (11), psychiatric (11), pancreatitis (1), volvolus (1), dystonia (1)	modest and temporary group improvement

Table 2. *Adrenal Medually Grafting Using Stereotactic Neurosurgery*

Center Authors	No. pat follow up/total	Follow up months	Transpl. site	Deaths surg. related/ not surg. related	Adverse effects (no. pat)	Evaluation	Clinical improvement
Karolinska institute Stockholm, Sweden Backlund *et al.* 1985	2/2	6–20	Caudate n. unilat.	0	Transient	own scoring	minor transient 2/2
Univ. Hospital Lund, Sweden Lindvall *et al.* 1987	2/2	6	Putamen unilat.	0	none	own scoring	minor shortterm 2/2
Beijing, China Jiao *et al.* 1989	9/10	8–27	Caudate n. unilat.	0	no major reported	Webster scale	50–60% in 4/8 30–40% in 4/8
Ospedale Maggiore Milan, Italy Pezzoll *et al.* 1990	2/2	6	Caudate unilat.	0	Hallucinations (2)	CURS	modest-moderate 2/2
Univ. Southern California Los Angeles, USA Apuzzo *et al.* 1990	8/10	16–20	Caudate n. unilat. 5 bilat. 4	0/1	Hallucinations (1), vivid dreams (1)	UPDRS H & Y Schwab-England	moderate in 4/8
Columbia Univ. New York, USA Fazzini *et al.* 1991	3/4	12	Caudate n. unilat. (3) Thalamus (1)	0/1	Hallucinations (4), dyskinesia (4), depression (1)	UPDRS	modest in 2/3 marked in 1/3 (died of mal. glioma)
Karolinska institute Stockholm, Sweden Olson *et al.* 1991	1/1	13	Putamen + NGF-infusion	0 0	none none	Own scoring	moderate transient initial modest longterm

to pharmacologic treatment and had disappeared at the time for CSF sampling.

All series of stereotactic adrenal medullary grafting include patients with some clinical improvements. However, the effects are minor and short term. Combining medullary grafting with NGF infusion in one patient may have prolonged the clinical improvement somewhat but long term follow up data are not reported.

It is unclear if the reported improvements relate to dopamine release from a surviving graft. First, repeated and long term clinical assessments before surgery, to compensate for fluctuations in symptomathology, have seldom been performed. Second, pre- and postsurgical comparisons are hampered by the fact that pharmacological treatment may have been changed during the follow up period. Third, and most importantly, there are no available *in vivo* data showing graft survival (Guttman *et al.* 1989).

The information on graft survival, therefore, relies only on autopsy cases (Table 3). Out of nine reported autopsies only two cases showed signs of few surviving cells in the grafted tissue, while no surviving cells were found in seven cases. The two patients with signs of graft survival were reported not to have any clinical improvements from the procedure, while improvements (transient in one and sustained in two) were reported in three out of the seven patients with nonsurviving grafts.

In one of the patients, operated in Mexico City 13 months before dying from severe complications, autopsy disclosed that the graft was inadequately placed in the thalamic region on the side contralateral to the intended caudate nucleus (Forno and Langston 1991).

Transplantation of Human Fetal Mesencephalic Tissue

The first human trials were started in 1987 in China, Mexico and Sweden. At present the exact number of patients operated worldwide is not known but can be estimated to be between 150–200, i.e. two to three times the number of published cases. Tables 4 and 5 summarize published results of 77 patients followed at least 6 months and at maximum 46 months after transplantation. Table 4 gives the data from 33 patients operated on in Sweden, USA, France and England using stereotactic techniques, while data from 44 patients who underwent open microneurosurgery in Mexico, Cuba, Spain and Poland are given in Table 5.

The age of the fetal donors varies quite widely between the different transplanting centres: from between 6–8th weeks (Lund, Sweden) to 11–19th weeks (Birmingham, England) after conception. Patients operated on stereotactically have received material from 4–8 fetuses in two of the surgical centres (Lund, Sweden and Tampa, USA), including patients grafted bilaterally and both in the putamen and caudate nucleus. In two of

Table 3. *Autopsy Findings in Patients Grafted with Adrenal Medulla*

Authors	No. pat.	Place of trpl. surgery	Cause of death	Trpl. technique	Trpl. site	Time lapse (months)	Reported clinical improvement	Graft survival	TH-staining in graft
Dohan *et al.* 1988	1	Memphis USA	Multiple complic.	n.r.	Caudate unilat	4	none	none	n.r.
Frank *et al.* 1988	1	Bologna Italy	Leucemia	stereot.	inadequate	5	n.r.	none	—
Peterson *et al.* 1989	1	Mexico City Mexico	Cardiac	open	Caudate unilat	4	initial improvement	none	no
Hurtig *et al.* 1989	1	New York, USA N.Y. Univ.	Spinal abscess	open	Caudate unilat	4	none	small no. of surviv. cells	no
Jancovic *et al.* 1989	1	Houston USA	Cardiac	open	Caudate unilat	8	mild sustained improvement	none	no
Waters *et al.* 1990	1	Los Angeles USA, Univ. of S. Calif.	Cardiac	stereot.	Caudate bilat	$1\frac{1}{2}$	none	few surviv. cells	no

Authors	No. pat.	Place of trpl. surgery	Cause of death	Trpl. technique	Trpl. site	Time lapse (months)	Reported clinical improvement	Graft survival	TH-staining in graft
Hirsch *et al.* 1990	1	Mexico City Mexico	Aspiration pneumonia multiple complic.	open	Caudate unilat	4	none	none	no
Forno and Langston 1991	1	Mexico City Mexico	Pneumonia multiple complic.	open	inadequate	13	none	none	no
Fazzini *et al.* 1991	1	New York USA, Columbia Univ.	Glioblastoma	stereot.	Caudate unilat	12	sustained improvement	none	no

n.r. not reported.

Table 4. *Stereotactic Grafting of Human Fetal Mesencephalic Tissue to the Brain*

	Lund Sweden Lindvall *et al.* 1989 1990, 1992, 1994a Widner *et al.* 1993	Yale USA Spencer *et al.* 1992	Denver USA Feed *et al.* 1992	Tampa USA Freeman *et al.* 1994 Snow *et al.* 1994	Paris France Peschanski *et al.* 1994	Birmingham U.K. Henderson *et al.* 1991
No. of patients	6	4	7	2	2	12
Follow up period (max)	36 months	18 months	46 months	6 months	17 months	12 months
Fetal age (postconception)	6–8 w.	7–11 w.	7–8 w.	6.5–9 w.	6–9 w.	11–19 w.
No. of fetuses	4–8	1	1–2	6–8	2–3	1
Tissue material	acute Diss. cell susp.	cryopreserved fragments	cultured < 7 days Diss. + strands	acute fragments	acute Diss. cell susp.	acute Tissue susp.
Volume/trpl. site	20–22.5 μl	not rep.	not rep.	not rep.	24 μl	0.5–2.0 ml
Cannula diam.	2.5 and 1.0 mm	1.0 mm	1.0–0.46 mm	not rep.	0.8 mm	0.9 mm
Transpl. length	8–14 mm	8 mm	10 mm	not rep.	7 mm	spot injection
Immunosuppr.	all	all	4/7	not rep.	all	no
Surg. compl.	none	none	none	none	none	none
Adverse effects	none	epilepsia 1 (transient)	none	none	minor psyk.	none
Pre- and postop. PET	6/6	1/4	1/7	2/2	2/2	not pref.

	Lund, Sweden; Lindvall *et al.* 1989, 1990, 1992, 1994a; Widner *et al.* 1993			Yale, USA; Spencer *et al.* 1992	Denver, USA; Feed *et al.* 1992		Tampa, USA; Freeman *et al.* 1994; Snow *et al.* 1994	Paris, France; Peschanski *et al.* 1994		Birmingham, U.K.; Henderson *et al.* 1991
Trpl. site	*caud.+put* unilat	*caud.+put* bilat	*put* unilat	*caud.* unilat	*caud.+put* unilat	*put* bilat	*caud.+put* bilat	*caud.+put* unilat	*put* unilat	*caud.* unilat
No. pat.	2	2	2	4	2	5	2	1	1	12
Increase in FD-PET uptake	— in 0/2	marked in 2/2	marked in 2/2	modest in 1/1	not perf.	— in 0/1	marked in 2/2	marked in 1/1	marked in 1/1	not perf.
Clinical improvements	2/2	2/2	2/2	3/4	1/2	5/5	2/2	1/1	1/1	3/12
Motor perform.	modest	marked	moderate	modest	modest	moderate	moderate	moderate	moderate	moderate
Time spent in "on"	no	yes	yes	nr	yes	yes	yes	yes	yes	yes
Rigidity	no	yes	yes	yes	nr	nr	nr	yes	yes	nr
Bradykinesia	yes	yes	yes	yes	yes	yes	nr	yes	yes	yes
Posture	yes	yes	yes	nr	nr	nr	nr	nr	nr	nr
Gait	yes	yes	yes	yes	yes	yes	nr	yes	yes	nr
Dyskinesia	no	yes	—	nr	nr	yes	yes	yes	yes	yes

n.r. not reported.

Table 5. *Open Microneurosurgical Grafting of Human Fetal Mesencephalic Tissue to the Brain*

	Mexico city Mexico Madrazo *et al.* 1990	Havanna Cuba Molina *et al.* 1991	Madrid Spain Lopez-Lozano *et al.* 1991	Warsaw Poland Zabeck *et al.* 1994
No of patients	4	30	7	3
Follow up (months)	19–32	24	7	30
No. of fetuses per operation	1	1	1	1
Fetal age (postconceptional)	12–14	6–12	6–15	9–10
Tissue material	fragments	fragments	fragments	fragments
Immunosuppr.	permanent	6 months	permanent	6 months
Transplantation site	right caudate	right caudate	right caudate	left caudate 1 right caudate 2
Surgical complications	brain abscess	none	none	none
Adverse effects	"frontal lobe syndromes"	"postsurg. syndrome" 1–3 months	none	stupor 1 paranoia 1 frontal lobe syndr.
Evidence of graft survival	none	none	none	none
Reported improvement no. pat.	4	30	7	3
Motor performance	moderate	moderate	modest	modest
Increased "on"-time	yes	yes	not reported	yes
Rigidity	yes	yes	"	yes
Bradykinesia	yes	yes	"	yes
Posture	yes	yes	"	not reported
Gait	yes	yes	"	yes
Tremor	no	yes	"	yes
Dyskinesia	not reported	yes	yes	yes

the centres (Yale, USA and Birmingham, England) fetal material from one single donor was transplanted routinely to each patient with the caudate nucleus as the only target. The outer diameters of the different transplant cannulas used have for most of the cases been close to 1 mm, but a 2.5 mm instrument was used for the first two operated patients in Lund, and a cannula diameter of 0.7 mm was used in some of the cases transplanted in Denver. Sixteen patients received only transplants in the caudate nucleus (Yale, Birmingham), while the putamen or putamen + caudate was the main target in 17. Lengths of the transplants have varied between 7–14 mm except for patients operated in Birmingham, where the grafts have been injected in a single spot in the caudate (Henderson *et al.* 1991). All patients operated with the open microneurosurgical technique have recieved tissue grafts prepared in small pieces from one single donor and placed in the caudate nucleus.

The majority of the patients were given immunosuppressive therapy, except for those operated on by the Birmingham group and some of the patients operated on in Denver.

No surgical complications and only few and minor adverse effects (epileptic seizure in one and transient mental disturbance in one patient) were reported after stereotactic fetal brain cell grafting. However, after open microneurosurgical grafting more severe side effects of the "frontal lobe syndrome" type have been noticed in a considerable number of patients by several authors.

Graft Survival

Of crucial importance is to validate the long term survival of grafted tissue and to correlate this with thorough observations of clinical effects. At present the only valid *in vivo* method available is to measure and image the uptake of (^{18}F)fluorodopa with positron-emission tomography (PET), see Fig. 3. The uptake of fluorodopa in striatum may depend mainly on three factors: the number of dopamine terminals in the region; the activity of the L-aromatic aminoacid decarboxylase enzyme (L-AAAD); the permeability of the blood-brain barrier. Since grafts to the brain do not change the L-AAAD activity and the blood-brain barrier is closed shortly after stereotactic grafting procedures, it can be concluded that changes in striatal fluorodopa uptake as measured by PET before and after grafting represent changes in the number of dopamine terminals (for references see Lindvall 1994b). Therefore, a significant increase in fluorodopa uptake in the transplantation region above everything is a measure of graft survival, but may also be sensitive to induced sprouting from remaining endogenous fibers. The latter possibility cannot be totally ruled out but is less likely since marked fluorodopa uptake was found after fetal grafting to patients

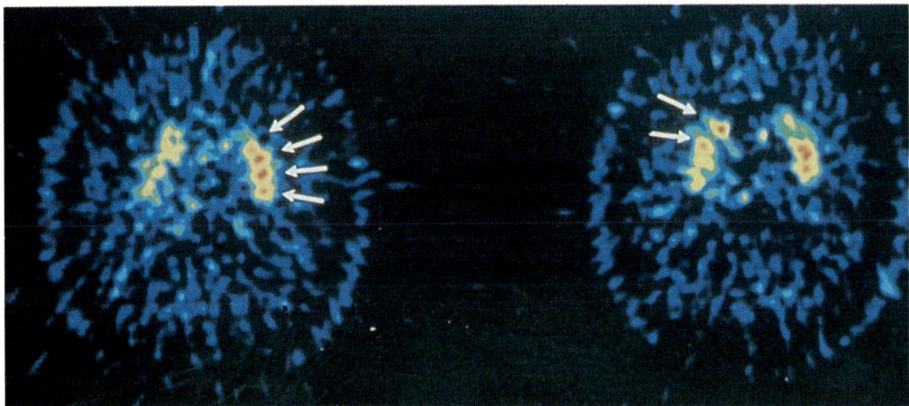

Fig. 3. PET-images showing the postengraftment uptake of (^{18}F)-fluorodopa in a patient with MPTP induced severe parkinsonism. The patient was transplanted bilaterally 3 years before the scanning and detailed clinical as well as complete pre- and postengraftment PET-data are given elsewhere (Widner *et al.* 1992, 1993). The patient received 3 implants in each putamen and one in each caudate nucleus. Surgery was performed in two sessions with a 14 days interval and material from 3 or 4 human fetuses was used for each side. The two scans clearly visualize the fluorodopa uptake in individual grafts corresponding to the intended transplantation sites. (PET-scanning was performed at the University of British Columbia, Vancouver, M.D. Barry Snow)

with MPTP induced parkinsonism (Widner *et al.* 1993). These patients had extremely low fluorodopa uptake before transplantation, indicating the absence of a significant endogenous fibre source for sprouting. Furthermore, autopsy of a patient 18 months after fetal cell grafting showed graft survival with massive fibre extensions as correlated to fluorodopa uptake on PET, but no signs of host derived axonal sprouting (Kordower 1995).

Only few centres have validated graft survival in humans with Parkinson's disease. Twelve out of the 77 grafted patients, referred to in Tables 4 and 5, have undergone fluorodopa PET scanning before as well as after transplantation. In 8 of these cases PET demonstrated a marked increase in fluorodopa uptake corresponding to the sites of grafting (Lindvall *et al.* 1990, 1994a, Widner *et al.* 1993, Peschanski 1994, Snow *et al.* 1994). The uptake in one patient was modest (Spencer *et al.* 1992) and in three of the patients PET scanning failed to show any significant increase in fluorodopa uptake after transplantation as compared with the preoperative scanning (Lindvall *et al.* 1989, Freed *et al.* 1992). Clinical effects in these four patients seem to have been considerably less conspicuous than in the patients with markedly increased fluorodopa uptake.

One patient receiving human fetal mesencephalic grafts died from pulmonary embolism 18 months later, unrelated to the transplantation surgery. Autopsy revealed well preserved viable grafts with outgrowths of numerous extensions reinnervating gross areas of the striatum (Kordower *et al.* 1995). Since earlier PET scanning of the same patient showed increased fluorodopa uptake it is tempting to conclude that PET is the method of choice for estimation of graft survival and growth.

Attempts to estimate graft viability and function by measurements of monoamine metabolites in the cerebrospinal fluid have been unsuccessful (Molina *et al.* 1991).

Clinical Results

Evaluations of and comparisons between different reported results are difficult since the data given are often incomplete, most series are small and based on individual case reports, preoperative evaluation periods are often short and, finally, pharmacological treatment may have been changed at surgery or during the postoperative follow up period. Such obstacles are quite natural at the very beginning of a new therapeutic strategy, but render the evaluation of the clinical value of the procedure in a more general sense impossible. The largest clinical series operated using a stereotactic technique is reported from Birmingham (Henderson 1991). All patients received unilateral grafts to the caudate only. Each graft was prepared as a tissue suspension in rather big total volumes (ranging from 0.5–2.0 ml) from one single fetal mesencephalon. Of the 12 originally included patients 9 were available for complete follow up after 1 year. Only three of these patients showed moderate improvements in motor performance and an increase in the time spent in "on". Since no estimates of graft survival were conducted it is impossible to conclude whether the improvements reported are results of graft function or not. With respect to the small number of patients improved and the fact that the mesencephalic tissue used for grafting had gestational ages above 11 weeks it seems highly unlikely that the transplantation method used resulted in surviving, dopamine producing and pysiologically integrated grafts.

Three transplanting centres (Lund, Tampa and Paris) have reported PET-scan data that clearly indicate graft survival (Lindvall *et al.* 1990, 1994a, Widner *et al.* 1992, 1993, Jacques *et al.* 1994, Peschanski *et al.* 1994). The clinical follow up evaluations of these patients have shown moderate and marked improvements in motor performance, increased time spent in "on", decreased rigidity and bradykinesia and a decrease in L-dopa provoked dyskinesias (see Table 4). The effect on tremor is however unclear since none of the patients transplanted had any obvious tremor symptoms prior to (or after) surgery.

The first two patients operated at the University Hospital in Lund (putamen and caudate unilaterally), showed only a possible, but insignificant uptake of fluorodopa on postoperative PET scanning (Lindvall *et al.* 1989). A similar result was reported from the group at Yale University, using cryopreserved tissue fragments from one fetus for transplantation to the caudate nucleus unilaterally (Spencer *et al.* 1992). Clinically these patients only showed modest improvements in motor performance and in some symptoms. Taken together the data of these three patients indicate a graft effect, but insufficient number of surviving cells to give improvements of therapeutic value.

Relating the different clinical neurologic results to the PET evaluations of individual cases, it can be concluded that there is a correlation between fluorodopa uptake and the clinical functional effects of human fetal mesencephalic grafts.

The reports on patients receiving fetal transplants in the caudate nucleus using the open surgical approach (Table 5) all describe modest or moderate clinical improvements but none of the authors have verified transplant survival. It is, therefore, impossible to conclude whether the reported effects are due to function of the graft or relate to some other (unknown) mechanism .

Transplantation of Other Dopamine Cells

Since some aspects of transplantation of fetal material are and will remain controversial and the source is limited, other possibilities for grafting to the central nervous tissue are being explored. These include cells that are genetically modified to produce dopamine, chromaffin cells from the superior cervical ganglion as an alternative to adrenal medullary tissue and, finally xenotransplants of dopaminergic neurons prepared from animals.

Rapid advances in molecular and cell biology have opened the possibility of altering cell function by gene transfer. The genetically modified cells are able to express the function of the transgene and fibroblasts modified to produce L-dopa or dopamine have been characterized and grafted to experimental animals (Horellou *et al.* 1990a, 1990b, Kawaja *et al.* 1991, Fisher *et al.* 1991). However many questions remain to be answered before this technique is ready to be tested in human trials (Gage *et al.* 1991).

Autotransplants of the superior cervical ganglion into the caudate nucleus of monkeys were shown to ameliorate MPTP induced Parkinsonism (Itakura *et al.* 1988, Nakai *et al.* 1990). Since a sympathetic ganglion contains both norepinephrine- and dopamine producing cells the mechanism may be similar to the experimental effects found with adrenal medullary grafts. The authors speculate that ganglion cells might be more capable of extending axons into the brain parenchyma, but the method has not been used in humans. Furthermore, resection of the superior cervical ganglion is complicated by Horner's syndrome.

Two weeks before completion of the present review it was reported that the first clinical experiment with xenografting using pig-derived dopamine producing brain cells to a patient with Parkinson's disease had been performed in Boston (Schumacher, Isacson, Personal communication). Even if xenotransplantation to the human brain must raise a lot of new ethical questions the result of this experiment is interesting and there is no doubt that xenografts in animals with experimental parkinsonism are functional (see above).

Brain Cell/Tissue Transplantation in Other Diseases

Stimulated by the first reports of clinical grafting in Parkinson's disease, less well founded, and premature, human experiments with brain tissue grafting were instituted to treat psychiatric disorders. On a disputable scientific basis and without clinical justification two patients with schizophrenia were bilaterally implanted with human embryonic brain tissue in the septal area (Kolarik *et al.* 1990). Psychiatric follow up and evaluations of these patients as well as of patients receiving grafts for Alzheimer's disease and posttraumatic brain atrophy by the same group, failed to show any success and the authors warn against excessive publicity and optimistic appraisal of the procedure (Starkova *et al.* 1991). There should be no controversy about this concluding warning and it should be thoroughly emphasized that human experiments with grafting to the central nervous system must be preceded by and rely on solid scientific data and methods.

Huntington's chorea is a genetic disease transmitted by a single autosomal dominant gene. It is characterized by progressive degeneration of neurons mainly in the striatum, ventrolateral thalamus, and brain stem as well as in the cortex (Lange *et al.* 1976). The involvement of striatal neurons and their projections to pallidum and substantia nigra leads also to cell loss and atrophy in these areas, probably due to the loss of afferent pathways. The exact pathogenic mechanism(s) underlying the disease are unknown and no effective treatment is available. Clinically, Huntington's disease leads to severe involuntary movements (chorea) and dementia, before death within 10–15· years after onset. Most animal models of the disease are based on excitotoxic lesioning of the striatum using either kainic or ibotenic acids (Coyle and Schwartz 1983). Fetal striatal grafts implanted in rat striatum have been shown to reinnervate the host globus pallidus, entopeduncular nucleus and substantia nigra and, also to be innervated by host derived afferent nerve fibers (e.g. Wictorin *et al.* 1989). Furthermore, striatal implants have functional effects both on behavioral deficits and at least on some of the motor disturbances in similar models (for reviews see Dunnett 1990, Dunnett and Svendsen 1993).

Two publications describe clinical experiments with implants prepared from fetal striatum in Huntington patients. The authors have used either a stereotactic technique (Sramka *et al.* 1992) or open surgery (Madrazo 1993) to place grafts either bi- or unilaterally in the caudate nucleus. None of these works give any evidences of graft survival or graft-induced clinical effects.

Alzheimer's disease is a neurodegenerative disorder with a more diffuse and generalized loss of cells with projections covering widespread areas. Cholinergic neuronal transmission in forebrain regions is especially affected, with reduction in choline acetyltransferase activity as well as cell loss in cortical areas and hippocampus (Frances *et al.* 1985, Katzman 1986); serotoninergic and noradrenergic systems are also involved (Bondareff *et al.* 1982, Yamamoto *et al.* 1985). Research aiming at repairing cell loss for restitution particularly of cholinergic transmission is hampered by a lack of adequate experimental models mimicking the disease; aged animals are aged and do not have Alzheimer's disease. At present interest in new therapeutic strategies for Alzheimer's disease centres on the administration of nerve growth factors into the central nervous system, and at least one clinical experiment with intracranial NGF infusion has recently been performed (Hefti and Schneider 1991, Olson 1993, Seiger *et al.* 1993). This research is, however, beyond the scope of this review.

Discussion and Perspectives

The brain transplantation paradigm aims at repairing the brain by replacement of lost cells to reanimate lost neurological functions. At least theoretically, it may be the only curative therapeutic strategy in many disorders involving brain cell loss.

The present clinical experience of transplantation to the human brain comes almost exclusively from trials with Parkinson's disease using either autologous adrenal tissue or allografts of fetal dopamine producing cells from the ventral mesencephalon. It is, therefore, pertinent first to discuss mechanisms of graft function and compare the different types of grafts before discussing methodological aspects and, finally, possibilities for future developments and applications.

Functional Interactions Between Grafts and Host Brain: Fetal Mesencephalic Versus Adrenal Tissue Grafts

Since the majority of adrenal medullary and fetal brain transplantations were performed with different surgical techniques the results do not lend themselves to direct comparisons. Most adrenal grafts have been placed in the head of the caudate nucleus due to the fact that other striatal regions are inaccessible to open surgery without taking unjustified surgical risks.

The main target for stereotactic fetal transplantations has instead been the putamen supplemented with grafts to the head of the caudate nucleus. The basic principal difference between fetal brain tissue and adreno-medullary grafts is that the former, by its neuronal origin, has the capacity to be better physiologically integrated in the neuronal circuits of the host brain and to display specific synaptic dopamine release. Chromaffin cells from the adrenal medulla may certainly transform into a more noradrenergic neuronal phenotype if isolated from the influence of adrenal corticosteroids (Olson 1970) but integration with host brain neurons is less obvious. Thus autopsies of patients after adrenal medullary transplantation have failed to give evidences for graft integration (see above). Furthermore, the release of adrenomedullary catecholamines is less specific and includes both adrenalin and noradrenalin together with dopamine. Therefore, an effect, if any, of adrenomedullary grafts is more likely to be mediated by non-synaptic catecholamine release and simple transmitter diffusion.

Both types of grafts have in common the possibility to induce sprouting from host neurons (Bankiewicz *et al.* 1990, Plunkett *et al.* 1990). Even if the occurrence of such trophic mechanisms hardly can be excluded, clinical results with fetal grafting do not favour this hypothesis. Thus PET using fluorodopa as a tracer, showed massive uptake in caudoputaminal transplantation sites in patients with MPTP-induced parkinsonism despite a close to complete loss of dopaminergic innervation before grafting (see above). The possibility that the surgical trauma induces sprouting in patients with idiopathic Parkinson's disease seems less likely since we found better clinical effects and substantially increased fluorodopa uptake on PET using a smaller and less traumatic implantation instrument. Finally, no signs of sprouting from host neurons were found on autopsy in a patient with massive reinnervation of the striatum from fetal mesencephalic grafts (Kordower *et al.* 1995).

The most dramatic clinical improvements after *adrenal grafting* were reported by Madrazo, who found good and moderate overall effects on rigidity, bradykinesia, posture as well as gait in about half of his series of patients available for follow up (34 out of 42) (Madrazo 1990). Similar results were reported by López-Lozano (López-Lozano *et al.* 1991) and the "Hispanic Registry of Graft Procedures for Parkinson's Disease" (Madrazo 1989). Taken together, however, the mortality was well above 10% with a very high morbidity rate in these series.

Other series (a total of 61 patients) as summerized by Goetz *et al.* (1990, 1991) and Olanow *et al.* (1990), including both stereotactic and open surgical procedures, show considerably less marked clinical improvements. They report a moderate increase of the time spent in "on" and reduction of some symptoms in the "off-phase" as the main findings. Also these series show a high mortality rate, with 10% surgery related deaths and, a high incidence of persistent morbidity, e.g. above 20% persistent psychiatric morbidity two years after surgery.

Even if mild, transient and sporadic it seems clear that adrenal transplants to the Parkinsonian brain may induce improvements. Since none of the groups have been able to present any evidence for long term survival of the grafts *in vivo*, or correlation between cell survival upon autopsy and clinical effects, it must be concluded that reported improvements must relate to other mechanisms than those originally intended. Thus, the acute, but modest and transient effects in the patients operated on by Backlund (Lindvall *et al.* 1987) may be explained by diffuse release of dopamine and other amines by dying and disintegrating adrenal cells. By the same token some of the acute effects of open microneurosurgical transplantation may be explained, but not the more persistent improvements seen in some cases. Since for about fifty years neurosurgeons have used various central lesions to treat Parkinsonian symptoms, and the Madrazo technique is quite traumatic to the brain, it is tempting to conclude that similar mechanisms may be operating (cf. Meyers 1942, Browder 1948).

Whatever may be the mechanism behind the reported clinical effects of adrenal autografting, it seems clear that improvements are small and do not justify the high risks for mortality, morbidity and side effects of the procedure.

Several groups working with human *fetal brain* grafts have reported clear and marked clinical improvements. There is strong evidence that these clinical effects are due to surviving and functioning grafts. First, graft survival has been established with PET in at least 9 patients (out of 12 investigated). Second, the clinical effects typically start and can be assessed around 3–4 months after surgery and the time course of improvements parallel the increase in fluorodopa uptake on PET. Third, the time course of clinical improvement also follows the expected time course as compared to the development and integration of fetal grafts in experimental animals. Fourth, the improvement of motor performance in patients with idiopathic Parkinson's disease transplanted unilaterally is most marked on the side contralateral to the transplant. Fifth, long term follow up (36 months) has shown stable fluorodopa uptake in the grafted regions and persistent clinical effects. Sixth, as recently reported, neuropathological examination demonstrated the survival of fetal brain grafts in a patient who died from unrelated causes (Kordower *et al.* 1995).

Methodological Aspects on Fetal Brain Tissue Grafting

Different methods have been used for grafting by different research groups. Unfortunately only few of the groups have studied and verified survival of the grafts and, therefore, detailed comparisons between the techniques are difficult. However some tentative conclusions can be drawn. With respect to the increased risks and the limitations of possible target sites for grafting, there should be no justification to use the open surgical approach. In fact the experience with stereotactical placements of grafts points to an inverse relationship between the diameter of the transplantation instrument on one hand and the clinical effect and PET results on the other, indicating a negative effect of tissue trauma. Thus, results improved after the diameter of the cannula was reduced from 2.5 mm to 1.0 mm after patient number 2 in our series. Probably the increased tissue trauma inflicted by a larger instrument induces an increased and perhaps deleterious inflammatory reaction (cf. Brundin *et al.* 1989). However, other methodological changes may be of equal importance. The cell medium used for our first two transplantations was an unbuffered saline-glucose solution rendering the fetal tissue suspension acidotic (a fall in pH to below 6.0) presumably due to anaerobic glycolysis (Rehncrona, Unpublished observation). This medium was exchanged for a buffered and pH-stable Hank's solution. Furthermore, the time lapse between abortions and transplantation was decreased by 2–3 hours and the mechanical dissociation of the tissue to be grafted was done immediately before implantation.

As recently emphasized by Lindvall (1994b) none of the patients receiving human fetal dopaminergic transplants has been cured from Parkinson's disease despite demonstrations of graft survival. The clinical therapeutic effects reported in the patients with PET-verified graft survival are still incomplete and methodological improvements have to be made before the procedure can be used as a clinical routine. There are several possible reasons for ineffective therapeutic results: 1. The population of surviving grafted cells in the host brain may be too small; 2. Reinnervation by graft derived extensions may not cover enough of the tissue volume to be reinnervated; 3. The pathogenic factor(s) causing Parkinson's disease may also affect the grafted cells and prevent their development; 4. Grafts to more targets than the putamen and caudate alone, might be necessary for more than partial clinical effects.

In view of the fact that 70% or more of the normal innervation to striatum must be lost before clinical symptoms of the disease become obvious a 30% reinnervation of striatum by grafts should be enough to give significant clinical improvements. Estimates from experiments with human fetal grafts to the rat indicate that only 5–10% of the original yield of dopaminergic cells survive and develop in the recipient's brain after transplantation (Frodl *et al.* 1994, Lindvall 1994b). The real cell survival rate after grafting to the human brain is unknown, but the experimental figures are corroborated by autopsy findings (Thomas B. Freeman, Personal communication). Thus, combined grafts from at least three embryos should be enough to compensate for unilateral cell loss in Parkinson's disease. Therefore, other explanations for incomplete recovery should be sought in respect to those centres using material from 3 or more fetuses for unilateral transplantation, while the modest or absent effects reported from other groups may be explained by the fact that material from only one or maximally two fetal mesencephalons was used.

Graft derived extensions may grow 2–7 mm to reinnervate the host brain tissue and graft deposits separated by 5 mm may therefore provide confluent innervation (Kordower *et al.* 1995). The density of reinnervation is best in close vicinity to the graft and sparse in the periphery (cf. Fig. 3). Considering the anatomical geometry of the striatum none of the transplantation techniques used may give a total and uniform reinnervation, which may be a prerequisite for an optimal clinical effect.

Since the etiology of idiopathic Parkinson's disease is unknown and cell degeneration progressive it could not be excluded that pathogenic factors also may affect transplanted dopaminergic neurons. In order to elucidate this possibility we decided to perform only unilateral transplantations in two of our first patients with idiopathic Parkinson's disease to be able to compare the transplanted with the non-transplanted side on long term follow up (Lindvall *et al.* 1994). Repeated PET scanning of these patients during a three year follow up period showed a progressive increase in fluorodopa uptake to stable levels in the grafted putamen. At the same time there was a fall in tracer uptake in the corresponding regions on the contralateral non-transplanted side (Fig. 4). These data give evidence for long term survival of fetal mesencephalic grafts despite progression of the

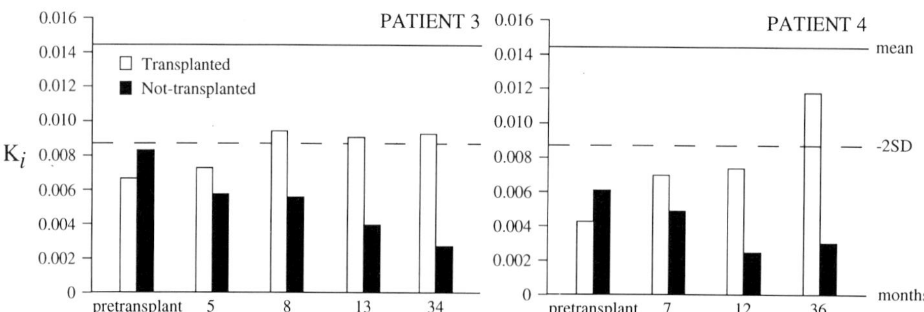

Fig. 4. Putaminal changes in (^{18}F)-fluorodopa uptake in two patients (numbers 3 and 4 in our own series) with idiopathic Parkinson's disease after unilateral fetal transplantation. For comparisons the normal mean value and -2SD is given for 17 normal subjects. In both patients the sequentially performed PET scans show a progressive and stable increase in fluorodopa uptake in the transplanted side (unfilled bars), while there is a decrease at the same time in the corresponding but not transplanted putamen (filled bars). Data from Lindvall *et al.* 1994a

disease with ongoing degeneration of the patient's "own" dopaminergic system. These data indicate that the grafted tissue remains unaffected by, or is less sensitive to the disease process and it may be speculated that differences in genetic codes between the cells of the parkinsonian brain and the transplanted cells might be responsible. If so, genetic factors together with other extrinsic-factors may be involved in the pathogenesis of Parkinson's disease.

Finally, even if the main pathophysiological changes in Parkinson's disease affect substantia nigra and its dopaminergic innervation of the striatum, other areas such as locus coeruleus, ventral tegmentum, nucleus basalis and the raphe nuclei may also be involved (Gaspar and Gray 1984, Jellinger 1987 a and b). Therefore, even a complete dopaminergic reinnervation of the striatum by the transplant may not be enough to cure all symptoms.

Will Transplantation be a Future Neurosurgical Routine in the Treatment of Parkinson's Disease?

As emphasized above the data on adrenal autografting give no scientific basis for any further clinical experiments with transplantation of chromaffin cells. Evidences for symptomatic therapeutic effects due to graft-host interactions are few and the evidences for long term graft survival are nonexistent.

On the other hand, fetal mesencephalic grafts clearly survive, integrate and may exert clinical effects of undisputable therapeutic value for extended time periods. However, even if promising, the reported effects are far from optimal and further research with clinical trials on selected patient groups in parallel with experimental research is needed before the technique can be used as a routine neurosurgical procedure. The main scientific issues pertinent to the development of transplantation into a future clinically useful therapy for Parkinson's disease are: to increase the survival of grafted neurons; to modify the surgical technique in order to induce a more homogeneous and complete dopaminergic reinnervation; to study possibilities for long term preservation of cells and tissues for later grafting and; finally, to explore other suitable sources for grafting than fetal tissue.

The reason why about 90% of the original yield of fetal dopamine cells is lost after the grafting procedure is unclear. The low survival rate of grafted cells necessitates that material from at least 3 fetuses is needed for unilateral transplantation with currently used techniques. This constitutes a serious limit to general clinical use of the method to treat extended groups of patients. Ongoing experimental studies aiming at increasing cell survival include the use of free-radical scavengers of the lazaroid type (Nakao *et al.* 1994) and administration of neurotrophic factors either as an addition to the cell suspension or directly into the grafted striatum (Mayer *et al.* 1993). Others have emphasized the importance of minimizing tissue trauma and inflammation by using microinjection techniques (Nikkah *et al.* 1994).

From the practical point of view preservation of fetal tissue/cells for later transplantation should be of great value in the neurosurgical practice. However, clinical results with cryopreserved tissue have given inferior results as compared with freshly obtained grafts (Redmond *et al.* 1990; Kordower 1995).

Experimental results on hibernation of human fetal material are promising and preservation of tissue at 4 °C for at least 3 days showed graft survival similar to acute grafting (Sauer and Brundin 1991). This observation may have a definite practical implication. If hibernation of the tissue can be prolonged to more than a week with undisturbed cell survival this will allow harvesting of fetal material over several days and also the transport of transplantation material.

Since the use of human fetal material is and will be limited and may remain a controversial issue it is important to explore other sources for future transplantations into the central nervous system. Such an alternative source may be cells that are genetically modified to produce and release dopamine. Thus, genetically modified cell lines from primary fibroblasts and myoblasts expressing tyrosine hydroxylase were shown to partially reverse some of the effects of striatal denervation in rats (Horellou *et al.* 1990b, Jiao *et al.* 1993, Anton *et al.* 1994). The stability of the inserted transgene, long-term effects, and the capacity for these cells to integrate in the new host brain to restore a well-regulated neuronal type of circuits are however still unknown and remain to be settled.

Future Transplantation Therapy in Other Neurologic Disorders

Brain tissue and cell loss due to trauma or vascular disease has stimulated several researches to devote some effort to studying the behaviour of tissue grafts in focal lesions. In 1983 Labbe and collaborators found amelioration of learning deficits in rats after cavitation of the prefrontal cortex and subsequent grafting with fetal frontal cortex (Labbe *et al.* 1983). The effect was only transient and, since similar effects were described also after glial cell grafting some acute trophic action of the procedure may be the underlying mechanism (Kesslak *et al.* 1986). Survival of fetal neocortical grafts transplanted to infarcted areas in rat models of focal ischemia was also demonstrated (Hadani *et al.* 1987, Mampalan *et al.* 1988, Grabowski *et al.* 1995) and hippocampal grafts may integrate structurally after global ischemic lesions (Tönder *et al.* 1989). From experiments with middle cerebral occlusions it seems clear that afferent connections from host neurons can innervate the graft but efferent connections from grafted neurons are less obvious (Grabowski *et al.* 1992, Grabowski *et al.* 1995). Functional clinical effects of grafts to the ischemically lesioned brain have not yet been demonstrated and a possibility for future transplantation therapy after stroke is still only a matter of speculation.

Most brain cell grafting procedures and experiments have centered around neuronal grafting. However, the very promising results with glial cell grafting should be emphasized. This research aims at remyelinating fibres to reanimate function in demyelination disorders like multiple sclerosis (MS), adrenoleucodystrophy (ALD) and adrenomyeloneuropathy (AMN). Transplanted oligodendrocytes have been shown to remyelinate widespread areas of demyelinated fibers in lysolecithin and X-ray induced focal lesions as well as in mutant mice, rats and dogs (Blakemore and Franklin 1991, Baron-Van Evercooren 1992, Duncan *et al.* 1992, Tontsch *et al.* 1994). Oligodendrocytes injected into the spinal cord may migrate quite long distances to exert their effect and, recently improvement in nerve fibre conduction time was demonstrated in fibres remyelinated in this way (Utzschneider 1994). These data strongly favour the possibility of future glial cell transplantation therapy in these currently intractable and devastating disorders.

General Conclusions

Of greatest importance is the central fact that neural transplantation to the human central nervous system is possible and that grafts can integrate, survive and improve lost neurological functions for extended time periods. Therefore, the concept of central nervous transplantation to treat severe and intractable disorders should no longer be regarded as wishful thinking, but a reality with great future clinical potential. At present, available data clearly show that tissue taken from aborted human fetuses has this capacity. This does not however mean that other sources are or should be excluded. On the contrary the development of clinically useful transplantation therapies in a general sense probably must rely on other sources than acutely aborted fetuses.

It should be thoroughly emphasized that current clinical data pertain only to Parkinson's disease, with MPTP-induced parkinsonism as a bridge between experimental and clinical research, and that this experience cannot be directly transferred to other disorders. Thus, methods and surgical techniques have to be modified and scientifically tested in order to suit other clinical disorders. It should also be pointed out that only small series of grafted patients with Parkinson's disease have been published and few of them include complete follow up data with validation of graft survival. None of these series demonstrate any patient that is cured from the disease and relatively few with major recovery. Therefore, clinical transplantation as a routine therapy even in Parkinson's disease still has to wait further scientific progress and developments to optimize the technique.

Of other disorders discussed here, Huntington's disease and demyelination disorders seem to be close to qualifying as candidates for clinical trials. In such future trials it is of incontrovertible importance to learn from the experiences with the earlier transplantation trials, and base all steps to be taken on solid scientific data, and to concentrate the efforts in centres with neurosurgical experience of neurotransplantation, facilities for thorough clinical follow up and validation as well as facilities for basic transplantation research. The desire to be able to write "for the first time" must not be the main objective of human trials.

References

1. Allen GS, Burns RS, Tulipan NB, Parker RA (1989) Adrenal medullary transplantation to the caudate nucleus in Parkinson's disease; initial results in 18 patients. Arch Neurol 46: 487–491
2. Anton R, Kordower JH, Maidment NT, Manaster JS, Kane DJ, Rabizadeh S, Scheuller SB, Yang J, Edwards RH, Markham CH, Bredesen DE (1994) Neural-targeted gene therapy for rodent an primate hemiparkinsonism. Exp Neurol 127: 207–218
3. Apuzzo MLJ, Neal JH, Waters CH, Appley AJ, Boyd SD, Couldwell WT, Wheelock VH, Weiner LP (1990) Utilization of unilateral and bilateral stereotactically placed adrenomedullary-striatal autografts in Parkinsonian humans: rationale, techniques, and observations. Neurosurgery 26: 746–757
4. Backlund E-O, Granberg P-O, Hamberger B, Knutsson E, Mårtensson A, Sedvall G, Seiger Å, Olson L (1985) Transplantation of adrenal medullary tissue to striatum in parkinsonism; first clinical trials. J Neurosurg 62: 169–173
5. Bakay RAE, Fiandanca MS, Barrow DL, Schiff A, Collins DC (1985) Preliminary report on the use of fetal tissue transplantation to correct MPTP-induced Parkinson-like syndrome in primates. Appl Neurophysiol 48: 358–361
6. Bakay RAE, Barrow DL, Fiandanca MS, Iuvone PM, Schiff A, Collins DC (1987) Biochemical and behavioral correction of MPTP Parkinson-like syndrome by fetal cell transplantation. Ann NY Acad Sci 495: 623–638
7. Bankiewicz KS, Plunkett RJ, Jacobowitz DM, Porrino L, Di Porzio U, London WT, Kopin IJ, Oldfield EH (1990) The effect of fetal mesencephalon implants on primate MPTP-induced parkinsonism. J Neurosurg 72: 231–244
8. Baron-Van Evercooren A, Clerin-Duhamel E, Lapie P, Glansmüller A, Lachapelle F, Gumpel M (1992) The fate of Schwann cells tansplanted in the brain during development. Dev Neurosci 14: 73–84
9. Benabid AL, Pollak P, Gervason C, Hoffman D, Gao DM, Hommel M, Perret JE, de Rougemont J (1991) Long-term suppression of tremor by

chronic stimulation of the ventral intemediate thalamic nucleus. Lancet 337: 403–406

10. Benabid AL, Pollak P, Seigneueret E, Hoffman D, Perret J (1993) Chronic VIM thalamic stimulation in Parkinson's disease, essential tremor and extrapyramidal dyskinesias. Acta Neurochir (Wien) [Suppl] 58: 39–44

11. Björklund A, Stenevi U, Svendgaard N-A (1976) Growth of transplanted monoaminergic neurons into the adult hippocampus along the perforant path. Nature 262: 787–790

12. Björklund A, Stenevi U (1979) Reconstruction of the nigrostriatal pathway by intracerebral nigral transplants. Brain Res 177: 555–560

13. Blakemore WF, Franklin RJM (1991) Transplantation of glial cells into the CNS. TINS 14: 323–327

14. Blond S, Caparros-Lefebvre D, Parker F, Assaker R, Petit H, Guieu J-D, Christaens J-L (1992) Control of tremor and involuntary movement disorders by chronic stereotactic stimulation of the ventral intermediate thalamic nucleus. J Neurosurg 77: 62–68

15. Bondareff W, Mountjoy CQ, Roth M (1982) Loss of neurons of origin of the adrenergic projection to the cerebral cortex (nucleus locus ceruleus) in senile dementia. Neurology 32: 164–168

16. Browder EJ (1948) Section of the fibers of the anterior limb of the internal capsule in parkinsonism. Am J Surg 75: 264

17. Brundin P, Strecker RE, Widner H, Clarke DJ, Nilsson OG, Åstedt B, Lindvall O, Björklund A (1988) Human fetal dopamine neurons grafted in a rat model of Parkinson's disease: immunological aspects, spontaneous and drug-induced behaviour, and dopamine release. Exp Brain Res 70: 192–208

18. Brundin P, Widner H, Rehncrona S, Björklund A, Lindvall O (1989) Influence of the size of the implantation instrument on the survival of dissociated fetal neural grafts. IIIrd International symposium on neural transplantation. Restor Neurol Neurosci [Suppl] 1: P200

19. Calne DB (1994) Neurodegenerative diseases. Saunders, Philadelphia

20. Clarke DJ, Brundin P, Nilsson OG, Strecker RE, Björklund A, Lindvall O (1988a) Human fetal dopamine neurons grafted in a rat model of Parkinson's disease: ultrastructural evidence for synapse formation using tyrosine hydroxylase immunocytochemistry. Exp Brain Res 73: 115–126

21. Clarke DJ, Dunnett SB, Isacson O, Sirinathsinghji DJS, Björklund A (1988b) Striatal grafts in rats with unilateral neostriatal lesions: ultrastructural evidence of afferent synaptic inputs from the host nigrostriatal pathway. Neuroscience 24: 791–801

22. Cooper IS, Bravo GJ (1958) Anterior choroidal artery occlusion, chemopallidectomy and chemothalamectomy in Parkinsonism: a consecutive seris of 700 operations. In: Fields WS (ed) Pathogenesis and treatment of Parkinsonism. Thomas, Springfield, pp 325–352

23. Coyle JT, Schwartz R (1983) The use of excitatory amino acids as selective neurotoxins. In: Björklund A, Hökfält T (eds) Handbook of chemical neuroanatomy. Elsevier, Amsterdam, pp 508–527

24. Dohan FC, Robertson JT, Feler C, Schweitzer J, Hall C, Roberson JH (1988) Autopsy findings in a Parkinson's disease patient treated with adrenal medullary to caudate nucleus transplant. Soc Neurosci Abstr 7(4): 8

25. Duncan ID, Paino C, Archer DR, Wood PM (1992) Functional capacities of transplanted cell-sorted adult oligodendrocytes. Dev Neurosci 14: 114–122

26. Dunnett SB (1990) Functional analysis of neural grafts in the neostriatum. In: Björklund A, Aguayo AJ, Ottosson O (eds) Brain repair. Wenner-Gren International Symposium Series, vol 56. McMillan, London, pp 355–373

27. Dunnett SB, Annett LE (1991) Nigral transplants in primate models of parkinsonism. In: Lindvall O, Björklund A, Widner H (eds) Intracerebral transplantation in movement disorders, experimental basis and clinical experience. Elsevier, Amsterdam, pp 27–51

28. Dunnett SB, Svendsen CN (1993) Huntington's disease: animal models and transplantation repair. Curr Opin Neurobiol 3: 790–796

29. Dunnett SB, Bjöklund A (eds) (1994) Functional neural transplantation. Advances in neuroscience, vol 2. Raven, New York

30. Fazzini E, Dwork AJ, Blum C, Burke R, Cote L, Goodman RR, Jacobs TP, Naini AB, Pezzoli G, Pullman S, Solomon RA, Truong D, Weber JC, Fahn S (1991) Stereotaxic implantation of autologuos adrenal medulla into caudate nucleus in four patients with Parkinsonism. Arch Neurol 48: 813–820

31. Fearnley J, Lees A (1994) Pathology of Parkinson's disease. In: Calne DB (ed) Neurodegenerative diseases. Saunders, Philadelphia, pp 545–554

32. Fisher LJ, Jinnah HA, Kale LC, Higgins GA, Gage FH (1991) Survival and function of intrastriatally grafted primary fibroblasts genetically modified to produce L-dopa. Neuron 6: 371–380

33. Forno LS, Langston JW (1991) Unfavorable outcome of adrenal medullary transplant for Parkinson's disease. Acta Neuropathol 81: 691–694

34. Francis PT, Palmer AM, Sims NR, Bowen DM, Davison AN, Esiri MM, Neary D, Snowden JS, Wilcock GK (1985) Neurochemical studies of early-onset Alzheimer's disease. Possible influence on treatment. N Engl J Med 313: 7–11

35. Frank F, Sturiale C, Gaist G, Manetto V (1988) Letter to the editor: adrenal medullary autograft in human brain for Parkinson's disease. Acta Neurochir (Wien) 94: 162–163

36. Freed W, Morihisa J, Spoor E, Hoffer B, Olson L, Seiger Å, Wyatt R (1981) Transplanted adrenal chromaffin cells in rat brain reduce lesion-induced rotational behaviour. Nature 292: 351–352

37. Freed WJ, Cannon-Spoor HE, Krauthamer E (1986) Intrastriatal adrenal medulla grafts in rats: long-term survival and behavioral effects. J Neurosurg 65: 664–670

38. Freed CR, Breeze RE, Rosenberg NL, Schneck SA, Wells TH, Barrett JN, Grafton ST, Huang SC, Eidelberg D, Rottenberg DA (1990) Transplantation of human fetal dopamine cells for Parkinson's disease. Arch Neurol 47: 505–512

39. Freed CR, Breeze RE, Rosenberg NL, Schneck SA, Kriek A, Qi Jx, Lone T,

Zhang Yb, Snyder JA, Wells TH, Ramig LO, Thompson L, Maziotta JC, Huang SC, Grafton ST, Brooks D, Sawle G, Schroter G, Ansari AA (1992) Survival of implanted fetal dopamine cells and neurologic improvement 12 to 46 months after transplantation for Parkinson's disease. N Engl J Med 327: 1549–1555

40. Freeman TB, Hauser R, Sanberg P, Snow B, Vingerhoets JG, Olanow CW (1994) Fetal transplantation in Parkinson's disease. Neurology 44 [Suppl 2]: 324 (Abstract 783S)

41. Freeman TB, Sanberg PR, Nauert GM, Boss BD, Spector D, Olanow CW, Kordower JH (1995) The influence of donor age on the survival of solid and suspension intraparenchymal human embryonic nigral grafts. Cell Transpl 4: 141–154

42. Freund TF, Bolam JP, Björklund A, Stenevi U, Dunnett SB, Powell JF, Smith AD (1985) Efferent synaptic connections of grafted dopaminergic neurons reinnervating the host neostriatum: a tyrosine hydroxylase immuno-cytochemical study. J Neurosci 5: 603–616

43. Frodl EM, Duan W-M, Sauer H, Kupsch A, Brundin P (1994) Human embryonic dopamine neurons xenografted to the rat: effects of cryopreservation and varying regional source of donor cells on transplant survival, morphology and function. Brain Res 647: 286–298

44. Gage FH, Friedmann T, Fisher LJ, Jinnah HA (1991) Genetically modified cells: potential therapeutic application to Parkinson's disease. In: Lindvall O, Björklund A, Widner H (eds) Intracerebral transplantation in movement disorders. Elsevier, Amsterdam, pp 259–266

45. Gaspar P, Gray F (1984) Dementia in idiopathic Parkinson's disease. Acta Neuropathol 64: 43–52

46. Goetz CG, Olanow CW, Koller WC, Penn RD, Cahill D, Morantz R, Stebbins G, Tanner CM, Klawans HL, Shannon KM, Comella CL, Witt T, Cox C, Waxman M, Gauger L (1989) Multicenter study of autologous adrenal medullary transplantation to the corpus striatum in Patients with advanced Parkinson's disease. N Engl J Med 320: 337–341

47. Goetz CG, Tanner CM, Penn RD, Stebbins III, Gilley DW, Shannopn KM, Klawans HL, Comella CM, Wilson RS, Witt T (1990) Adrenal medullary transplant to the striatum of patients with advanced Parkinson's disease: 1-year motor and psychomotor data. Neurology 40: 237–276

48. Goetz CG, Stebbins III, Klawans HL, Koller WC, Grossman RG, Bakay RAE, Penn RD (1991) United Parkinson Foundation Neurotransplantation Registry on adrenal medullary transplants: Presurgical, and 1- and 2-year follow up. Neurology 41: 1719–1722

49. Grabowski M, Brundin P, Johansson BB (1992) Fetal neocortical grafts implanted in adult hypertensive rats with cortical infacts following a middle cerebral artery occlusion: Ingrowth of afferent fibers from the host brain. Exp Neurol 116: 105–121

50. Grabowski M, Johansson BB, Brundin P (1995) Neocortical grafts placed in the infarcted brain of adult rats: few or no efferent fibers grow from transplant to host. Exp Neurol 134: 273–276

51. Guttman M, Burns RS, Martin WRW, Peppard RF, Adam MJ, Ruth TJ, Allen G, Parker RA, Tulipan, Calne DB (1989) PET studies of Parkinsonian patients treated wit autologous adrenal implants. Can J Sci 16: 305–309

52. Hadani M, Freeman T, Pearson J, Young W, Flamm E (1987) Embryonic cortical transplants survive in middle cerebral artery territory after permanent arterial occlusion in adult rats. Ann NY Acad Sci 495: 711–714

53. Hefti F, Schneider LS (1991) Nerve growthfactor and Alzheimer's disease. Clin Neuropharmacol 14 [Suppl]: S62–S76

54. Henderson BTH, Clough CG, Hughes RC, Hitchcock ER, Kenny BG (1991) Implantation of human fetal ventral mesencephalon to the right caudate nucleus in advanced Parkinson's disease. Arch Neurol 48: 822–827

55. Hirsch EC, Duyckaerts C, Javoy-Agid F, Hauw J-J, Agid Y (1990) Does adrenal graft enhance recovery of dopaminergic neurons in Parkinson's disease? Ann Neurol 27: 676–682

56. Hitchcock ER, Henderson BTH, Kenny BG, Clough CG, Hughes RC, Detta A (1991) Stereotactic implantation of foetal mesencephalon. In: Lindvall O, Björklund A, Widner H (eds) Intracerebral transplantation in movement disorders. Elsevier, Amsterdam, pp 79–86

57. Horellou P, Brundin P, Kalén P, Mallet J, Björklund A (1990a) In vivo release of DOPA and dopamine from genetically engineered cells grafted to the denervated striatum. Neuron 5: 393–402

58. Horellou P, Marlier L, Privat A, Mallet J (1990b) Behavioral effect of engineered cells that synthesize L-dopa or dopamine after grafting into the rat neostriatum. Eur J Neurosci 2: 116–119

59. Hurtig H, Joyce J, Slafek JR, Trojanowski JQ (1989) Postmortem analysis of adrenal-medulla-to-caudate autograft in a patient with Parkinson's disease. Ann Neurol 25: 607–616

60. Itakura T, Kamei I, Nakai K, Naka Y, Nakakita K, Imay H, Komai N (1988) Autotransplantation of the superior cervical ganglion into the brain, a possible therapy for Parkinson's disease. J Neurosurg 68: 955–959

61. Jankovic J, Grossman R, Goodman C, Pirizzolo F, Schneider L, Zhu Z, Scardino P, Garber AJ, Jhingran SG, Martin S (1989) Clinical, biochemical, and neuropathologic findings following transplantation of adrenal medulla to the caudate nucleus for treatment of Parkinson's disease. Neurology 39: 1227–1234

62. Jacques D, Kopyov OV, Markham CH, Rand RW, Snow B, Vingerhoets F, Lieberman A (1994) One-year follow-up of six Parkinson's patients with fetal ventral mesencephalon grafts. Neurology 44 [Suppl 2]: A223 (Abstract 780S)

63. Jellinger K (1987a) Neuropathological substrates of Alzheimer's disease and Parkinson's disease. J Neural Transm [Suppl] 24: 109–129

64. Jellinger K (1987b) Quantitative changes in some subcortical nuclei in aging, Alzheimer's disease and Parkinson's disease. Neurobiol Aging 8: 556–561

65. Jiao S, Ding Y, Zhang W, Cao J, Zhang G, Zhang Z, Ding M, Zhang Z, Meng J (1989) Adrenal medullary autografts in patients with Parkinson's disease. N Eng J Med 321: 324–325

66. Jiao S, Gurevich V, Wolff (1993) Long-term correction of rat model of Parkinson's disease by gene therapy. Nature 362: 450–453
67. Katzman R (1986) Alzheimer's disease. N Engl J Med 314: 964–973
68. Kawaja MD, Fagan AM, Firestein BL, Gage FH (1991) Intracerebral grafting of cultured autologous skin fibroblasts into the rat striatum: an assessment of graft size and ultrastructure. J Comp Neurol 308: 2–13
69. Kelly PJ, Ahlskog JE, van Heerden JA, Carmichael SW, Stoddard SL, Bell GN (1989) Adrenal medullary autograft transplantation into the striatum of patients with Parkinson's disease. Mayo Clin Proc 64: 282–290
70. Kesslak JP, Nieto-Sampedro M, Globus J, Cotman CW (1986) Transplants of purified astrocytes promote behavioral recovery after frontal cortex ablation. Exp Neurol 92: 377–390
71. Kolarik J, Nadvornic P, Rozhold O (1990) Transplantation of embryonal nerve tissue into the brain under experimental and clinical conditions. Rozhl Chir 69(9): 569–574
72. Kordower JH, Freeman TB, Snow BJ, Vingerhoets FJG, Mufson EJ, Sanberg PR, Hauser RA, Smith DA, Nauert GM, Pearl DP, Olanow CW (1995) Neuropathological evidence of graft survival and striatal reinnervation after the transplantation of fetal mesencephalic tissue in a patient with Parkinson's disease. N Engl J Med 332: 1118–1124
73. Labbe R, Firl A, Mufson EJ, Stein DG (1983) Fetal brain transplants: reduction of cognitive deficits in rats with frontal cortex lesions. Science 221: 470–472
74. Laitinen LV, Bergenheim AT, Hariz MI (1992) Leksell's posteroventral pallidotomy in the treatment of Parkinson's disease. J Neurosurg 76: 53–61
75. Lange HW, Thörner GW, Hopf A, Schröder KF (1976) Morphometric studies of the neuropathological changes in choreatic diseases. J Neurol Sci 28: 401–425
76. Lindvall O, Backlund E-O, Farde L, Sedvall G, Freedman R, Hoffer B, Nobin A, Seiger Å, Olson L (1987) Transplantation in Parkinson's disease: two cases of adrenal medullary grafts to the putamen. Ann Neurol 22: 457–468
77. Lindvall O, Rehncrona S, Brundin P, Gustavii B, Åstedt B, Widner H, Lindholm T, Björklund A, Leenders KL, Rothwell JC, Frackowiak R, Marsden CD, Johnels B, Steg G, Freedman R, Hoffer BJ, Seiger Å, Bygdeman M, Strömberg I, Olson L (1989) Human fetal dopamine neurons grafted into the striatum in two patients with severe Parkinson's disease. Arch Neurol 46: 615–631
78. Lindvall O, Brundin P, Widner H, Rehncrona S, Gustavii B, Frackowiak R, Leenders KL, Sawle G, Rothwell JC, Marsden CD, Björklund A (1990) Grafts of fetaldopamine neurons survive and improve motor function in Parkinson's disease. Science 247: 574–577
79. Lindvall O, Widner H, Rehncrona S, Brundin P, Odin P, Gustavii B, Frackowiak R, Leenders KL, Sawle G, Rothwell JC, Björklund A, Marsden CD (1992) Transplantation of fetal dopamine neurons in Parkinson's disease: one year clinical neurophysiological observations in two patients with putaminal implants. Ann Neurol 31: 155–165

80. Lindvall O, Sawle G, Widner H, Rothwell JC, Björklund A, Brooks D, Brundin P, Frackowiak R, Marsden CD, Odin P, Rehncrona S (1994a) Evidence for long term survival and function of dopaminergic grafts in progressive Parkinson's disease. Ann Neurol 35: 172–180

81. Lindvall O (1994b) Neural transplantation in Parkinson's disease. In: Dunnett SB, Björklund A (eds) Functional neural transplantation. Raven, New York, pp 103–137

82. López-Lozano JJ, Bravo G, Brera B, Uría J, Dargallo J, Salmean J, Insausti J, Cerrolaza J (1991) Can an analogy be drawn between the clinical evolution of Parkinson's patients who undergo autoimplantation of adrenal medulla and those of fetal ventral mesencphalon transplant recipients? In: Lindvall O, Björklund A, Widner H (eds) Intracerebral transplantation in movement disorders; experimental basis and clinical experience. Elsevier, Amsterdam, pp 87–98

83. López-Lozano JJ, Bravo G, Abascal J (1991) Grafting of perfused adrenal medullary tissue into the caudate nucleus of patients with Parkinson's disease. J Neurosurg 75: 234–243

84. López-Lozano JJ, Bravo G, Abascal J, Brera B, Santos H, Gomez-Angulo C (1992) Co-transplantation of peripheral nerve and adrenal medulla in Parkinson's disease. Lancet 339: 430

85. Madrazo I, Drucker-Colín R, Diaz V, Martinez-Mata J, Torres C, Becerril JJ (1987) Open microsurgical autograft of adrenal medulla to the right caudate nucleus in two patients with intractable Parkinson's disease. N Engl J Med 316: 831–834

86. Madrazo I, Franco-Bourland R, Aguilera M, Ostrosky-Solis F (1989) Hispanic registry of graft procedures for Parkinson's disease. Lancet ii: 751–752

87. Madrazo I, Franco-Bourland R, Ostrosky-Solis F, Aguilera M, Cuevas C, Zamorano C, Morelos A, Magallon E, Guizar-Sahagun G (1990) Fetal homotransplants (ventral mesencephalon and adrenal tissue) to the striatum of Parkinsonian subjects. Arch Neurol 47: 1281–1285

88. Madrazo I, Franco-Bourland R, Ostrosky-Solis F, Aguilera M, Cuevas C, Alvarez F, Magallon E, Zamorano C, Morelos A (1990) Neural transplantation (auto-adrenal, fetal nigral and fetal adrenal) in Parkinson's disease: the Mexican experience. In: Dunnett SB, Richards SJ (eds) Neural transplantation: from molecular basis to clinical application. Progr Brain Res 82: 593–602

89. Madrazo I, Cuevas C, Castrejon H, Guizar-Sahagun G, Franco-Bourland RE, Ostrosky-Solis F, Aguilera M, Magallon E (1993) Primer homotransplante fetal homotopico de estrediado para el tratamiento de la enfermedad de Huntington. Gac Med Max 129(2): 109–117

90. Mahalik TJ, Finger TE, Stömberg I, Olson L (1985) Substantia nigra transplants into the denervated striatum of the rat: ultrastructure of graft and host interactions. J Comp Neurol 240: 60–70

91. Mampalam TJ, Gonzales MF, Weistein P, Sharp FR (1988) Neuronal changes in fetal cortex transplanted to ischemic adult rat cortex. J Neurosurg 69: 904–912

92. Mayer E, Fawcett JW, Dunnett SB (1993) Basic fibroblast growth factor promotes the survival of embryonic ventral mesencephalic dopaminergic neurons-II. Effects on nigral transplants in vivo. Neuroscience 56: 389–398
93. Meyers R (1942) The modification of alternating tremor, rigidity and festination by surgery of the basal ganglia. Res Publ Assoc Nerv Ment Dis 21: 602–655
94. Molina H, Quinones R, Alvarez L, Galarraga J, Piedra, Suárez C, Rachid M, García JC, Perry TL, Santana A, Carmenate H, Macías R, Torres O, Rojas MJ, Córdova F, Munos JL (1991) Transplantation of human fetal mesencephalic tissue in caudate nucleus as treatment for Parkinson's disease: the cuban experience. In: Linvall O, Björklund A, Widner H (eds) Intracerebral transplantation in movement disorders. Experimental basis and clinical experiences. Elsevier, Amsterdam, pp 99–110
95. Morihisa JM, Nakamura RK, Freed Wj (1987) Transplantation techniques and the survival of adrenal medulla autografts in the primate brain. Ann NY Acad Sci 495: 599–605
96. Nakai M, Itakura T, Kamei I, Nakai K, Naka Y, Imai H, Komai N (1990) Autologous transplantation of the superior cervical gangleon into the brain of parkinsonian monkeys. J Neurosurg 72: 91–95
97. Nakao N, Frodl EM, Duan W-M, Widner H, Brundin P (1994) Lazaroids improve the survival of grafted rat embryonic dopamine neurons. Proc Natl Acad Sci USA 91: 12408–12414
98. Narabayashi H, Okuma, T, Shikiba S (1956) Procaine-oil blocking of the globus pallidus. Arch Neurol 75: 36–48
99. Nikkhah G, Cunningham MG, Jödicke A, Björklund A (1994) Improved graft survival and striatal reinnervation by microtransplantation of fetal nigral cell suspensions in the rat Parkinson model. Brain Res 633: 133–143
100. Nyberg P, Nordberg A, Wester P, Winblad B (1983) Dopaminergic deficiency is more pronounced in putamen than in nucleus caudatus in Parkinson's disease. Neurochem Pathol 1: 193–202
101. Olanow CW, Koller W, Goetz CG, Stebbins GT, Cahill DW, Gauger LL, Morantz R, Penn RD, Tanner CM, Klawans HL, Shannon HM, Comella CL, Witt T (1990) Autologous transplantation of adrenal medulla in Parkinson's disease; 18-month results. Arch Neurol 47: 1286–1289
102. Olson L (1970) Fluoroscence histochemical evidence for axonal growth and secretion from transplanted adrenal medullary tissue. Histochemie 22: 1–7
103. Olson L, Seiger Å, Freedman R, Hoffer B (1980) Chromaffin cells can innervate brain tissue: evidence from intraocular double grafts. Exp Neurol 70: 414–426
104. Olson L, Backlund E-O, Ebendal T, Freedman R, Hamberger B, Hansson P, Hoffer B, Lindblom U, Meyerson B, Strömberg I, Sydow O, Seiger Å (1991) Intraputaminal infusion of nerve growth factor to support adrenal medullary autografts in Parkinson's disease; one year follow up of first clinical trial. Arch Neurol 48: 373–381
105. Olson L (1993) NGF and the treatment of Alzheimer's disease. Exp Neurol 124: 5–15

106. Penn RD, Goetz CG, Tanner CH, Klawans HL, Shannon KM, Comella CL, Witt TR (1988) The adrenal medulla transplant operation for Parkinson's disease: clinical observations in five patients. Neurosurgery 22: 999–1004
107. Perlow MJ, Freed WJ, Hoffer BJ, Seiger Å, Olson L, Wyatt RJ (1979) Brain grafts reduce motor abnormalities produced by destruction of the nigrostriatal dopamine system. Science 204: 643–647
108. Peschanski M, Defer G, N'Guyen JP, Ricolfi F, Monfort JC, Remy P, Geny C, Samson Y, Hantraye P, Jeny R, Gaston A, Kéravel Y, Degos JD, Cesaro P (1994) Bilateral motor improvement and alteration of L-dopa effect in two patients with Parkinson's disease following intrastriatal transplantation of foetal ventral mesencephalon. Brain 117: 487–499
109. Peterson DI, Price ML, Small C (1989) Autopsy findings in a patient who had an adrenal-to-brain transplant for Parkinson's disease. Neurology 39: 235–238
110. Pezzoli G, Motti E, Zecchenelli A, Ferrante C, Silani V, Falini A, Pizzuti A, Mulazzio D, Baratta P, Vegeto A, Villani R, Scarlato G (1990) Adrenal medulla autograft in 3 parkinsonian patients: results using two different approaches. In: Dunnett SB, Richards S-J (eds) Neural transplantation: from molecular basis to clinical application. Progr Brain Res 82: 677–682
111. Plunkett RJ, Bankiewicz KS, Cummins AC, Miletich RS, Schwartz JP, Oldfield EH (1990) Long-term evaluation of hemiparkinsonian monkeys after adrenal autografting or cavitation alone. J Neurosurg 73: 918–926
112. Redmond Jr DE, Leranth C, Spencer DD, Robbins R, Vollmer T, Kim JH, Roth RH (1990) Fetal neural graft survival. Lancet 336: 820–82
113. Sauer H, Brundin P (1991) Effects of cool storage on survival and function of intrastriatal ventral mesencephalic grafts. Restor Neurol Sci 2: 123–135
114. Seiger A, Nordberg A, von Holst H, Bäckman L, Ebendal T, Alafuzoff I, Amberla K, Hartvig P, Herlitz A, Lilja A et al (1993) Intracranial infusion of purified nerve growth factor to an Alzheimer patient: the first attempt of a possible future treatment strategy. Behav Brain Res 57: 255–261
115. Snow BJ, Vingerhoets FJG, Schulzer M, Calne DB (1994) Fluorodopa PET evolution of bilateral striatal fetal mesencephalic graft for idiopathic Parkinsonism. Neurology 44 [Suppl 2]: A281 (Abtract 609P)
116. Spencer DD, Robbins RJ, Naftolin F, Marek KL, Vollmer T, Leranth C, Roth RH, Price LH, Gjedde A, Bunney BS, Sass KJ, Elsworth JD, Kier EL, Makuch R, Hoffer PB, Redmond ER (1992) Unilateral transplantation of human fetal mesecephalic tissue into the caudate nucleus of patients with Parkinson's disease. N Engl J Med 327: 1541–1548
117. Sramka M, Rattaj M, Molina H, Vojtassak J, Belan V, Ruzicky E (1992) Stereotactic technique and patophysiological mechnisms of neurotransplantation in Huntington's chorea. Stereotactic Funct Neurosurg 58: 79–83
118. Starkova L, Mrna B, Bartosova S (1993) Neurotransplantation—a new method of treatment in psychiatry? Acta Univ Palacki Olomuc Fac Med 136: 33–35
119. Strecker RE, Sharp T, Brundin P, Zetterström T, Ungerstedt U, Björklund A (1987) Autoregulation of dopamine release and metabolism by intrastriatal nigral grafts as revealed by intracerebral dialysis. Neuroscience 22: 169–178

120. Strömberg I, Herrera-Marschitz M, Hultgren L, Ungerstedt U, Olson L (1984) Adrenal medullary implants in the dopamine-denervated rat striatum. 1. Acute catecholamine levels in grafts and host caudate as determined by HPLC-electrochemistry and fluorescence histochemical image analysis. Brain Res 297: 41–51

121. Strömberg I, Herrera-Marschitz M, Ungerstedta U, Ebendal T, Olson L (1985) Chronic implants of chromaffin tissue into the dopamine-denervated striatum. Effects of NGF on graft survival, fiber outgrowth and rotational behavior. Exp Brain Res 60: 335–349

122. Svennilson E, Torvik A, Lowe R, Leksell L (1960) Treatment of parkinsonism by stereotactic thermolesions in the pallidal region. Acta Psychiatr Scand 35: 358–377

123. Takeuchi J, Takebe Y, Sakakura T, Hara Y, Yasuda T, Imai T (1990) Adrenal medulla transplantation into the putamen in Parkinson's disease. Neurosurgery 26: 499–503

124. Tontsch U, Archer DR, Dubois-Dalcq M, Duncan ID (1994) Transplantation of an oligodendrocyte cell line leading to extensive myelination. Proc Natl Acad Sci 91(24): 11616–11620

125. Tönder N, Sörensen T, Zimmer J, Jörgensen MB, Johansen FF, Diemer NH (1989) Neural grafting to ischemic lesions of the adult rat hippocampus. Exp Brain Res 74: 512–526

126. Utzschneider DA, Archer DR, Kocsis JD, Waxman SG, Duncan ID (1994) Transplantation of glial cells enhances action potential conduction of amyelinated spinalcord axons in the myelin-deficient rat. Proc Natl Acad Sci 91(1): 53–57

127. Waters C, Itabashi HH, Apuzzo LJ, Weiner LP (1990) Adrenal to caudate transplantation—postmortem study. Mov Disord 5: 248–250

128. Wictorin K, Simerly RB, Isacson O, Swanson LW, Björklund A (1989) Connectivity of striatal grafts implanted into the ibotenic acid-lesioned striatum-III. Efferent projecting graft neurons and their relation to host afferents within the grafts. Neuroscience 30: 313–330

129. Widner H, Tetrud J, Rehncrona S, Snow B, Brundin P, Gustavii B, Björklund A, Lindvall O, Langston W (1992) Bilateral fetal mesencephalic grafting in two patients with parkinsonism induced by 1-methyl-4-phenyl-1,2,3,6-tetrahydropyridin (MPTP). N Engl J Med 327: 1556–1563

130. Widner H, Tetrud J, Rehncrona S, Snow B, Brundin P, Björklund A, Lindvall O, Langston JW (1993) Fifteen month's follow up on bilateral embryonic mesencephalic grafts in two cases of severe MPTP-induced parkinsonism. Adv Neurol 60: 729–733

131. Yamamoto T, Hirano A (1985) Nucleus raphe dorsalis in Alzheimer's disease: neurofibrillary tangles and loss of large neurons. Ann Neurol 17: 357–361

132. Zabek M, Mazurowski W, Dymecki J, Stelmachów J, Zawada E (1994) A long term follow-up of fetal dopaminergic neurons transplantation into the brain of three parkinsonian patients. Restorative Neurol Neurosci 6: 97–106

133. Zetterström T, Brundin P, Gage FH, Sharp T, Isacson O, Dunnett SB, Ungerstedt U, Björklund A (1986) In vivo measurement of spontaneous release and metabolism of dopamine from intrastriatal nigral grafts using intracerebral dialysis. Brain Res 362: 344–349

Editorial Comment

One aspect of possible development in this field has not been covered: that is the transplantation of cells genetically engineered to produce neurotrophic factors. To avoid immune rejection, these cells can be encapsulated in a polymer. The implanted cells are surrounded by a biocompatible semipermeable membrane permissive to passage of oxygen, nutrients, electrolytes and cell products, but restrictive to transport of the larger agents of the body's immune defense system. Cell lines offer several advantages for potential clinical uses. They can be banked, screened prior to transplantation for the presence of pathogens and efficiently enginereed to express and release neurotrophic factors using recombinant DNA technologies. Transplantation of cells isolated within a permselective polymer capsule restricts cell growth to the capsule space and protects them from immune destruction while allowing exchange of molecules between the entrapped cells and host tissue. In the event of capsule breakage, cells from a xenogenic origin are rejected by the host immune system.

The transplantation of genetically engineered cells is an active domain of research and clinical applications are already in view.

The Editors

The Normal and Pathological Physiology of Brain Water

K. G. Go

Department of Neurosurgery, University of Groningen, Groningen
(The Netherlands)

With 21 Figures

Contents

Summary

The physicochemical properties of water enable it to act as a solvent for electrolytes, and to influence the molecular configuration and hence the function—enzymatic in particular—of polypeptide chains in biological systems. The association of water with electrolytes determines the osmotic regulation of cell volume and allows the establishment of the transmembrane ion concentration gradients that underlie nerve excitation and impulse conduction.

Fluid in the central nervous system is distributed in the intracellular and extracellular spaces (ICS, ECS) of the brain parenchyma, the cerebrospinal fluid, and the vascular compartment—the brain capillaries and small arteries and veins. Regulated exchange of fluid between these various compartments occurs at the blood-brain barrier (BBB), and at the ventricular ependyma and choroid plexus, and, on the brain surface, at the pia mater. The normal BBB is relatively permeable to water, but considerably less so to ions, including the principal electrolytes. Brain fluid regulation takes place within the context of systemic fluid volume control, which depends on the mutual interaction of osmo-, volume-, and pressure-receptors in the hypothalamus, heart and kidney, hormones such as vasopressin, renin-angiotensin, aldosterone, atriopeptins, and digitalis-like immunoreactive substance, and their respective sites of action. Evidence for specific transport capabilities of the cerebral capillary endothelium, for example high Na^+K^+-ATPase activity and the presence at the abluminal surface of a Na^+—H^+ antiporter, suggests that cerebral microvessels play a more active part in brain volume regulation and ion homoeostasis than do capillaries in other vascular beds. The normal brain ECS amounts to 12–19% of brain volume, and is markedly reduced in anoxia, ischaemia, metabolic poisoning, spreading depression, and conventional procedures for histological fixation. The asymmetrical distributions of Na^+, K^+ and Ca^{2+} between ICS and ECS underlie the roles of these cations in nerve excitation and conduction, and in signal transduction. The relatively large volume of the CSF, and extensive diffusional exchange of many substances between brain ECS and CSF, augment the ion-homoeostasing capacity of the ECS. The choroid plexus, in addition to secreting CSF principally by bio*chemical* mechanisms (there is an additional small component from the extracellular fluid), actively transports some substances from the blood (e.g. nucleotides and ascorbic acid), and actively removes others from the CSF. In contrast with CSF secretion, CSF reabsorption is principally a bio*mechanical* process, passively dependent on the CSF-dural sinus pressure gradient.

Pathological increases in intracranial water content imply development of an intracranial mass lesion. The additional water may be distributed diffusely within the brain parenchyma as brain oedema, as a cyst, or as an increase in ventricular volume due to hydrocephalus. Brain oedema is classified on the basis of pathophysiology into four categories, vasogenic, cytotoxic, osmotic and hydrostatic. The clinical conditions in which brain oedema presents the greatest problems are tumour, ischaemia, and head injury. Peritumoural oedema is predominantly vasogenic and related to BBB dysfunction. Ischaemic oedema is initially cytotoxic, with a shift of Na^+ and Cl^- ions from ECS to ICS, followed by osmotically obliged water; this shift can be detected by diffusion-weighted MRI. Later in the evolution of an ischaemic lesion the oedema becomes vasogenic, with disruption of the BBB. Recent imaging studies in patients with head injury suggest that the development of traumatic brain oedema may follow a biphasic time course similar to that of ischaemic oedema. Hydrocephalus is associated in the great majority of cases with an obstruction to the circulation or drainage of CSF, or, occasionally, with overproduction of CSF by a choroid plexus papilloma. In either case, the consequence is a rise in intracranial pressure (ICP) due to increased ventricular volume. *Ex vacuo* hydrocephalus is a consequence of atrophy and does not disturb ICP; the same applies to some intracranial cysts, whereas those arachnoid or neuroepithelial cysts which do not have free communication in both directions with the CSF may cause rises in ICP. Intratumoral cysts resulting from necrosis or liquefaction within the tumour will usually also behave as mass lesions.

Introduction

Water constitutes a major proportion of brain tissue mass, and under pathological conditions increase of brain water may occur as brain oedema. Although greatly subdued at the present time, the spectre of brain oedema still looms in the background of neurosurgical management as one of the space-occuping lesions. Like tumours, haematomas, abscesses, cysts, and hydrocephalus, it may raise intracranial pressure or cause herniation of the brain. Moreover, brain oedema often accompanies these lesions, greatly contributing to their mass effect. In conditions such as brain trauma and infarction, however, brain oedema may even be the main space-occupying component.

Not only at the bedside, in which brain oedema may be responsible for obtundation and increasing neurological impairment, but also during operation and in conjunction with vasoparalysis, brain oedema may present itself as acute brain swelling. This is a dramatic condition in which the brain fills up all available space needed for surgical manoeuvring; the brain may protrude massively through the craniotomy opening, eventually preventing closure of the dura, replacement of the bone flap or even closure of the skin.

It is because of the potential of the brain to swell through water accumulation, that the physiology of brain water and of its disturbances is important for neurosurgery.

Brain Water, its Origin and Significance

Brain water, as all other forms of tissue water, should be regarded as a structural constituent of the tissue, pertinent to tissue function and integrity. To seek the origin of tissue water one must go back in evolutionary history, even beyond the origin of tissues and multicellular organisms, to the very beginnings of the cell itself, in which water constitutes an essential component of its protoplasm. Undoubtedly one will come upon the properties of water, as these determine what Henderson (1913) referred to as the "fitness" of an aqueous environment to play an essential role in the genesis and evolution of life.

A primary function of water is that of a solvent for many substances involved in cell physiology. In many respects it is an exceptional solvent. By its molecular mass, water should be a gas under terrestrial conditions, such as CO_2 or H_2S. However, in the water molecule the oxygen atom exerts a strong attraction upon electrons of the hydrogen atoms, providing the oxygen atom with a negative and the hydrogen atoms with a positive charge. This results in the formation of "hydrogen bonds" between the hydrogens and oxygens of adjoining water molecules, thus composing a polymeric network which is so tight, that the boiling point of water is high in comparison to that of substances of similar molecular mass (Fig. 1). An example of such a substance is H_2S in which no hydrogen bonds are formed as the S atom does not exert such a strong attraction upon the electrons of the hydrogen atoms. Moreover, water molecules can form hydrogen bonds to —OH, —NH, and —SH groups of other organic molecules, which thus may become soluble in water (Back 1993).

The asymmetrical distribution of positive and negative electrical

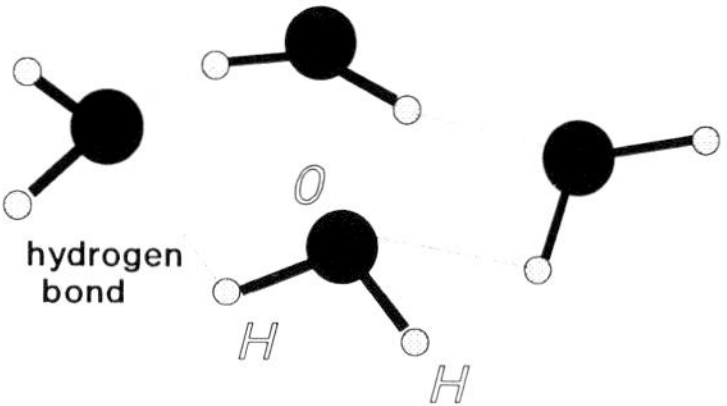

Fig. 1. Water molecules forming polymeric network by hydrogen bonds

charges in the water molecule results in a large dipole moment and a high dielectric constant, which facilitates the dissociation of soluble ionisable groups, both organic like —COOH and —NH$_2$ and inorganic, and opposes the reassociation of ions of opposite charge. It is by the solution and ionization of inorganic salts such as those of Na$^+$, K$^+$, Ca^{++}, Mg^{++}, Cl$^-$ and HCO$_3^-$ ions that the conductance of electricity becomes possible, a prerequisite for nerve conduction and excitation. It also allows the osmolar coupling of the predominant ions Na$^+$, K$^+$ and Cl$^-$ to water volume, constituting the basis of cell volume regulation, fluid secretion, and systemic fluid volume regulation.

For proteins in solution, hydrogen bonds between hydrophilic groups of their amino acid residues are among the forces which determine the way a protein's polypeptide chain will fold into the protein's so-called tertiary structure. Other forces which determine the tertiary structure of proteins are hydrophobic interactions. As pure hydrocarbon chains cannot form hydrogen bonds with water, hydrophobic amino acid residues of proteins tend to avoid contact with water molecules by self-aggregation. The tertiary structure of a protein in solution is pertinent to the protein's function as it determines the way in which the active site of an enzyme or the ligand binding site of a receptor is spatially presented. In the cleft of an enzyme molecule giving access to its active site, removal of water molecules surrounding a substrate molecule may favour reactions that involve a hydrophobic environment (Wolfenden 1983). Hydrophobic interaction also explains why the hydrophobic domains of certain proteins (e.g. transporters, ion channels and receptors) tend to be located within the lipid membrane, thus anchoring the protein in its strategic position (Fig. 16).

As a result of the small size of its molecules (0.1 nm), water readily penetrates most tissues (except the tight epithelia). Consequently, most tissues tend to have the same osmolarity, as differences of osmolarity would induce shifts of water that can freely move between the tissues and soon cancel the osmolarity differences. It also implies that movements or accumulations of water in tissues have to be attributed to osmotic forces (being osmotically obliged), following movements or accumulations of solutes, notably the prevailing electrolytes and proteins.

The epithelia tend to be impermeable to water, and certain epithelia possess specialized water channels, which are composed of proteins. An example is the membrane protein CHIP-28 with a molecular mass of 28 kDa which has been found in various parts of the nephron (Harris *et al.* 1993).

Therefore, it is incorrect to assume that accumulation of water in brain oedema is due to binding of water to certain tissue components. It is true that free and bound water fractions may be distinguished. The technique of differential scanning calorimetry allows determination of the amount of water in a tissue that is susceptible to freezing, which represents the fraction of free water. By subtraction from the total water content the fraction of bound water can be calculated. In normal brain the free water fraction was measured to be 88.9%, and the bound water fraction to be 11.1%. In brain tissue with cryogenic oedema, increase of the free water fraction parallelled the increase of total tissue water, although at a later phase of oedema there was also some increase of the bound water fraction (Furuse *et al.* 1984).

In fact, three fractions of tissue water may be postulated (Berendsen 1975): a fraction of free water, which is bulk water consisting of water molecules with great mobility; a fraction of hydration water loosely bound as a hydration mantle to macromolecules of the tissue (such as proteins or proteoglycans); and a very small fraction of crystalline water, which is specifically and tightly bound to the structural elements (Fig. 4). On the basis of this model, a fast proton exchange model has been developed by Fullerton (1982), in which the composition of the various fractions accounts for the magnetic resonance behaviour of the tissue.

Normal Brain Water Content: Effect of Maturation

The average water content of the human brain is about 85% of tissue fresh weight for grey matter and 70% for white matter, with some differences among the various grey matter structures (cerebral cortex 84.3, thalamus 75.1) and white matter areas (centrum ovale 70.7, corpus callosum 75.7, cerebellar white matter 70.6) (Stewart-Wallace 1939). The relatively lower water content of cerebral white matter is undoubtedly related to its content of myelinated fibers, and is reflected by its content of lipids: cholesterol 4%, phospholipids 9%, glycolipids 3%, versus proteins 14% and water 70%. Nevertheless, the proton magnetic resonance signal of cerebral white matter originates from water, in contrast to fatty tissue in which triglycerides constitute the majority of total proton density (Kamman *et al.* 1984).

There is a progressive decrease of brain water content with age, both in animals and in humans, of which the most pronounced decrease in early infancy is obviously related to maturation (Graves and Himwich 1955). In rat, brain water content measures around 87% at birth, and decreases to 80% in 6 weeks (De Souza and Dobbing 1971). The decrease of brain tissue water in early infancy forms part of a general pattern of decreasing total tissue water. Before birth there is a high content of tissue water (as well as sodium), which is mobilized and excreted in the first days of life (Friis-Hansen 1961). It has been suggested that prolactin plays a role in these events; prolactin has been shown to cause retention of water and salt, and fetal prolactin levels increase in the final third period of gestation (Coulter 1989, Lorenzo *et al.* 1983).

Measurement of Brain Water Content

Gravimetry

Gravimetry is the classical standard method of measuring brain water content by weighing fresh and dried brain tissue. On the assumption that the loss of weight is caused by the evaporation of water, brain water content is obtained as the difference between fresh and dry tissue weight, usually expressed as a percentage of fresh tissue weight.

$$\% \text{ Water content} = \frac{(\text{Fresh tissue weight} - \text{Dry tissue weight})}{\text{Fresh tissue weight}} \times 100\%$$

$$\% \text{ Dry weight} = \frac{\text{Dry tissue weight}}{\text{Fresh tissue weight}} \times 100\%$$

The percentage water content gives an idea of the water content of brain tissue. It can be used to express changes of water content as in oedema. However, it does not indicate the absolute amount of water per unit amount of tissue. To this end it is preferable to express water content as:

$$\text{g water}/100 \text{ g dry tissue} = \frac{\% \text{ Water content}}{\% \text{ Dry weight}} \times 100\%$$

It allows calculation of changes of tissue volume in oedema. For example, with 70% water content, normal white matter has 30% dry weight, and expressed per 100 g dry weight, it contains $70/30 \times 100 = 233$ g water. If its water content increases to 80%, 100 g dry tissue contains $80/20 \times 100 = 400$ g water, which implies a volume increment of $400 - 233 = 167$ ml.

Determination of Tissue Specific Weight

This technique which has been introduced by Nelson *et al.* (1971), allows estimation of brain oedema in small pieces of tissue by the use of a liquid gradient column. The column is made up of liquids that are not miscible with water, such as bromobenzene and kerosene. By means of an appro-

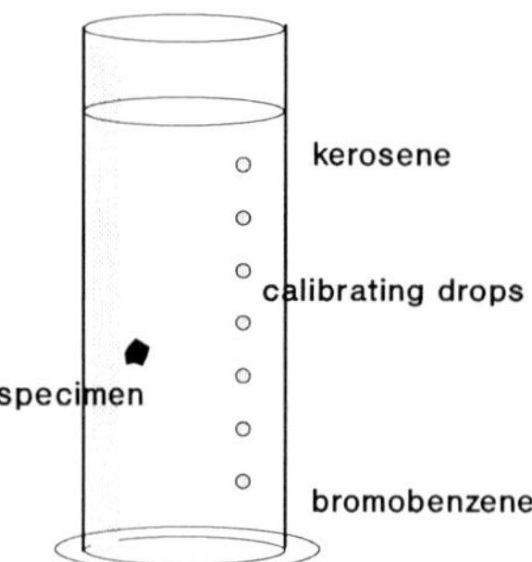

Fig. 2. Liquid gradient column for determination of tissue specific weight

priate technique of pouring the liquids, the bottom layer of the column consists only of the heavier bromobenzene, with higher layers gradually containing less bromobenzene and more kerosene. The tissue sample is deposited into the column, and the depth to which it has sunk after 2 minutes is observed. The relation between depth and specific gravity has been calibrated previously by deposition of drops of standard salt solutions of various densities (Fig. 2). Human cerebral cortex e.g. has a specific gravity of 1.0356, and human white matter 1.038 (Takagi *et al.* 1981). The specific gravity of the tissue diminishes as its water content increases. If desired, tissue water content can be calculated from tissue specific gravity by means of the following equations:

$$\text{g water}/g_t = 1 - (sg_t - 1)/(1 - 1/sg_s)sg_t$$

where sg_t is the particular tissue specific gravity to be measured, and sg_s is the specific gravity of tissue solids, which can be determined by:

$$sg_s = 1/(1 - (sg_t - 1)g_t/g_s \cdot sg_t$$

where g_t is the tissue weight and g_s the weight of tissue solids.

A correction should be introduced into the equation when the oedema fluid contains protein, as this changes the specific gravity of the tissue solids (Marmarou *et al.* 1982). The equation then becomes:

$$\text{g water}/g_t = \frac{(H_{nb} - H_{sr}) \cdot sg_{nb} \cdot sg_{sr} + sg_t \cdot (H_{sr}sg_{sr} - H_{nb}sg_{nb})}{(sg_{sr} - sg_{nb}) \cdot sg_t}$$

where H_{nb} is the normal tissue water content, H_{sr} the normal water content of serum, sg_{nb} the normal specific gravity of fresh tissue and sg_{sr} the normal specific gravity of serum (1.0248 in the cat); for serum the actual specific gravity of oedema fluid may be taken: 1.0213 ± 0.003, as determined in cats with a freezing injury (Go 1988c).

Computerized tomography (CT) has provided a method to determine tissue water content in a noninvasive, nondestructive fashion.

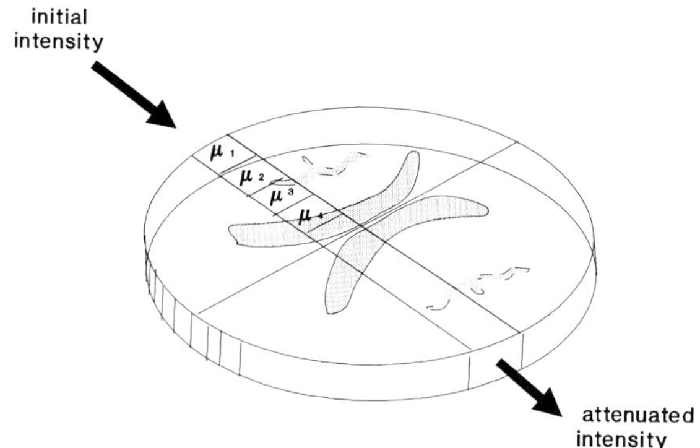

Fig. 3. Brain slice passed by scanning X-ray beam. Volume elements in the ray path have attenuation coefficients μ

On the CT-scan the signal intensity in each picture element (pixel) represents the attenuation coefficient or density μ of the corresponding volume element (voxel) of the depicted organ section. These densities are currently expressed in Hounsfield-units (HU) on a scale in which 0 was assigned to water, positive values to structures with a higher density than water, and -1000 to air. On this scale the following attenuation values have been measured for white matter: $+32$ HU, grey matter: $+39$ HU, CSF: $+15$ HU, whole blood: $+56$ HU, red blood cells: $+98$ HU, and plasma: $+33$ HU.

As brain tissue displays a higher attenuation than water, low densities on brain CT-scans may be correlated with an increase of brain water content (Hounsfield and Ambrose 1973). Thus it was found that with perifocal white matter oedema (after histological fixation of the brain), there was an attenuation of 12.6 ± 2.9 HU, corresponding to a water content of $79.9 \pm 4.77\%$ and a specific gravity of 1.044 ± 0.005, as compared to control values of 18.2 ± 1.5 HU, $70.5 \pm 1.40\%$, and 1.048 ± 0.0026, respectively (Torack *et al.* 1976).

Complicating the correlation with water content, however, is the dependence of attenuation upon other tissue components, such as tissue lipids with a 10% lower attenuation than water, and blood with its iron content. In spite of its higher water content, cerebral cortex has a higher attenuation number than white matter, on account of its higher content of oxygen instead of carbon, while oxygen with its higher atomic number causes greater absorption of X-rays than carbon. Moreover, in a lesion the normal relative proportions of water, lipids, blood and solids may be altered, causing changes of density which may be different from those expected from differences in water content alone.

Also, methodological and technical factors may interfere with the accuracy of the measurements. Among X-rays of various wave-lengths, those with the longest wave-lengths tend to be absorbed during their passage across materials with high atomic numbers, such as bone and iodine-containing contrast agents. This so-called beam-hardening effect causes errors in reconstruction and produces incorrect attenuation numbers. System-dependent factors such as the reconstruction algorithm used, the detector efficiency and the signal-to-noise ratio may affect measurement, as well as changes of positioning and movements of the patient, and the so-called partial-volume effect, which means that with the use of a matrix of large pixels, the density in a certain pixel may represent the average of widely differing attenuation of the tissue elements contained within the corresponding voxel.

Proton Magnetic Resonance

Magnetic resonance imaging (MRI) is another technique that allows the *in vivo* measurement of brain water content. Shortly summarized, tissue water protons, which may be considered to behave like small magnets, tend to align along the direction of a stationary static magnetic field, to which the tissue is subjected. They also perform a precession movement with a frequency v (in MHz), which is governed by the relation $v = \gamma B_0$, where B_0 is the magnetic field strength (in Tesla), and γ the gyromagnetic ratio (for protons, 42.6 MHz/T). Application of an additional rotating magnetic field perpendicular to the steady field gives rise to resonance, when the frequency of the rotating field equals the precession frequency. During resonance this net magnetic moment executes a precession movement around the transverse field; i.e. the magnetic moment progressively tilts to 90° or even 180° (the flip angle) with respect to the original alignment; (the exciting radiofrequency pulses are accordingly termed 90° and 180° pulses, respectively). The precession of the magnetic moment induces an electrical potential in a receiving coil, which is the signal. At the end of the pulse the magnetization M of the spins returns to its original alignment; in this *relaxation* process the amplitude of the signal decays according to an exponential function. The process of relaxation can be resolved into a return of the longitudinal vector of M (the vector M_z along the direction of the steady field), and an independent decay of a transverse component (M_{xy} in the transverse plane X—Y) due to dephasing of the proton spins, all of which had been aligned in phase during excitation. The relaxation of M_z is characterized by a time constant T_1, also called the *spin-lattice* relaxation time as this component of relaxation is assumed to be caused by interaction with neighbouring molecules (the lattice). The transverse relaxation time T_2, or *spin-spin* relaxation time, characterizes the dephasing of spins due to spin-spin interaction.

In biological tissues, the proton spins exhibit shorter relaxation times than in pure water, where T_1 and T_2 amount to about 2500 ms. A T_1 of around 400 ms was found for rat cerebral cortex and 350 ms for white matter, while T_2 amounted to about 80 ms for both tissues in an NMR spectroscopic study at 14 MHz. The behaviour of water protons in tissue may be explained by a model, in which the water protons in the vicinity of tissue macromolecules are assumed to interact with the macromolecules, to which the proton spins readily transfer their energy, quickening their relaxation to the equilibrium state. In brain oedema of various origins, a linear correlation is observed between the relaxation times and tissue water content. In oedematous tissue, the greater quantity of water may be assumed to resemble an environment like that of pure water, in which the proton spins show longer relaxation times (Go and Edzes 1975).

As focal lesions of the brain tend to be associated with brain oedema, and various cerebral structures have different water contents, these differences in water content may be reflected as differences in signal intensity in MRI, particularly when T_1 and T_2 effects are included into the signal. Thus, for reconstruction of the image in MRI, the signal must encode for relaxation parameters of the tissue to provide the differences in signal intensity, as well as for spatial coordinates. Modulation of T_1 and T_2 into the signal is accomplished by the application of various pulse sequences. Sequences which result in a T_1-dependent signal are called T_1-weighted, whereas those in which T_2 is predominant in determining signal intensity, are called T_2-weighted. Furthermore, the signal is retrieved from a plane or a volume, which is defined and selected by means of selective gradients of the magnetic field, with the aim that the field strength at the site of detection should fulfil the requirements for resonance posed by the reso-

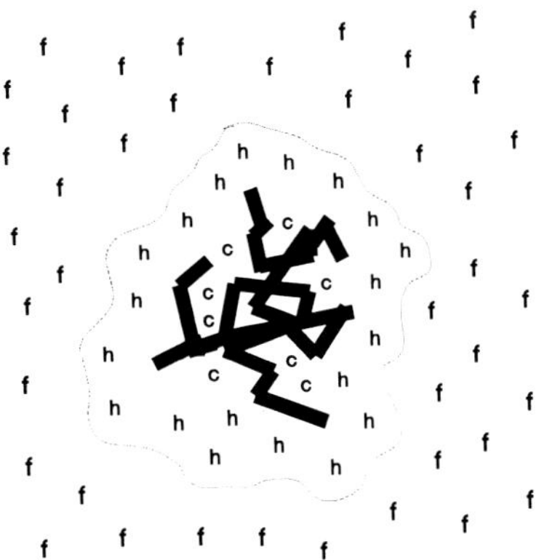

Fig. 4. Fractions of tissue water, c crystalline water tightly bound within macromolecule, h hydration water as a mantle around the macromolecule, f free water

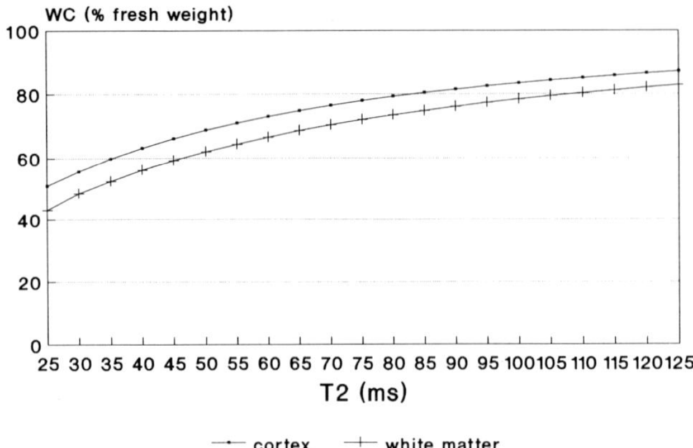

Fig. 5. Relation between water content WC in % of tissue fresh weight and relaxation time T_2 in milliseconds, for human cortex and white matter

nance frequency. Therefore, the proton signal is influenced by motion of the proton with respect to the plane or volume of detection; this allows the measurement or visualization of blood flow in magnetic resonance angiography (MRA), as well as that of flow and pulsations of the CSF by the choice of appropriate sequences. On a microscopic scale, motion of water protons by diffusion may also be visualized by the technique termed diffusion-weighted MRI. Furthermore, the signal is determined by the chemical environment of the proton, e.g. when the proton is part of a —CH_2 group; this results in a shift of its resonance frequency called chemical shift, which finds its application in magnetic resonance spectroscopy (MRS). In the spectrum, several proton-containing substances or groups, including important tissue metabolites like lactate, creatine and choline, are represented by resonance peaks along the frequency axis according to their chemical shift. MRS may also be applied to other atomic nuclei, such as ^{31}P which is characterized by its own gyromagnetic ratio, and is a constituent of the nucleotides ATP, ADP and phosphocreatine; therefore ^{31}P-MRS allows the study of tissue energy balance, while ^{23}Na MRS can be used to investigate lesions which are associated with sodium accumulation. The water proton signal is also influenced by the presence of paramagnetic substances in its vicinity, such as gadolinium which finds its application as an MRI contrast agent. Another technique, called magnetization transfer contrast (MTC), may visualize the rate of exchange of magnetization between a free water and a bound water fraction. Exchange can be observed by the decrease in the steady-state magnetization, and the relaxation times of the free water pool by irradiation of the bound water pool with a slightly off-resonance pulse (Wolff and Balaban 1989). This results in a change of the (apparent) T_1 of tissues such as muscle and brain which contain a significant proportion of free water; in this way white matter may by its myelin content be differentiated from grey matter.

Intracranial Fluid Compartments

The fluid within the cranial (and spinal) cavity comprises the cerebrospinal fluid (CSF), which is discernible as free fluid located within the ventricles, cisterns and subarachnoid spaces, but also the fluid contained within the brain tissue.

In the ventricles and other CSF-spaces the fluid is freely mobile, and therefore the pressure is equal everywhere in the compartment (Pascal's law), since any pressure differences are readily abolished by fluid shifts. On the other hand, in the brain tissue the pressure may show regional differences. In this respect the tissue may be envisaged as a network of membranes and fibres with the tissue fluid being located within the mazes. In the propagation of pressure through the fluid, the network offers resistance against the flow of fluid, and therefore regional tissue pressure is progressively reduced downstream, allowing pressure gradients to exist.

Brain tissue lacks a true lymphatic system which in other tissues drains the excess of tissue fluid formed in transcapillary fluid exchange. The CSF more or less fulfills this function, and moreover, maintains homoeostasis of the constituents of tissue fluid by extensive diffusional exchange.

Tissue fluid may be considered to be located in an extracellular and an intracellular compartment. In the extracellular fluid (ECF) Na^+ is the prevailing cation, whereas in the intracellular fluid (ICF) it is K^+. Moreover, in ECF Ca^{++} occurs in a millimolar (10^{-3} M) concentration, whereas the intracellular concentration of Ca^{++} amounts to 10^{-7} M, which pertains to its function as a second messenger.

An additional compartment in the brain is the vascular compartment; its fluid content constitutes part of the body's systemic fluid, and has the electrolyte composition of extracellular fluid. Although it occupies only 5% of total brain volume (the cerebral blood volume), it is important as a pathway through which fluid and solutes enter and leave the system. The other pathway is the CSF, as it is produced by the choroid plexus and reabsorbed into the blood by the arachnoid villi.

Intercompartmental Exchanges

The various compartments maintain mutual exchanges of fluid and solutes through their respective interfaces (see Fig. 6). Exchange between blood and brain is governed by the blood-brain barrier situated in the cerebral capillary endothelium. Exchange between CSF and brain tissue (ECF) proceeds through the ependyma lining the ventricles and through the pia

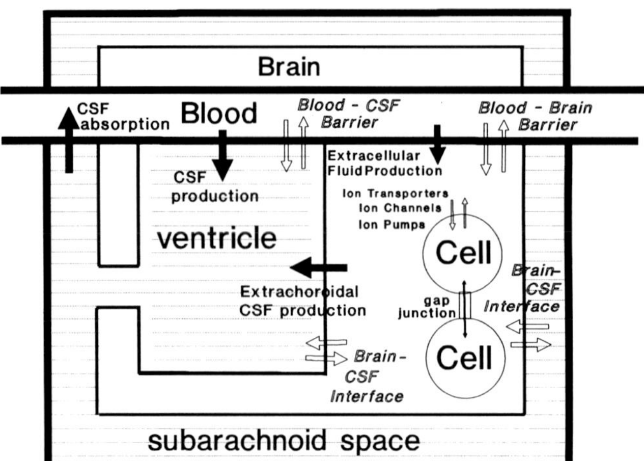

Fig. 6. Cerebral fluid compartments and their mutual exchanges

mater at the brain convexity. Therefore the interface between blood and CSF (the blood-CSF barrier) is dually represented by the choroid plexus and the blood-brain barrier via the brain-CSF interface. Finally, exchange between extra- and intracellular fluid proceeds through the plasma membrane of the cellular elements, in which ion channels, ion exchange mechanisms, and ion-pumps (ATP-ases) govern the exchange of electrolytes.

Fluid Volume: The Coupling of Water to the Prevailing Electrolyte NaCl: Regulation of Systemic Fluid Volume

Regarding the origin of body fluids, again it has been pointed out by Henderson (1913), that in many animals the electrolyte composition of blood plasma and other body fluids shows a great similarity to that of sea water, suggesting that sea water might be the original fluid environment bathing the ancestral cells, with its composition being reflected at the present time by the body fluids of modern animals. As to the origin of cerebrospinal fluid, it may be relevant that in some Prochordata, such as Ptychodera bahamensis, which may be considered close to the ancestral line of the Vertebrates, and in the larva of the protochordate Amphioxus, the neural tube is still in open communication with the ambient marine environment (Ariëns-Kappers 1929).

In blood plasma and tissue extracellular fluids, NaCl is the prevailing osmolar electrolyte. On the systemic level, the osmolar coupling of water and NaCl allows regulation of fluid volume by the regulation of water and salt balance, either separately or in conjunction. Influx of water is generally by oral ingestion, while its efflux proceeds by renal excretion, or as losses

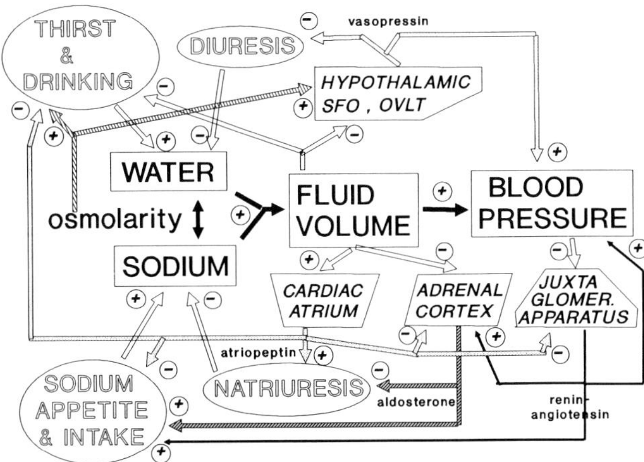

Fig. 7. Complex of regulations in the maintenance of systemic fluid homoeostasis. (+ stimulating influence; − inhibitory influence; stimulation of an inhibitory influence results in inhibition: + × − = −; inhibition of an inhibitory influence results in stimulation: − × − = +)

by way of the digestive tract, the respiratory tract, and perspiration. Uptake of NaCl also proceeds by oral ingestion, while efflux takes place through the urinary tract and by perspiration.

Systemic fluid volume is paramount in the maintenance of blood volume, and indirectly, of blood pressure as well (Fig. 7). Regulation of systemic blood pressure is not only accomplished by vascular tone and cardiac action, but also requires the maintenance of systemic fluid volume. Sodium loading is capable of raising arterial blood pressure, and increases the blood pressure response to catecholamines, while restriction of dietary salt intake which reduces fluid volume, tends to lower blood pressure (Weinberger 1987). Therefore, maintenance and regulation of systemic fluid volume, systemic blood pressure, and body fluid osmolarity are closely interrelated. It is reflected by the multiple actions of the various factors involved in the control of fluid balance, e.g. vasopressin not only raises blood pressure by inducing vasoconstriction, but also accomplishes conservation of water.

The homoeostatic control of fluid balance depends upon the release of these factors regulating water and salt excretion, and on an efficient thirst mechanism. Thirst is a strong emotional drive resulting in behaviour to seek and consume water. For salt, animals may exhibit a similar drive called salt appetite, to seek and consume salty foods and fluids. Thirst seems to be elicited by reduction of plasma volume, as resulting from haemorrhage, dehydration, or experimentally, by the subcutaneous injection of colloidal macromolecular solutions. Salt appetite can also be induced in rats by measures that reduce plasma volume (Stricker and Verbalis 1988). In patients with hypothalamic lesions the loss of the capacity to experience thirst has proved lethal because of the lack of the appropriate drive to consume water.

The renal excretion of water is controlled by the secretion of vasopressin or anti-diuretic hormone, which tends to reduce diuresis. Renal excretion of sodium is inhibited by aldosterone, and stimulated by atriopeptins (atrial natriuretic factor). Decrease of plasma volume not only induces thirst, but also stimulates the release of vasopressin, which tends to conserve water (Verney 1947). Increase of plasma osmolarity also induces thirst and the release of vasopressin, inhibiting diuresis, but in addition there is increased natriuresis. Loss of plasma volume also induces the secretion of aldosterone by the adrenal cortex, which tends to inhibit renal sodium excretion, but also elicits salt appetite in rats. Sodium appetite may also be induced by angiotensin II, acting synergistically with aldosterone. Angiotensin II, on the other hand, stimulates aldosterone release by the adrenal gland (Goodfriend *et al.* 1984). The renin-angiotensin system comprises the juxtaglomerular apparatus in the kidney, which, more precisely, is located in the walls of afferent arterioles as these enter the glomeruli. The juxtaglomerular cells secrete renin as a response to decrease of pressure in the renal vascular bed; in the blood circulation renin results in the formation of angiotensin I from angiotensinogen, a component of the plasma α_2-globulin fraction (Skeggs *et al.* 1967). Finally, angiotensin I is converted into angiotensin II by the angiotensin converting enzyme (also called kininase II).

The atriopeptins constitute a family of peptides with molecular weights of 2.5 to 13 kDa, which induce dramatic increases of renal sodium excretion. They are secreted by cardiocytes of the atrium as a response to atrial distension by the expansion of blood volume, obviously serving to prevent hypervolaemia. Moreover, they may inhibit the secretion of aldosterone and of renin (De Bold 1986). Brain also appears to secrete a natriuretic peptide (BNP), which shows a close structural resemblance, but is not identical, to atriopeptin; upon intravenous administration BNPs exerted natriuretic as well as hypotensive effects in hypertensive rats (Kita *et al.* 1989). Carbachol stimulation of the anteroventral region of the third ventricle (AV3V) could increase plasma levels of atriopeptin, part of which may originate from the brain (Baldissera *et al.* 1989).

Regarding the site of the regulating centres, experiments on goats have demonstrated that drinking behaviour, natriuresis, and release of vasopressin, could also be induced by infusion of hypertonic NaCl solutions into the third cerebral ventricle (Andersson and Westbye 1970). The osmoreceptors seem to be localized in the subfornical organ (SFO) and the organon vasculosum laminae terminalis (OVLT). These are circumventricular organs located around the third ventricle, from which efferent projection fibres mediate the effects, passing by way of the AV3V to the paraventricular nucleus, which is stimulated to secrete vasopressin and oxytocin. The subfornical organ and the OVLT are also the morphological substrates of drinking behaviour and the central pressor action elicited by angiotensin II administration (Simpson and Routtenberg 1973). On the other hand, microinjection of atriopeptin into the third ventricle or the subfornical organ inhibited water and salt intake. Chronic lesions of the hypothalamic region cause disturbances of fluid balance, such as hypernatraemia and a reduced natriuretic response to sodium loading (Brody *et al.* 1986).

In the syndrome of inappropriate antidiuresis there is hyponatraemia with concentration of urine and renal sodium wasting due to sustained production of vasopressin in spite of increased water intake and hypervolaemia (Schwartz 1957). The syndrome of inappropriate antidiuresis has also been suggested to explain the hyponatraemia in patients who exhibited dilatation of the third ventricle and alleged hypothalamic damage following subarachnoid haemorrhage; measurement of blood volume in these patients, however, demonstrated hypovolaemia, natriuresis and the presence of digoxin-like immunoreactive substance (DLIS) in the blood plasma (Wijdicks *et al.* 1987). DLIS is an endogenous factor isolated from bovine hypothalamus (Haupert and Sancho 1979) with the structure of digitalisglycosides, and which has the capacity to inhibit Na^+K^+-ATPase and to cause natriuresis by inhibition of tubular reabsorption (Hallaq and Haupert 1989). Its presence in human CSF has been shown to reduce choroid CSF production in an animal experiment (Lorenzo *et al.* 1989). Following subarachnoid haemorrhage or severe head injury, however, elevation of plasma atriopeptin levels and decrease of serum aldosterone levels have been measured as well (Diringer *et al.* 1988, Kiwit *et al.* 1988).

Apart from these well known factors, prolactin has been implicated as an antidiuretic factor, involved in the maintenance of the high tissue water content of preterm and newborn individuals (Lorenzo *et al.* 1983). In rabbits, prolactin has been shown to cause a reduction of urine volume and renal sodium excretion, whereas antidiuretic hormone only caused a reduction of urine volume but no change of sodium excretion, and aldosterone only caused a reduction in renal sodium excretion (Burstyn 1978).

The various factors usually exert their actions in the target tissues by interaction with specific receptors on the cell surface, followed by the activation of one or more of the intracellular signal transduction systems. For example, the aldosterone secretory response of adrenal glomerulosa cells to angiotensin II depends on receptor-mediated calcium influx and activation of the inositolphospholipid messenger system with consequent release of diacylglycerol (Isales *et al.* 1989). In the hypothalamus, high-affinity binding sites for atriopeptins have been demonstrated in the AV3V and the subfornical organ, which showed up-regulation in dehydration (Saavedra *et al.* 1986, Saavedra 1988, Saper *et al.* 1985). The mechanism of action of vasopressin on the nephron appears to involve the increase in water permeability of the epithelium due to fusion of water channel containing vesicles with the luminal plasma membrane (Harris *et al.* 1993). On the other hand, reabsorption of sodium through (epithelial) sodium channels of the distal part of the nephron is regulated by vasopressin and aldosterone (Canessa *et al.* 1993).

As will be mentioned in the appropriate section, the blood-brain barrier constitutes a veritable barrier to the passage of ions from the blood circulation into the brain, thus separating the systemic fluid compartments from those of the brain.

Blood-Brain Exchanges: The Blood-Brain Barrier and the Blood-CSF Barrier

The vascular system is one of the pathways by which fluid enters the brain. In Mongolian gerbils unilateral carotid occlusion resulted in the development of increasing amounts of cerebral oedema (demonstrated by the decrease of tissue specific gravity), as blood flow was progressively reduced below 20 ml/100 g/min. At zero flow values following bilateral carotid occlusion, however, no oedema was observed, obviously because no blood could enter the system to contribute to the fluid accumulation (Crockard *et al.* 1980). But even in the absence of any blood circulation, there is an indication that brain tissue may derive some fluid from the CSF in postmortem brain swelling, since the postmortem size of the ventricular system appeared to be reduced when compared with the size on ventriculograms made during life (Messert *et al.* 1972).

Exchange, i.e. influx and efflux, of fluid and solutes between blood and brain tissue is governed by the blood-brain barrier. It seems to be the function of the blood-brain barrier to optimize the biochemical environment of the neuronal elements in the brain by eliminating external perturbing influences, so as to allow the fine tuning of intrinsic regulatory mechanisms. It may be compared with providing delicate electronic equipment with a constant source by keeping out large fluctuations of voltage.

The following rules apply to the action of the blood-brain barrier: gases and neutral small-molecular substances pass readily, especially when they are lipid-soluble. From a molecular weight of ~ 500 onward, even lipophilic substances pass less easily. Conceivably, large-molecular substances such as proteins and polysaccharides pass with difficulty. An exception is the passage of substances that may qualify as vital to the tissue, such as glucose and some other sugars, amino acids, and nucleosides, which pass by way of a saturable transport system. The passage of ions is restricted, and for some inorganic ions, modulated by transport as described below.

Although it is a small molecule, water does not exhibit the greatest permeability across the blood-brain barrier. As expressed by the so-called permeability-surface area (PS) product, permeability across the blood-brain barrier was calculated for a number of alcohols from the fraction of injected substance extracted by the brain during single capillary passage; this was accomplished in a non-invasive way by external recording of positron emitting tracers; it demonstrated that the PS product (370 ml/min/100 g) of isopropanol, for example was higher than that of water (Raichle *et al.* 1976). The movement of water across the capillary wall may be envisaged to consist of (1) a diffusional component, and (2) a convective or bulk flow component. The diffusional component is subject to the influence of CBF according to the relation: $\ln(1 - E) = -PS/CBF$ (Renkin 1959, Crone 1963), in which E is the fraction of water extracted from the capillary during single transit (Fig. 8). On the other hand, the convective component is subject to hydrostatic and osmotic forces according to the Starling relationship of transcapillary fluid exchange. Measurement of the ^{15}O-water extraction fraction during a single capillary passage through rat brain demonstrated that extraction was only determined by the CBF according to the Renkin (1959)-Crone (1963) relation, whereas no effect of osmotic or hydrostatic forces could be established. This implies that the extraction of ^{15}O-water during single transit is almost entirely diffusional, and that the convective component apparently is far slower, eluding mea-

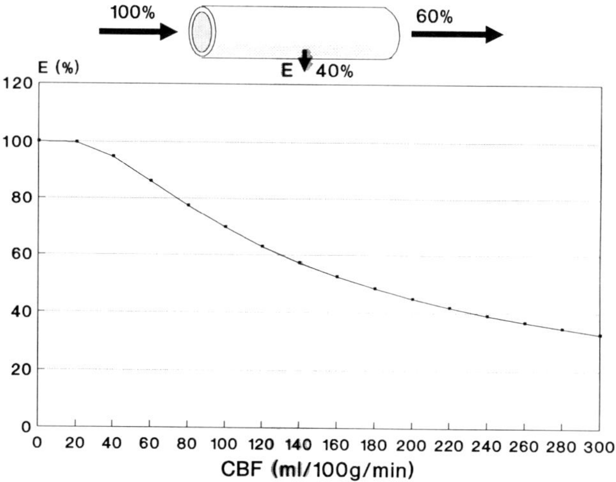

Fig. 8. Relation between extraction of water during single capillary passage and CBF

surement. With a PS product of 119 ml/min/100 g, only a fraction of 60% of the water flowing through the cerebral vascular system was extracted by the rat brain at a blood pressure of 130 mm Hg during single passage (Go *et al.* 1981). Notably, intraventricular administration of vasopressin to Rhesus monkeys increased the PS-product for water from ~ 120 to ~ 150 ml/100 g/min (Raichle and Grubb 1978).

The restricted passage of the prevailing ions Na^+ (and Cl^-) also implies a restriction of the passage of fluid in transcapillary fluid exchange. Generally, in most organs the capillaries are only impervious to proteins, but not to ions, and transcapillary fluid exchange proceeds according to the Starling fluid flux equation:

$$J_v = L_p(\Delta P - \sigma \Delta\Pi)$$

in which J_v represents the volume of fluid passing, L_p the so-called hydraulic conductivity of the capillary wall, i.e. a coefficient characterizing the mechanical filtration capacity of the capillary wall for fluid, ΔP the pressure difference between capillary and tissue, σ the so-called Staverman reflection coefficient, i.e. a coefficient reflecting the permeability of the capillary wall for the solute, reducing the effect of $\Delta\Pi$, the difference of colloid-osmotic pressure between capillary and tissue fluid.

Since there is restricted blood to brain passage for proteins as well as ions, the equation of transcapillary fluid exchange should include a term representing the osmotic pressure difference resulting from sodium (Habers and Berendsen, as cited by Go 1991):

$$J_V = L_P\Delta P + L_{PDs}\Delta\Pi_s + L_{PDp}\Delta\Pi_p$$

$$J_{DS} = L_{DsP}\Delta P + L_{Ds}\Delta\Pi_s + L_{DsDp}\Delta\Pi_p$$

$$J_{Dp} = L_{DpP}\Delta P + L_{DpDs}\Delta\Pi_s + L_{Dp}\Delta\Pi_p$$

where J_v is volume flow, J_{Ds} the diffusional flow for sodium and J_{Dp} the diffusional flow for proteins. Apart from the hydrostatic pressure difference ΔP, the other forces involved are the osmotic pressure difference $\Delta\Pi_s$ resulting from sodium concentration differences, and the colloid-osmotic pressure difference $\Delta\Pi_p$ resulting from protein concentration differences. The coefficients L_P, L_{Ds} and L_{Dp} are respectively the hydraulic conductivity of the capillary wall, and the diffusional mobilities of sodium and of protein per unit of osmotic pressure. The coupling coefficients are:

$$L_{PDp} = (J_v/\Delta\Pi_p)_{\Delta P=0,\,\Delta\Pi s=0}, \text{ and } L_{PDs} = (J_v/\Delta\Pi_s)_{\Delta P=0,\,\Delta\Pi p=0}$$

expressed in reflection coefficients $\sigma_i = -L_{PDi}/L_P$, the volume flow can be written as:

$$J_V = L_P(\Delta P - \sigma_s\Delta\Pi_s - \sigma_p\Delta\Pi_p).$$

In spite of the restricted passage of sodium through the blood-brain barrier, there are arguments favouring the validity of the Starling relationship. It may be envisaged that during filtration of fluid across the capillary wall driven by the hydrostatic pressure difference, a quantity of Na^+ is carried with the fluid, as much as is allowed by barrier permeability. When the cerebral uptake of sodium from the blood was measured following intravenous administration of radioactive Na^+; there appeared to be a linear relationship between the Brain Sodium Uptake from the blood (BSU, in μl blood equivalents/min/g) and the arterial blood pressure P_a (in mm Hg): BSU $= 1.6 + 0.03\ P_a$ (Go and Pratt 1975). The sodium taken up by the brain seemed to be of dual origin, with a blood pressure-dependent component, allegedly representing filtration across the capillary wall, and a component corresponding to the intercept on the BSU-axis (Fig. 9). The latter might well represent the diffusional component from the CSF as it decreased when the temperature was lowered (0.34 μl blood equivalents/g/min at 15° C, as compared to 1.6 μl blood equivalents/g/min at 33° C) in accordance with the behaviour of an active transport mechanism such as CSF secretion, while it also decreased following removal of the choroid plexuses (Go *et al.* 1979a). Another argument for the validity of the Starling relationship is the phenomenon of hydrostatic brain oedema resulting from elevation of arterial blood pressure. The significance of the colloid-osmotic pressure is demonstrated by the influence of extracellular protein upon absorption of fluid: after the infusion of saline into cerebral white matter, the fluid was retained much longer when it contained protein (Marmarou *et al.* 1984).

The restricted passage of Na^+ also implies that brain extracellular space is in fact segregated from systemic extracellular space, and unless the blood-brain barrier is disrupted, inflation of systemic extracellular space

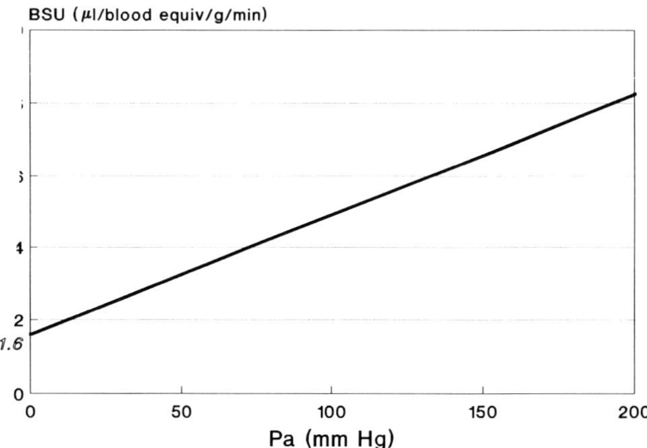

Fig. 9. Brain sodium uptake in the rat as a function of arterial blood pressure at 33° C

by isotonic hyperhydration with saline is not followed by expansion of cerebral extracellular space, as in other organs not possessing a barrier. In other words, isotonic hyperhydration cannot initiate brain oedema, but it can aggravate existing vasogenic brain oedema, as the blood-brain barrier is disrupted (Go *et al.* 1972a, Gerschenfeld *et al.* 1959). On the other hand, the integrity of the blood-brain barrier is necessary for the efficacy of therapeutic dehydration of the brain by hyperosmolar solutions, as well as for osmotic brain oedema to develop, since disruption of the barrier readily abolishes the osmotic gradient between blood plasma and brain responsible for the osmotic effects.

An alternative mechanism for transcapillary fluid passage would be active transport of Na^+ across the capillary wall with osmotically obliged water (similar to the process of CSF secretion by the choroid plexus). There are arguments for this mechanism, such as the high Na^+K^+-ATPase activity of cerebral capillary endothelium (amounting to 500 times that of peripheral capillary endothelium) (Eisenberg and Suddith 1979), and which appears to be localized in the abluminal plasma membrane of the endothelial cells (Betz *et al.* 1980). The enzyme may accomplish Na^+ transport from the blood to the cerebral extracellular space, associated with a K^+ countertransport from the extracellular space into the blood. It may subserve regulation of extracellular K^+ content by transport into the blood. The K^+ transport by isolated brain capillary fractions can be inhibited by corticosteroids (Chaplin *et al.* 1981). Other ion exchange mechanisms involved in the transport of Na^+ from blood to brain include a sodium channel sensitive to amiloride, and a Na^+-Cl^- cotransport mechanism sensitive to furosemide (Betz 1983a, Goldstein and Betz 1983). Furthermore, a Na^+/H^+ antiporter may be present in the abluminal membrane, as indicated by the pH-sensitivity of sodium uptake by isolated brain capillary fractions; it may be involved in the pH-regulation of the cerebral extracellular fluid (Betz 1983b). Patch-clamp studies on membrane patches from isolated cerebral microvascular endothelium have shown amiloride-sensitive cation channels with a conductance of 23 pS, and a selectivity for Na^+ over K^+ of 1.5/1; the pharmacological profile for their binding of various amiloride analogues resembled that of epithelial Na^+ channels (Vigne *et al.* 1989).

Another cation transport mechanism that, moreover, would account for blood pressure dependence of Na^+-influx may consist of the stretch-activated non-selective cation channels that have been found in the anti-luminal membrane of porcine cerebral capillaries (Popp *et al.* 1992).

Pertinent to its function in the passage of fluid and electrolytes, brain capillary endothelium has been reported to contain receptors for atrio-peptins, angiotensin II, and vasopressin (Chabrier *et al.* 1987, Speth and Harik 1985, Zlokovic *et al.* 1990).

Morphologically, the blood-brain barrier consists of the luminal (apical) plasma membrane of the cerebral capillary endothelium, together with the tight junctions occluding the clefts between the endothelial cells.

Tight junctions, or zonulae occludentes, are junctions that tightly occlude the intercellular clefts between adjacent cerebral capillary endothelial cells, choroid plexus epithelial cells, and barrier cells of the arachnoid mater. Transmission electron microscopy visualizes the tight junction as a five-layered structure in cross section, with its middle layer being formed by coalescence of the apposed external layers of the usual three-layered plasma membranes of adjoining cells (Fig. 10). The freeze-fracturing technique displays the tight junction as an area characterized by a network of more or less parallel ridges, consisting of fibrils of 10 nm diameter.

Studies on the passage of substances through endothelium have indicated that the passage of water and small hydrophylic solutes takes place through a small-pore system (in bovine cerebral endothelium calculated to measure 8 μm (Van Bree *et al.* 1988). This small-pore system has allegedly been identified as the intercellular clefts between endothelial cells, also called the paracellular pathway. The large pore system, through which larger molecules such as those of proteins may pass, has been identified in the cerebral capillary endothelium as the pinocytotic transport pathway, in which pinocytotic vesicles are formed by invagination and subsequent sequestration of the luminal plasma membrane, while engulfing the substance to be transported; after passage through the endothelial cytoplasm, they release their contents upon arrival at the basal plasma membrane, with which they merge again (Fig. 10).

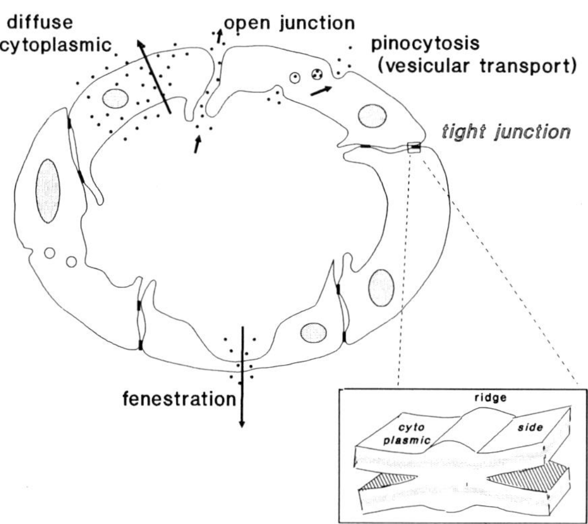

Fig. 10. Mechanisms of protein tracer passage through brain capillary endothelium. Inset shows detail of tight junctional structure

The finding of the contractile proteins actin and myosin in brain capillary endothelium (Le Beux and Willemot 1978) may bear upon the paracellular pathway. In other epithelial tissues tight junction permeability has been shown to be influenced by the cytoskeleton. Intestinal epithelium contains a perijunctional ring of actin and myosin, which is associated with the plasma membrane at a site just below the tight junction belt. Exposure to cytochalasin induced contraction of the perijunctional ring with alteration of tight junction structure and enhanced permeability (Madara *et al.* 1987).

Pathology: Breakdown of the Blood-Brain Barrier and Vasogenic Brain Oedema

Breakdown of the blood-brain barrier, which is associated with focal cerebral lesions, causes leakage of plasma constituents into the brain parenchyma as vasogenic brain oedema (Klatzo *et al.* 1958). Reversible and discrete impairments of blood-brain barrier permeability occur during hypercapnia and epileptic seizures, but are usually not associated with brain oedema. Gross blood-brain barrier disruption and inherent vasogenic brain oedema generally occur with focal lesions of the brain.

In the laboratory, blood-brain barrier disruption may be studied by the systemic administration of indicators, such as the dyes Evans blue, trypan blue, fluorescein, and their exudation into the brain parenchyma noted upon killing the animal. A more sophisticated indicator substance is the synthetic amino acid α-aminobutyric acid (AIB), usually given as a ^{14}C-tracer, which is not metabolized by the tissue and therefore remains in situ after its extravasation. For electron microscopical investigation of the barrier, tracers are employed which are either electron-dense, such as ferritin, or which produce an electron-dense reaction product, such as the enzyme horse radish peroxidase (HRP). Clinically, e.g. in meningitis, blood-brain (-CSF) barrier breakdown may be verified by analysis of CSF, in which plasma proteins appear in increased concentration. Normally, passage of plasma proteins as reflected by the ratio Q = plasma concentration/CSF concentration, is inversely proportional to the molecular weight of the protein. With barrier disruption there is increased entrance of the protein into the CSF, resulting in decrease of Q (Felgenhauer *et al.* 1976). The diagnostic imaging techniques, in particular, allow the clinical verification of barrier disruption. The technique of cerebral scintigraphy or isotope scanning was based upon visualization of cerebral lesions by the exudation of the radioactive tracer (usually [^{99m}Tc]-pertechnetate or [^{131}]I-radioiodinated serum albumin). The current techniques of CT and MRI still employ as an aid to diagnosis contrast enhancement, which is the result of exudation of the contrast agent.

Exudation of proteins, beside water and electrolytes, is a distinctive feature of vasogenic brain oedema. Morphological studies of the familiar experimental models of barrier disruption, using electron microscopy and HRP, have not unambiguously elucidated the mechanism of protein exudation in these models. In earlier studies it has seemed, that separation of tight junctions was responsible for protein exudation (Brightman *et al.* 1973). Later studies indicated an increase of vesicular transport as the relevant mechanism of passage (Westergaard 1975). However, on the basis of experiments, in which endogenous anti-HRP antibodies were induced by previous vaccination with HRP, it was demonstrated that the tracer passed diffusely through the endothelial cytoplasm, presumably by increased permeability of the endothelial cell membranes (Fig. 10) (Houthoff *et al.* 1982, Gazendam *et al.* 1984). In brain tumours, protein exudation and vasogenic oedema are apparently based on the presence of abnormalities of the capillary endothelium, such as fenestrations, separation of tight junctions, absence of basal lamina and the occurrence of tubular bodies and increased numbers of vesicles in the cytoplasm (Long 1970, Hirano and Matsui 1975).

The Blood-CSF Barrier

The choroid plexus not only secretes CSF, but in its function of blood-CSF barrier it performs the transport of a number of substances, such as nucleosides, that are not transported by the blood-brain barrier (Spector 1980), and ascorbic acid (Spector 1977). On the other hand, it also accomplishes the removal from the CSF by transport to the blood, of substances such as iodide, thiocyanate, amino acids and certain oligopeptides (Rapoport 1976, Lorenzo 1974, Banks *et al.* 1986).

The Cerebral Extracellular Space

The 1930s saw the emergence of the concept of extracellular space, in which a different distribution of various ions was observed with respect to the intracellular space. In the nervous system, the electrolyte composition of extracellular fluid has great relevance to the ionic shifts during nerve excitation and conduction. From the distribution of ions, which were predominantly extracellularly located, the size of the extracellular space of various tissues such as muscle, spleen and liver, was calculated (Harrison *et al.* 1936, Manery and Hastings 1939). Measurement of cerebral extracellular space has been conducted in vitro on brain slices using extracellular space (ECS)-indicators such as sucrose, inulin, thiocyanate, and sulfate. But measurements in vivo proved to be complicated by the blood-brain barrier which prevented many indicators from adequately entering the brain following their systemic administration. Administration into the CSF alone also had its limitations, as penetration of the indicator into the brain parenchyma depended on distance from the CSF, especially in larger animals. These difficulties had to be overcome by administration of the marker both into the blood and the CSF, and applying corrections for the decrease of tissue concentration with increasing distance from the CSF. After application of the corrections, values in the range of 12–19.4% were calculated for the fractional volume of cerebral extracellular space (Reulen *et al.* 1970a, Fenstermacher *et al.* 1970).

A controversy arose when observations with the novel technique of electron microscopy indicated close packing of cellular elements in the central nervous system, which only left an intercellular space of around 6%, far below the values provided by the methods using ECS-indicators. As recognized by Van Harreveld (1966), there was increase of tissue electrical impedance indicating reduction of extracellular space on account of cell swelling, during conventional fixation procedures of the tissue as a prelude to electron microscopic viewing. Only when the neural tissue was extremely rapidly frozen by contact with a silver plate cooled to a temperature of −207° C, and then subjected to freeze substitution with a fixative, interstitial clefts of 20–25 nm could be observed (Van Harreveld 1966).

Methods to Study Extracellular Space

As mentioned before, extracellular space may be measured by the use of ECS-indicators, both of brain slices in vitro, and in experimental animals by administration of the marker both into the blood and the CSF, with correction for the decrease of tissue concentration with increasing distance from the CSF.

Electron microscopy only visualizes markedly enlarged intercellular spaces in oedema of the vasogenic or hydrostatic types, whereas normal and less enlarged intercellular spaces tend to be obliterated by the cell swelling taking place during routine fixation. These methods are destructive, and require the taking of tissue samples for analysis.

Measurement of electrical tissue impedance may be used as a non-destructive technique in humans and animals to monitor changes of extracellular space, rather than to obtain absolute data on the size of extracellular space. It is based upon the concept that alternating current of low frequency passing through tissue is conducted predominantly through the extracellular fluid, since the cell membranes enveloping the cellular contents impede the participation of intracellular ions. Therefore, the electrical impedance of the tissue may be considered to reflect the size of the extracellular space (Van Harreveld 1966). Measurement of tissue impedance has been used to localize brain tumours, which show a decreased impedance due to expansion of the extracellular space in the oedematous tissue within and around the tumour (Organ *et al.* 1968). Decreased impedance has also been measured in oedematous contusional lesions, haemorrhages, and infarctions (Go *et al.* 1972b). Impedance measurement has found application in stereotactic neurosurgery and percutaneous chordotomy to identify neural structures passed by the probe (Robinson 1962).

In cats with vasogenic brain oedema caused by a cortical freezing injury, (extra-cellular) oedema fluid may be collected from the brain by the insertion of needles, with the shorter reaching into the cortex and the longer into the white matter. The needles contain a loose bundle of moistened nylon fibres at their tips to prevent clogging by tissue debris (Fig. 11). The oedema fluid accumulates into polyethylene tubes, connected to the needles and filled with a volatile kerosene fraction, to prevent evaporation of the accumulating oedema fluid (Patberg *et al.* 1977, Gazendam *et al.* 1979a). Analysis of the fluid provided data on the concentration of electrolytes and other solutes in the oedema fluid, and demonstrated that during hypoxia or following the intracerebral injection of ouabain there was an increase of protein content indicative of condensation due to shrinkage of the extracellular space (Go *et al.* 1979b, Gazendam *et al.* 1979b).

Microdialysis is a technique by means of which the concentrations of various extracellular fluid constituents may be monitored continuously. A microdialysis probe consisting of a U-shaped hollow-fibre dialysis tube is inserted into the brain, and perfused with artificial CSF at a rate of 10 μl/min; the substance to be monitored diffuses from the tissue extracellular fluid into the dialysate, which is then analysed, preferably on-line. It has not been possible to derive absolute extracellular concentrations from the

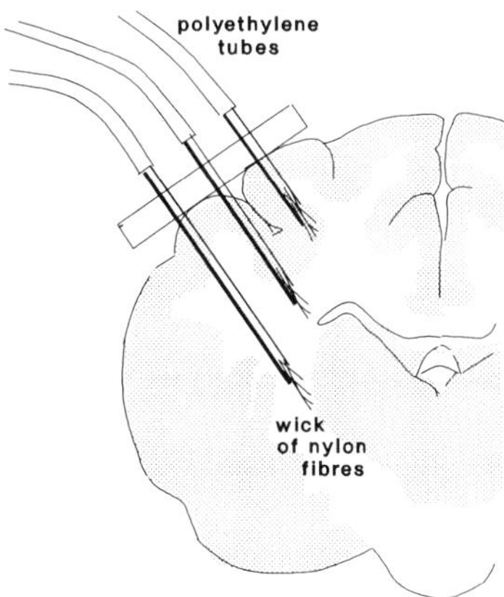

Fig. 11. Technique for isolation of oedema fluid in the cat

dialysate concentrations, since such variables as the diffusion of the substance through brain tissue and across the cellular membranes are difficult to estimate. The method has, for example, demonstrated the production of lactate by the brain under various physiological as well as ischaemic conditions (Korf 1989); it has also revealed decrease of extracellular glucose concentration during periods of repetitive hypoxia/ischaemia, followed by restoration of the levels during the intervals (Klein 1992).

The technique of ventriculo-cisternal perfusion has been used for the assessment of the exchange of various substances between CSF and brain, concomitant to the measurement of CSF formation and absorption rates. Through a needle, which is usually inserted into a lateral cerebral ventricle of the animal, artificial CSF (i.e. a fluid with the ionic composition of natural CSF) is infused into the ventricular system. Outflow of the fluid takes place through a needle which is inserted into the cisterna magna through the atlanto-occipital membrane. The rate of exchange between the various compartments (brain extracellular space, CSF, blood) can be calculated from the total material balance and the contributions of the compartments. In this way the exchange of ^{42}K between ventricular CSF and brain has been studied following the administration of ^{42}K into the perfusion fluid (Katzman and Pappius 1973).

The concentration of extracellular ions can be monitored on-line and in situ by the insertion of ion-selective microelectrodes. These electrodes consist of a double-barreled arrangement of glass capillaries, with one reference barrel containing a saline solution of the same osmolarity as tissue fluid, and the other being provided at its tip with a liquid membrane that is selective for the ion to be measured. Ion-selective microelectrodes have been developed to measure Na^+, K^+, Ca^{++}, Cl^- and H^+ (pH) concentrations. Problems that may be encountered during the use of ion-selective microelectrodes may arise from interference by other ions, breakdown of the liquid membrane and difficulties with calibration (Nicholson and Rice 1988).

Nuclear magnetic resonance techniques allow the in vivo investigation of several extracellular constituents or parameters.

Sodium-23 NMR and sodium-23 MRI are based on the odd number of nucleons in the nucleus of this prevalent sodium isotope, which exhibits four possible orientations of its magnetic moment, permitting three transitions in between. On account of its lower concentration in the tissue its signal is much weaker than that of hydrogen. Moreover, under certain conditions the ^{23}Na signal is invisible in tissue because of so-called quadrupolar interactions within the cell (Berendsen and Edzes 1973). Sodium-23 imaging typically shows high signal areas in structures with high water content, such as CSF spaces, vascular cavities and oedematous areas, in accordance with the predominant extracellular distribution of sodium (Hilal *et al.* 1985, Turski *et al.* 1988). Nevertheless, there is still a considerable intracellular distribution of tissue sodium, and several attempts have been made to distinguish extra- from intracellular sodium, e.g. by the use of the shift reagent dysprosium, which does not enter cells and consequently cause a shift of the extracellular sodium resonance frequency with respect to that of intracellular sodium. However, dysprosium exhibits some toxicity, its passage into brain is restricted by the blood-brain barrier and its uniformity of distribution in the tissue has been questioned (Burstein 1988).

Proton-NMR based measurement of water diffusion is a non-invasive MR technique employing the phenomenon that in a certain volume element of tissue, excited proton spins tend to display incoherent motions as a result of true molecular diffusion and microcirculatory flow which carry the spins in various directions. These intravoxel incoherent motions, which may be expressed mathematically in the form of an apparent diffusion coefficient (ADC), result in an attenuation of the signal. Diffusion-weighted imaging is essentially based upon the use of twin sequences, the first of which is a standard sequence in which the effects of intravoxel incoherent motions on the signal S_0 are negligible, and the second a sequence that contains additional gradient pulses to increase the effects of intravoxel incoherent motions on the signal S_1. From such pairs of images the ADC can be obtained on a voxel-by-voxel basis by: $\text{ADC} = \text{Log}(S_0/S_1)/(b_1 - b_0)$, where b_1 and b_0 are the gradient factors of the respective sequences. Separation of the diffusion and perfusion components is achieved by the use of a third sequence S_2, which is identical to the S_1 sequence except that the additional gradient pulses are stronger; this results in a greater attenuation due to diffusion in sequence S_2. As the contribution of flow is negligible in S_1 and S_2, the ADC image obtained from S_1 and S_2 is a pure diffusion image ($\text{ADC} = \text{D}$). Typical values for ADC are $(2.0 \pm 0.1) \cdot 10^{-3}$ mm^2/sec for grey matter and $(1.7 \pm 0.1) \cdot 10^{-3}$ mm^2/sec for white matter (Le Bihan *et al.* 1986, Le Bihan *et al.* 1988).

The Structure and Functional Significance of Cerebral Extracellular Space

Tissue extracellular space comprises the entire volume of tissue space located between the cellular elements. Measurements of tissue electrical impedance, water diffusion coefficients, and the pattern of spreading of vasogenic oedema fluid, have all indicated that in white matter, contrary to grey matter, there is anisotropy of extracellular space related to fibre architecture. The anisotropy favours fluid movement in the direction of the fibre tracts and impedes movement at right angles to the fibres, although its effect on small molecules is less apparent in some areas. Compartmentation of the extracellular space seems also to exist on a microscopic scale.

Cerebellum and thalamus contain glomerular synapses, i.e. capsules of glial processes surrounding a group of axonal and dendritic terminals (Szentágothai 1970). These are presumably intended to restrict inappropriate diffusion of released transmitters (Galambos 1971). The encapsulation of some circumventricular organs by the processes of tanycytes also tends to seggregate humoral influences from the mainstream of extracellular fluid (Krisch and Leonhardt 1978).

In the extracellular space diffusional processes take place, such as gas exchange, the transfer of metabolites between capillaries and cells, and the ionic movements in neuronal excitation and conduction of impulses.

Following their administration into the ventricular CSF, ions and small-molecular substances appear to penetrate readily across the ependyma of the ventricular wall into the surrounding tissue. The permeability of the ependyma is much lower to macromolecular substances, such as proteins and polysaccharides. A "sink-action" of the CSF has been found to be the basis of a diffusional movement of a substance toward the CSF-spaces, corresponding to a concentration gradient in the tissue toward the CSF. This may result from a greater influx of a substance across the blood-brain barrier compared to that across the blood-CSF barrier, from its endogenous formation within the brain parenchyma, or from its active excretion into the blood by the choroid plexus. A well-known example is that of sucrose, which shows a distribution into an apparent cerebral sucrose-space of 2.66% following its systemic administration. When the sink-action of the CSF was enhanced by ventriculo-cisternal perfusion with a sucrose-free fluid the sucrose space decreased to 1.76% while it increased to 9% when the perfusion fluid contained sucrose (Oldendorf and Davson 1967).

In view of the importance of the various inorganic ions, the existence of homoeostatic mechanisms is conceivable. Homoeostasis is achieved by the blood-brain and blood-CSF barriers, which protect the neural tissue from large fluctuations of systemic electrolyte levels, in addition to the buffering functions of the astroglia and of the large ionic reservoir formed by the CSF. This is illustrated by the homoeostasis of extracellular K^+, to the effect that accumulation of K^+ released during neural excitation is prevented by uptake into astrocytes, exchange with CSF, and possibly also by efflux through capillaries (Fig. 12).

Among neurotransmitters, glutamate that is released into the extracellular space during neural excitation and that may readily assume toxic concentrations, is soon taken up by astrocytes, in which it is converted to glutamine; this is subsequently released into the extracellular space, where it can be retrieved by neuronal elements (Van Gelder 1983). The uptake of glutamate by astrocytes seems to be dependent on external sodium, and possibly also on external potassium (Schousboe et al. 1977).

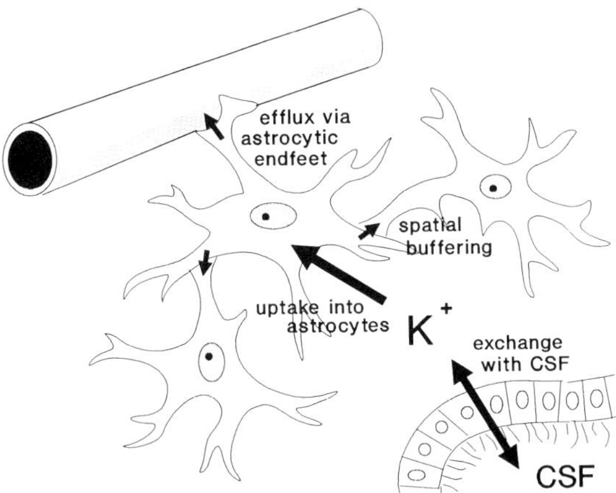

Fig. 12. Homoeostasis of extracellular K$^+$

Moreover, the high-affinity uptake of glutamate by astrocytes was found to be increased by the α_1-adrenergic agonist phenylephrine. Apart from glutamate, other amino acids such as aspartate, GABA and taurine may be taken up into astrocytes by way of high-affinity uptake mechanisms, which often are dependent on extracellular Na$^+$ and Cl$^-$, and are controlled by monoamine (α- and β-adrenergic agonists, dopamine, serotonine) receptor stimulation (Hansson and Rönnbäck 1991).

Apart from diffusion, movement of substances in the extracellular space may be due to bulk flow of interstitial fluid. Periventricular diffusion profiles of substances, that had been introduced into the ventricular CSF, did not indicate convective movement, as the diffusion profiles agreed well with theoretically calculated profiles in which the influence of convective flow was excluded (Rall 1968). It may be argued, however, that the study was conducted with small-molecular highly diffusible substances, for which the slow convective movements may be negligible with respect to the diffusional movements. Existence of bulk flow was suggested by studies in which a small amount of a macromolecular substance such as blue dextran or polyethylene glycol was introduced into the brain; the spreading of the substance from the site of injection was not concentric, as expected in diffusion, but excentric, following fibre tracts and perivascular spaces (Cserr et al. 1976). Study of the tissue penetration profiles of ^{3}H-sucrose, a molecule with extracellular distribution, demonstrated that in grey matter the apparent diffusion coefficients were similar at different times, as expected from diffusion, whereas in white matter they significantly decreased with time, suggesting bulk flow of interstitial fluid (Rosenberg et al. 1980). The maximal clearance of interstitial fluid was computed to amount 0.11 μl/min/g tissue. There are indications that part of the interstitial fluid drained into the deep cervical lymph nodes, via the olfactory bulb and the cribriform plate (Bradbury *et al.* 1981).

The existence of a physiological flow of extracellular fluid toward the ventricle would be consistent with the formation of extracellular fluid, either by transcapillary fluid filtration according to the Starling fluid flux relation, or alternatively by fluid secretion by the capillaries, and thus contributing to the formation of CSF as the so-called extrachoroidal component. Under pathological conditions, such as in the presence of vasogenic oedema, there is evidence for the existence of bulk flow of oedema fluid through expanded interstitial spaces.

The Extracellular Matrix

In many organs the extracellular space between cell bodies and cell processes is filled with extracellular matrix. The components of the extracellular matrix may be classified as glycoproteins, proteoglycans, and collagens. Glycoproteins are polypeptides that are linked to branched sugar chains. These complex carbohydrate structures are hydrophilic, and possess a great potential for encoding information on account of their large structural diversity, which is the result of the multitude of possible isomeric linkages between the sugars and the branching of the carbohydrate chains. The glycosylation sequence may be uniquely determined by the structure of the polypeptide chain. Glycoproteins of the extracellular matrix include laminin, fibronectin and nidogen (or entactin). Proteoglycans are complexes of glycosaminoglycans covalently linked to polypeptides. Glycosaminoglycans consist of repeating disaccharide units of glucosamine or galactosamine coupled to glucuronic acid or iduronic acid. Familiar proteoglycans are chondroitinsulfate proteoglycan and heparansulfate proteoglycan. (Heparin and hyaluronic acid are glycosaminoglycans that are not linked to proteins). The collagens comprise the types I to VI. Many of these proteins possess structural features that favour association to supramolecular assemblies, and association with other glycoproteins or proteoglycans. Fibronectin contains a site which seems to be essential for cell attachment and locomotion, and fibronectin may bind to heparin, which induces a conformational change of the fibronectin molecule affecting the locomotion of cells in the extracellular matrix. Many of the glycoproteins exhibit domains which show homology with the diffusible growth factors (epidermal growth factor and transforming growth factor α). They may also possess growth promoting functions (Engel 1991, Jackson *et al.* 1991).

Compared to other organs, however, the parenchyma of the brain is notable for its paucity of extracellular matrix. Generally, cerebral extracellular space clearly lacks collagen, except in the circumventricular organs. Furthermore, collagen IV occurs in basal laminas of capillaries and the pial membrana limitans. The extracellular matrix seems to be better represented in the developing brain, where it plays an important role in the migration of cellular elements. In the extracellular space of the developing postnatal rat cerebellum, immunocytochemistry has demonstrated the presence of chondroitinsulfate proteoglycan forming aggregates with hyaluronic acid (Ripellino *et al.* 1989). Glial cells have been shown to express proteoglycans which provide a barrier inhibiting the outgrowth of neurites. On the other hand, laminin exhibits neurite-promoting activity induced by interaction with heparansulfate proteoglycan. By their uronic acid residues proteoglycans of the extracellular matrix provide anionic sites which determine the movement of charged proteins through the extracellular space. In pathology, proteoglycans may control the growth and spreading of tumours, as well as their vascularization in several organs. In Alzheimer's disease, heparansulfate proteoglycan is typically deposited in the amyloid plaques.

The Cerebrospinal Fluid

Next to the tissue extracellular fluid which is contained within the brain parenchyma, the cerebrospinal fluid constitutes the second major reservoir of extracellular fluid. The studies of Cushing (1914), Dandy and Blackfan (1914) and Weed (1914), have provided the familiar picture of the CSF circulation. Following its production in the cerebral ventricles, the CSF flows through the ventricular system, exits into the cisterna magna, and then passes through the other basal cisterns to the subarachnoid spaces of the cerebral convexity, where it reaches the arachnoid villi and granulations to be absorbed into the blood circulation.

The formation and absorption rates of CSF can be measured by means of ventriculo-cisternal perfusion with artificial CSF containing an impermeant tracer. The CSF formation rate V_f is measured on the basis of the dilution of tracer concentration as a result of the addition of newly formed CSF, while the absorption rate V_a is obtained by the difference between inflowing volume V_{in} plus newly produced volume V_f and the outflowing volume V_{out}. Thus:

$$V_f = \frac{V_i(C_{in} - C_{out})}{C_{out}}; \; V_a = V_{in} + V_f - V_{out}$$

with V_{in} being the volume of inflowing perfusion fluid, C_{in} the concentration of tracer in the inflowing fluid, V_{out} the volume of outflowing fluid, and C_{out} the tracer concentration in the outflowing fluid (Heisey *et al.* 1962). Recommended tracers are [131]I- or ^{123}I-RISA or blue dextran which are truely impermeant and hardly enter surrounding brain, contrary to inulin, which has been used earlier, and proved to give rise to higher values of CSF formation rate (Martins *et al.* 1975).

In a method used by Masserman (1934) a volume ΔV of 10 to 60 ml of CSF was withdrawn by lumbar puncture in recumbent human subjects, and the time t was measured, required for the return of CSF pressure to its previous resting value. Calculated from $V_f = \Delta V/t$, the CSF formation rate V_f amounted to 0.319 ml/min. With a similar procedure Katzman and Hussey (1970) obtained a CSF formation rate of 0.323 ml/min in humans.

A proton NMR-based technique of measuring fluid flow through the Sylvian aqueduct has allowed the non-invasive assessment of total CSF production (excluding that in the fourth ventricle) in human volunteers. It amounted to a mean of 650 ml/day, and exhibited a circadian variation, with a maximum at 2.00 hr. a.m. and a minimum at 6 hrs p.m., which was 30% of the maximum (Nilsson *et al.* 1992).

Factors Determining Normal CSF Formation

These comprise osmolarity, pH, cerebral perfusion pressure, temperature, hormones, and certain drugs.

The *osmolarity* of CSF with respect to that of plasma strongly influences CSF formation rate. In the goat, ventriculo-cisternal perfusion with fluids of various osmolarities demonstrated increase of CSF formation rate with rising osmolarity of the perfusion fluid (Heisey *et al.* 1962), whereas elevating plasma osmolarity in cats diminished CSF formation rates (Hochwald *et al.* 1974). On the other hand, reduction of plasma osmolarity increased CSF production, associated with an increase of brain tissue water content (i.e. development of osmotic brain oedema). The increase of CSF production is apparently related to efflux of oedema fluid into CSF, as indicated by the increase of Na^+ efflux from the brain into the CSF (DiMattio *et al.* 1975). Therefore, in patients with untreated hydrocephalus and raised intracranial pressure, dehydration due to frequent vomiting may reduce CSF formation rate and check further elevation of intracranial pressure, whereas rehydration may increase CSF production with consequent intracranial pressure elevation.

As to the influence of *pH*, metabolic or respiratory alkalosis appeared to induce a reduction, whereas metabolic or respiratory acidosis caused no significant changes in CSF formation rate (Oppelt *et al.* 1963). It may pertain to the dual involvement of the enzyme carbonic anhydrase, which in the choroid plexus may subserve the mechanism of CSF production as well as the regulation of acid-base balance. Administration of acetazolamide, an inhibitor of carbonic anhydrase, therefore results in a reduction of CSF production (Tschirgi *et al.* 1954).

Concerning the significance of *cerebral perfusion pressure*, it has been observed that raising intracranial pressure in cats did not diminish CSF formation rate, provided that cerebral perfusion pressure was not reduced below a value of 70 mm Hg (Weiss and Wertman 1978). Reduction of arterial blood pressure to 62 mm Hg in dogs caused a 39% reduction of CSF formation rate with respect to normotensive animals (Carey and Vela 1974). Measurements of CSF formation rates in patients with hydrocephalus showed a decrease of CSF production rate amounting to 0.003 ml/min per mm CSF pressure elevation (Lorenzo *et al.* 1970). The influence of cerebral perfusion pressure is another argument for an extrachoroidal source of CSF formation, which should be the extracellular fluid from the surrounding brain parenchyma, and allegedly formed under the influence of cerebral perfusion pressure according to the Starling fluid flux equation.

The effect of endogenous *vasopressin* in decreasing CSF formation rate has been attributed to a decrease of *blood flow* to the choroid plexus induced by the peptide (Faraci *et al.* 1994). However, CSF production does not always have to be coupled to choroid plexus blood flow; simultaneous measurement in the rat of choroid plexus blood flow and of CSF formation rate has demonstrated that intraventricular administration of vasoactive intestinal polypeptide induced a reduction of CSF production by 30%, although blood flow was increased by 20% (Nilsson *et al.* 1991). In sheep, blood flow to the choroid plexus was increased by infusion of dopamine, and decreased by infusion of haloperidol, but remained unchanged by propranolol (Townsend *et al.* 1984).

Furthermore, *hypothermia* may result in an obvious suppression of CSF production of 11% per degree centigrade between $31°$ and $41°$ C (Snodgrass and Lorenzo 1972). Hypothermia also caused a decrease of ^{24}Na-turnover in the CSF (Davson and Spaziani 1962). From the reduction of a blood-pressure-independent component of brain ^{24}Na uptake by the lowering of brain temperature to $15°$ C in rats, the origin of this component was attributed to the contribution by CSF secretion (Go and Pratt 1975).

Sympathetic stimulation in rabbits with kaolin-induced hydrocephalus reduced CSF production significantly (Lindvall 1984).

Among the *drugs* that affect CSF production mention should be made of acetazolamide, which inhibits carbonic anhydrase, and in the rabbit suppresses CSF formation rate by 50% (Davson and Pollay 1963). The reduction of CSF formation rate was associated with a lower turnover rate of Na^+ and Cl^- in the CSF (Davson and Luck 1957, Maren and Broder 1970). In studies on the isolated choroid plexus, almost complete inhibition of CSF formation was observed when acetazolamide was administered in the vascular perfusion fluid (Pollay *et al.* 1972). Although in humans acetazolamide could achieve a 16–78% decrease of CSF formation rate (Rubin *et al.* 1966), the clinical use of acetazolamide for the treatment of hydrocephalus generally proved disappointing. *Diuretics* such as *ethacrynic acid* and *chlorthiazide* (Domer 1969), as well as *furosemide* in high doses (Reed 1969), and bumetanide (Javaheri and Wagner 1992) have been reported to cause a reduction of CSF production, indicating the involvement of a $Na^+K^+/2$ Cl^- cotransport mechanism in the secretion of CSF. *Transmitters*: Introduced into the ventricular system, serotonin appeared to decrease CSF production in the rabbit; this could be partly counteracted by the antagonist ketanserin (Lindvall-Axelsson *et al.* 1988).

As to hormones, *dexamethasone* in therapeutic doses accomplished a reduction of CSF production, which was attributed to inhibition of the Na^+K^+ ATPase (Mayman 1972). *Atriopeptins* appeared to diminish CSF production when added to the ventricular perfusion fluid.

In this context, *receptors* for atriopeptins have been demonstrated on the membrane bound guanylate cyclase of choroid plexus epithelium (Steardo and Nathanson 1987). Choroid plexus also contains vasopressin V_1 receptors, associated with the phospholipase C (PLC-A) signal transduction mechanism (Phillips *et al.* 1988, Ross *et al.* 1989). Moreover, choroid plexus appears to possess GABA-A receptors (Amenta *et al.* 1989), as well as receptors or binding sites for histamine (H_2) (Crook *et al.* 1986), vasoactive intestinal polypeptide, β-adrenergic agonists (Lindvall *et al.* 1985), and prolactin, the latter allegedly being involved in tissue water regulation especially in the fetus and the newborn (Lorenzo *et al.* 1983).

Generally, the *signal transduction mechanisms* underlying regulation of secretory processes are still poorly understood. Cholera toxin has been reported to induce a considerable increase of CSF formation (Epstein *et al.* 1977); as the toxin is known to bind to the G-regulatory protein of adenylate cyclase, it points to a role of the cAMP signal-transduction mechanism in CSF secretion. In cultured bovine choroid plexus epithelium, exposure to cholera toxin indeed increased cAMP levels 50-fold; elevation of cAMP levels could also be elicited by exposure to isoproterenol, PGE_1, histamine and serotonin, but not to prolactin, vasopressin and corticotrophin (Crook *et al.* 1984). Moreover, choroid plexus epithelium appears to contain two cAMP-regulated protein phosphatase-1 inhibitor proteins, namely inhibitor-1 and a dopamine- and cAMP-regulated phosphoprotein of 32 kDa molecular mass (DARPP-32); drugs and hormones that are known to alter epithelial fluid secretion and to increase cAMP or cGMP levels, such as forskolin, isoproterenol, vasoactive intestinal polypeptide, atriopeptin and serotonin, appeared to increase the phosphorylation of inhibitor-1 and DARPP-32, as demonstrated with phosphorylation-state specific monoclonal antibodies (Snyder *et al.* 1992). Vasopressin V_1 and serotonin 1C receptors have been found to be associated with phospholipase C in the choroid plexus, olfactory bulb and hippocampus, as shown by an in situ hybridization study using mRNA for PLC isozymes (Ross *et al.* 1989).

Intracellular signal transduction comprises mediation of the influence of external factors, such as transmitters, by so-called second messengers, in achieving an intracellular effect. This is ultimately accomplished by the phosphorylation and consequent activation of an effector protein, such as an enzyme, or by changing cytosol Ca^{++} concentration, which also influences the activity of enzymes. A well-known mechanism is the cAMP system, in which cAMP is formed by adenylate cyclase in the cell membrane, and then activates a cAMP-dependent protein kinase (type A) which phosphorylates the effector protein. Interaction of a β-adrenergic agonist with its receptor results in stimulation of adenylate cyclase via a guanine-nucleotide binding protein (G-protein), whereas binding of an α_2-adrenergic agonist results in inhibition of adenylate cyclase, also mediated by a G-protein. Another signal transduction mechanism involves membrane inositol phospholipids, e.g. when an α_1-adrenergic agonist binds to its receptor; the enzyme phospholipase C in the cell membrane is activated via a G-protein, and splits inositol phospholipids into diacylglycerols and inositoltriphosphate (IP_3), the diacylglycerol then activates protein kinase C, which phosphorylates the effector protein. Alternatively, IP_3 releases Ca^{++} from endoplasmic reticulum, raising cytosol Ca^{++}, which is the mechanism of vasopressin action. Other transmitters, like glutamate, may open receptor-gated Ca^{++}-channels, also raising cytosol calcium. Reduction of cytosol Ca^{++} concentration is a mechanism, by which atriopeptins act; upon binding to the receptor a membrane guanylate cyclase is activated, producing cGMP which then activates the membrane Ca^{++}-ATPase, and this enzyme causes Ca^{++} efflux.

Choroidal CSF Formation

Formation of CSF by the choroid plexus has been observed to take place on the bottom of an exposed cerebral ventricle in the cat (De Rougemont *et al.* 1960), and by the isolated feline choroid plexus in a closed chamber (Miner and Reed 1972). Moreover, the fluid collected directly from the plexus had an ionic composition (Na^+ 158, K^+ 3.28, Ca^{++} 1.67, Mg^{++} 1.47, and Cl^- 138 mM), which is different from that of plasma ultrafiltrate, clearly indicating active transport, i.e. secretion (Ames *et al.* 1964). The differences that occur downstream, such as higher Cl^- and lower K^+, Ca^{++} and Mg^{++}, in the CSF obtained from the cisterna magna (Na^+ 158, K^+ 2.69, Ca^{++} 1.50, Mg^{++} 1.33, Cl^- 144 mM), point to exchange with surrounding brain parenchyma during passage through the ventricular system.

The Mechanism of CSF Secretion by the Choroid Plexus

The ion movements across the plexus between ventricular and vascular sides have been studied in the frog by mounting the isolated choroid plexus between two lucite chambers. The movement of $^{22}Na^+$ from the vascular to the CSF side appeared to exceed the opposite movement by 1.6 μmol/ cm^2, and to be inhibited by ouabain. The net Na$^+$ transport to the CSF side could also be inhibited by removal of HCO$_3^-$ from the fluid media. There was a net ^{42}K$^+$ movement from the ventricular to the vascular side (Wright 1972). The active transport of Na$^+$ from blood across the choroid plexus epithelium presumably constitutes the driving force of CSF secretion, with the ouabain-sensitive Na$^+$K$^+$-ATPase on the CSF side of the plexus epithelial cells being responsible, exchanging Na$^+$ for K$^+$.

The isotonic character of the secreted CSF indicates coupling of water movement to Na$^+$ transport, which probably proceeds according to the model of the "standing osmotic gradient" (Diamond and Bossert 1967). The secreted Na$^+$ collects within clefts between microvilli of the choroid plexus, allowing local osmotic gradients to build up by the secreted Na$^+$, which then may attract fluid from the cells, resulting in the formation of an isotonic secretion.

The dependence of Na$^+$ transport on the presence of HCO$_3^-$ suggests that H$^+$ ions are involved. The Na$^+$ may have been acquired by exchange with H$^+$ via the Na$^+$/H$^+$ antiporter. The H$^+$ ions may be formed from CO$_2$ and H$_2$O in the carbonic anhydrase reaction. Choroid plexus epithelium has been shown to contain the isoenzyme CA II of carbonic anhydrase, which is different from the CA IV isoenzyme situated in cerebral capillary endothelium (Ghandour *et al.* 1992). Furthermore, the influence of furosemide and ethacrynic acid on CSF production rate indicates the involvement of the Na$^+$K$^+$/2 Cl$^-$ cotransport system, which performs the electroneutral transport of a Na$^+$ and a K$^+$ ion in conjunction with 2 Cl$^-$ ions.

Therefore, the following mechanism may be proposed for CSF formation by the choroid plexus. Secretion of Na$^+$ which is responsible for the osmotic gradient, proceeds by the Na$^+$K$^+$-ATPase of the plexus epithelial cell at the expense of ATP and in exchange for K$^+$. The Na$^+$ ion enters the CSF, accompanied by the anions Cl$^-$ and HCO$_3^-$. The cellular Na$^+$ is acquired by exchange for H$^+$ through the Na$^+$/H$^+$ antiporter. and Cl$^-$ is supplied by exchange against HCO$_3^-$. The contribution of carbonic anhydrase consists of the provision of H$^+$ and HCO$_3^-$ ions from H$_2$O and CO$_2$. Finally, K$^+$ ions, that have entered in exchange for Na$^+$, may leave the cell together with Na$^+$ and two Cl$^-$ ions by means of the Na$^+$K$^+$/2 Cl$^-$ cotransport system, and this is susceptible to inhibition by furosemide or bumetanide (Fig. 13).

Extrachoroidal CSF Formation

There are indications for the existence of a component of CSF formation that does not originate from the choroid plexus, but derives from the brain

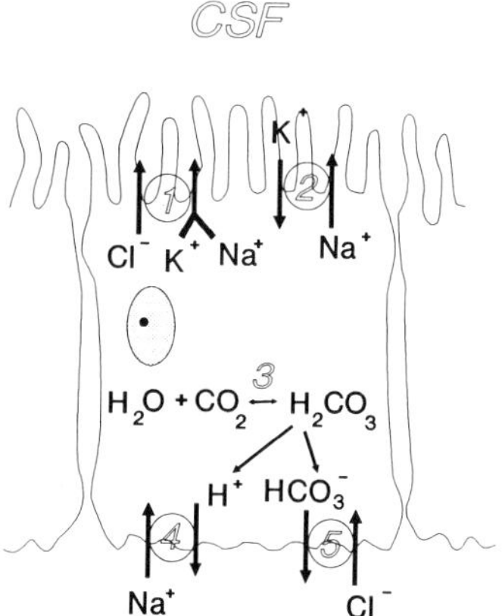

Fig. 13. Cerebrospinal fluid production by the choroid plexus, which involves the Na^+K^+/Cl^- cotransport mechanism *(1)*, Na^+K^+ ATPase *(2)*, carbonic anhydrase *(3)*, Na^+/H^+ *(4)* and Cl^-/HCO_3^- *(5)* antiporters

parenchyma. The necessary condition of a free exchange of fluid between brain parenchyma and CSF is consistent with the extensive diffusional exchange between CSF and tissue extracellular fluid. Other arguments are provided by experiments, in which resection of a choroid plexus in dogs apparently did not reduce the amount of CSF obtained from the ventricle from which the choroid plexus had been removed, compared to the other ventricle (Bering 1958). In monkeys, the blood to CSF transport of ^{24}Na only decreased by 40% after bilateral plexectomy, equivalent to a reduction of CSF production from 19.2 to 13.3 $\mu l/min$ (Milhorat *et al.* 1971). After bilateral plexectomy in a child for the treatment of hydrocephalus, CSF formation rate as measured by interventricular perfusion was perfectly normal (0.35 ml/min) (Milhorat *et al.* 1976).

CSF Absorption

The dynamics of CSF absorption have been well studied using ventriculo-cisternal perfusion, and can be expressed by the following equation: $J_a = (P - P_d) \cdot R_0$. In humans, it was found that CSF absorption (J_a) increases by 0.076 ml/min when CSF pressure rises 1 cm, this is the so-called outflow conductance $(C_0 = 1/R_0 = 0.076$ ml/min/cm; and $R_0 = 13.2$ cm CSF pressure/ml/min); R_0 being the outflow resistance, presumably representing the absorption characteristics of the arachnoid granulations. Moreover, CSF absorption only proceeds if CSF pressure exceeds an opening pressure of 6.8 cm H_2O, which corresponds to the pressure (P_d) in the dural sinuses (Cutler *et al.* 1968b). Assuming an average CSF formation rate of 0.35 ml/min in the human, formation rate equals absorption rate at a CSF

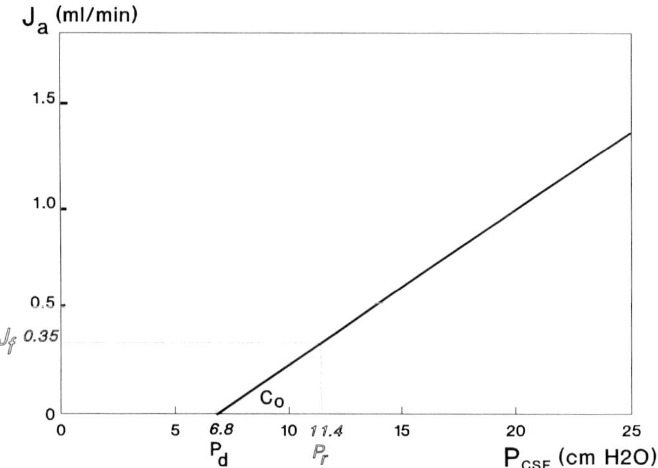

Fig. 14. Relation between CSF absorption rate J_a (ml/min) and CSF pressure (cm H_2O) in the human. To accomodate the normal CSF production rate J_f of 0.35 ml/min, requires a CSF pressure of 11.4 cm H_2O (the resting pressure P_r). P_d is the opening pressure, C_0 is the CSF outflow conductance, being J_a/P_{CSF}

pressure of $(0.35/0.076) + 6.8 = 11.4$ cm H_2O, and this is in good agreement with the measured equilibrium value of 11.2 cm (Fig. 14). Absorption and drainage of CSF into the dural sinuses occurs only if the pressure in the sinus is lower, or at most equal to the CSF pressure. Indeed in dogs, a pressure of 9 cm H_2O has been determined in the sagittal sinus at a CSF pressure of 14.7 cm H_2O (Shulman *et al.* 1964).

The pressure dependence of CSF absorption, as expressed by the equation, provides the link between cerebral fluid balance and intracranial pressure. Speaking of pressure, under physiological conditions a resting pressure exists which is determined by the balance between CSF production rate, the pressure in the dural sinus, and the absorption characteristics of the arachnoid granulations; in terms of fluid balance, there is a surplus of CSF, stored in the CSF compartment and reflecting its degree of filling. It is also a buffer of displaceable fluid volume which can be used up in the presence of space occupying lesions.

Morphological Aspects of CSF Absorption

The arachnoid villi which are responsible for CSF absorption in many animals, look like club-shaped structures of a size that is macroscopically hardly visible. They have a core of arachnoid space containing arachnoid cells, which protrude across the dura into the lumen of the sinus, abut on a vein within the dura, or into the subdural space (Andres 1967, Wolpow and Schaumburg 1972). Apart from villi, larger animals also possess Pacchionian arachnoid granulations that are visible to the naked eye and have the appearance of mushroom-shaped lobulated structures with a cauliflower-like surface. In the arachnoid granulation the subarachnoid space also extends through the stalk of the granulation into its interior. In this core the arachnoid cells form a loose lattice-work with large intercellular spaces interlaced by collagen fibres. The entire structure is covered by a lining that may be considered as specialized endothelium of the sinus (Fig. 15). According to other observations, the larger human granulations are covered by dura (with an underlying subdural space), except at the top, where there is an endothelial covering (Upton and Weller 1985). Morphologically, however, these endothelial cells are indistinguishable from the underlying cells of the villus. Tripathi (1977) denoted the covering cells as arachnoid mesothelial cells, while Andres (1967) and Rascol and Izard (1969) recognized three layers in the villus: an inner core of mesothelial cells, surrounded by an intermediate layer of neurothelial cells (the continuation of the subdural neurothelium, the outer layer of the arachnoid mater attached to the dura), and most superficially the lining of endothelium. The basal lamina of this endothelium is not continuous but occasionally interrupted, or even lacking.

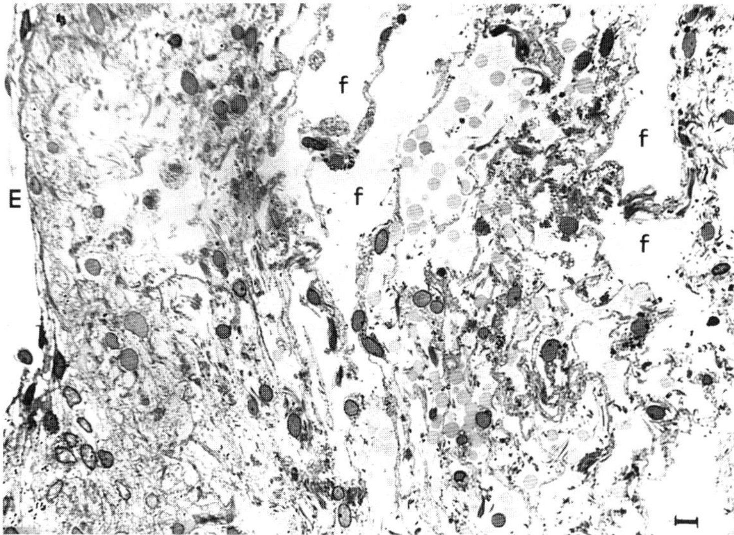

Fig. 15. Microphotograph of part of a human arachnoid granulation. Its interior consists of a meshwork of arachnoid mesothelial cells and collagen fibres, some larger mazes of which have presumably contained cerebrospinal fluid *(f)*. The side surface shows a covering of endothelial cells *(E)*. Toluidine blue stain. Scale bar: 10 μm

There are many controversies as to the mechanism of CSF absorption. Welch and Friedman (1960) observed microscopical tubular structures of 4–12 μm in diameter, leading from the core of the villus into the sinus lumen. However, other electronmicroscopical studies of arachnoid villi revealed an uninterrupted layer of endothelial cells (Andres 1967, Alksne and Lovings 1972, Alksne and White 1965), which impeded the passage of red blood cells from the subarachnoid space into the blood (Alksne and Lovings 1965). Tripathi (1977) observed that the endothelial cells covering arachnoid villi, contained large vacuoles when there was a CSF pressure gradient. Although this mesothelial covering of the villus was continuous, in the presence of a CSF pressure gradient the vacuoles could be observed to break through into the sinus lumen; the vacuoles thus constitute a dynamic system of transcellular channels that connect the subarachnoid spaces of the villus core with the sinus lumen. Gomez and Potts (1977) also reported such vacuoles in the endothelial covering of villi in the presence of a CSF pressure gradient, but these seemed to be extracellular rather than intracellular; in fact they also imply the formation of transendothelial channels. Potts and Gomez (1974) observed tubules of 10 μm diameter in the arachnoid granulations of sheep; these were lined with endothelium and constituted direct connections between the subarachnoid and sinus sides. Such endothelium-lined tubules have also been observed in human arachnoid granulations, both by transmission and scanning electronmicroscopy (Jayatilaka 1965, D'Avella *et al.* 1980, Upton and Weller 1985). It was pointed out by Go *et al.* (1984b) that the cells covering arachnoid granulations show a morphological similarity to the cells of the subdural neurothelium, as well as to the cells lining arachnoid cysts. By enzyme ultracytochemistry (on the basis of the p-nitrophenylphosphatase reaction), the presence of transport Na^+K^+-ATPase can be demonstrated in the plasma membrane of the cells lining arachnoid cysts, indicating their capacity to secrete CSF. In human arachnoid granulations, Na^+K^+-ATPase could also be demonstrated in the luminal plasma membrane of the endothelium, suggesting that in the process of CSF absorption a biochemical transport mechanism may play a role in addition to the biomechanical systems (including tubules or the formation of transendothelial channels) (Go *et al.* 1986). The reported effect of dexamethasone, which in perfusion studies of arachnoid villi proved to be capable of reducing the opening pressure, would also support a biochemical mechanism (Love *et al.* 1984). In this light it is notable that arachnoid granulations, and other derivatives of subdural neurothelium viz. meningiomas and the wall of arachnoid cysts, appear to possess progesterone receptors (Verhagen *et al.* 1994). Metabolites of progesterone have been reported to modulate the function of receptor-operated chloride channels in the nervous system (Majewska *et al.* 1986), an observation that may be relevant to ion, and possibly also, fluid transport. It may well bear upon the observed (mean 11.5 ml) increase of CSF volume in women in the premenstrual phase, according to an MRI study of CSF volume undertaken to investigate premenstrual complaints (Grant *et al.* 1988).

Alternative CSF Absorption Pathways

Apart from the familiar absorption mechanisms,the existence of other pathways have been postulated, such as absorption from the spinal subarachnoid space by arachnoid villi located in venous sinuses at the dural infoldings of spinal root sheaths (Woollam and Millen 1958, Welch and Pollay 1963).

The absorption of CSF in the brain parenchyma implies a bulk flow of fluid, which has to be directed from the ventricles, in conditions of elevated pressure within the ventricles such as in hydrocephalus. Alleged evidence for this mechanism was the observation of a deeper penetration of radioactive serum albumin in the periventricular tissue following its intraventricular injection, compared to a lesser depth of penetration in control dogs (Strecker *et al.* 1974). However, diffusional movement of the tracer cannot be excluded as an explanation for the difference in depth of penetration. The presence of oedema (of the hydrostatic type) in the periventricular tissue, visible on CT-scans as periventricular lucencies (Hopkins *et al.* 1977, Hiratsuka *et al.* 1982), has also been cited as evidence for transventricular CSF absorption, although this does not really constitute proof of the existence of bulk flow of fluid.

Many studies using the administration of dyes or radioactive tracers into the CSF have suggested the existence of drainage pathways along the sheaths of various cranial nerves, such as the olfactory or the optic nerves, eventually leading to the cervical lymph nodes (Faber 1937, Bradbury *et al.* 1981).

The Flow of CSF

The flow of CSF from the production sites in the ventricular system towards the basal cisterns and further down through the subarachnoid spaces, has been the subject of clinical studies using isotope-cisternography. In humans, the injection of radioactive serum albumin into lumbar CSF, is followed 4 hours later by the appearance of radioactivity in the cervical region, the cisterna magna and other cisterns around the lower brain stem, the Sylvian fissure, and the interhemispheric fissure. 24 hours later the radioactivity has arrived at the subarachnoid spaces of the cerebral convexity, and converges upon the sagittal sinus. The radioactivity decreases only after 48 hours (Penning and Front 1975). Under normal circumstances, no filling of the ventricles is observed. The ventricles show up when there is obstruction of the subarachnoid spaces of the cerebral convexity or of the absorption sites, such as in communicating hydrocephalus, including the normal pressure type.

The forces driving the movement of CSF include in the first place the ventricular fluid pressure, as a consequence of CSF production being in excess of CSF absorption; secondly, there are the changes of CSF pressure, resulting mainly from the arterial pulsations but also from respiratory movements and changes of posture; finally, there is the movement of the ependymal cilia, which probably only have a very local action and are intended to prevent sedimentation of debris on the ventricular walls and to achieve thorough mixing of fluid.

Non-invasive MRI techniques exist which may depict the low velocities of CSF flow, and especially the pulsatile CSF movements. It could be observed that during the systolic phase of the CSF pulse there was caudally directed CSF flow in both the foramen of Monro and the aqueduct. Caudad motion of the brain stem produces a CSF wave through the spinal canal. In diastole, the direction of flow reverses to cephalic (Feinberg and Mark 1987). The techniques are currently also applied especially for the diagnosis of flow obstructions in the spinal canal.

The Cerebral Intracellular Space

In considering brain water compartments, the cell is usually regarded as a single intracellular space, although it is clearly compartmentalized, with the cytoplasm and the nucleus as the main compartments; other compartments are the various organelles, such as the mitochondria and endoplasmic reticulum, which are separated from the cytoplasmic compartment by enveloping membranes. Compartmentation also applies to energy metabolism, with glycolysis proceeding in the cytoplasm, and oxidative phosphorylation in the mitochondria, and mutual exchange of substrates and metabolites across the mitochondrial membrane.

Exchanges between organelle compartments also take place in intracellular calcium signal transduction; calcium may be released into the cytosol by the endoplasmic reticulum under the influence of inositoltriphosphate (IP_3), which is formed from membrane inositolphospholipids when certain transmitter receptors are activated; in other circumstances cytosol calcium may be taken up by the endoplasmic reticulum and the mitochondria. By means of calcium-specific indicators such as aequorin the cytosolic calcium movements have been elucidated as waves traveling with speeds of 5–30 μm/s in fast waves, and 1 μm/s in slow waves (Jaffe 1993).

There are also solute movements within the intracellular space in the context of intercellular communication. Astrocytes maintain extensive mutual contacts through gap junctions, which allow dispersal of various constituents such as potassium from one cell to many neighhouring astrocytes. This process, which has been called spatial buffering, is involved in the homoeostasis of extracellular potassium: an elevation of extracellular K^+ concentration such as may occur after massive neuronal discharges, will induce ingestion of the K^+ by local astrocytes, followed by intracellular dispersal across a larger part of the astrocytic population (Fig. 11). It seems that calcium also may be dispersed across astrocytes through gap junctional contacts (Hertz 1978, Orkand 1966, Trachtenberg and Pollen 1970). In hippocampal slices, it was found that neuronal activity as well as application of glutamate triggered intracellular Ca^{++} elevation in astrocytes, which moreover, propagates as waves across the astrocytic population at velocities of 7–27 μm/sec (Dani *et al.* 1992).

Gap junctions are junctions between adjoining cells, in which the intercellular space is narrowed, but not obliterated. This narrowed intercellular space is bridged by a system of tubules, called connexons, that connect the contents of both cells. In freeze-fracture studies the connexons are depicted as more or less densely packed units, arranged in a hexagonal lattice. The connexon may be envisaged as being composed of six rod-shaped subunits (2.5 nm in diameter and 7.5 nm long), each of which consists of a single protein, called connexin. These are aggregated to form the hollow connexon cylinder of 7 nm diameter, containing a cavity of 2 nm.

In nerve cells, in which excitation is a main function, the initiation and propagation of the action potential involves the exchange of the ions Na^+, K^+, and Cl^- of the cell with the extracellular space through respective ion selective channels in the plasma membrane. Restoration of membrane potential and recovery of excitability are again based upon exchanges between the cell and the extracellular space, driven by ion pumps viz. the Na^+ K^+ ATPase. When the action potential arrives at the nerve terminal, the depolarization induces the opening of voltage-gated Ca^{++} channels in the presynaptic membrane, and the resulting Ca^{++} influx and elevation of cytosolic Ca^{++} triggers the release of neurotransmitter (Zucker and Lando 1986). Normalization of intracellular Ca^{++} again involves an ion pump, the Ca^{++} ATPase.

Shifts of inorganic ions also occur during osmotically induced changes of cellular volume, and during the regulatory processes for its maintenance, which mainly comprise electroneutral ion movements through counter-transport mechanisms (like the Na^+/H^+ and Cl^-/HCO_3^- antiporters) or co-transport mechanisms (such as the Na^+ $K^+/2$ Cl^- cotransport mechanism) and the Na^+ K^+ ATPase.

As the various ion transport mechanisms subserve excitation, as well as maintenance and regulation of cell volume and intracellular pH, it is conceivable that these processes are interrelated. Electrical stimulation of spinal nerve roots in rats elicited—in addition to an increase in extracellular

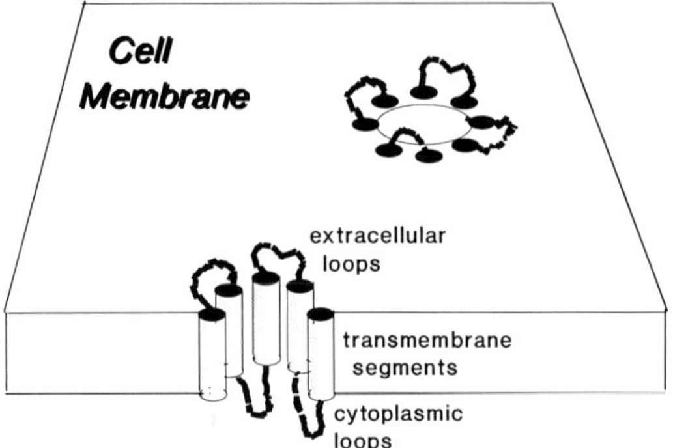

Fig. 16. General configuration of channel, transporter or receptor, with transmembrane segments spanning the cell membrane

K^+ concentration—shifts of extracellular pH, which could be influenced
by various compounds such as acetazolamide, amiloride and DIDS, indicating that the Na^+/H^+ and Cl^-/HCO_3^- exchange mechanisms are
involved (Sykova *et al.* 1992).

Ion channels such as Na^+, K^+, Cl^-, and Ca^{++} channels are transmembrane proteins, the molecules of which span the entire thickness of the cellular plasma
membrane (Fig. 16). They are usually characterized by their conductance as measured biophysically, and by their susceptibility to blocking by certain toxins or
inhibition by certain drugs. Some are activated by an electrical potential, others
are receptor operated. By cloning of complementary DNA the amino acid
sequence of some of them has been deduced, and usually shows a number of
transmembrane domains that allegedly form the channel. In nerve and skeletal
muscle, the voltage-gated Na^+ *channel* is responsible for the action potential: the
channel can be blocked by tetrodotoxin. It consists of an α-subunit of 260 kDa,
and 2 smaller β-subunits. The α-subunit from rat brain has an amino acid
sequence with 4 repetitive homology units, each containing 6 putative transmembrane segments, one of which (S_4) is charged and presumably is involved in
the voltage-dependent activation of the channel. Epithelial Na^+ channels subserve
fluid secretion or sodium absorption in glands, intestine and kidney, and are
inhibitable by the diuretic amiloride. There is a multitude of K^+ *channels*, even in
brain, many of which are voltage-gated and are important for repolarization of the
membrane. A voltage-gated K^+ channel from Drosophila showed a predicted
sequence of 616 amino acids (70 kDa) with 7 putative membrane spanning segments, one of which (S_4) was positively charged, and showed homology that of the
Na^+ channel. There is also a K^+ channel that is Ca^{++}-dependent and is found in
acinar cells of exocrine glands; a K^+ channel that is ATP-dependent is found in
cardiac tissue. Ca^{++} *channels* occur in various organs, and also exist in several
types: L-type channels are sensitive to blocking by dihydropyridines such as
nimodipine, N-type channels show activation by strong depolarisation and are
blocked by ω-conotoxin, and P-type channels are both dihydropyridine and ω-

conotoxin insensitive. In rabbit skeletal muscle 4 tightly coupled subunits, α_1, α_2, β, and γ, compose a voltage-gated Ca^{++} channel complex. The largest subunit of 170 kDa is a receptor for dihydropyridine, and contains 6 transmembrane segments, one of which is a positively charged segment (S_4), exhibiting structural features similar to the sodium channel. An NMDA glutamate receptor-operated Ca^{++} channel in hippocampus is physiologically involved in the phenomenon of long term potentiation, and pathologically in ischaemic cell damage. *Cl^--channels* that are voltage-dependent play a role in the generation of the membrane potential; the voltage-gated Cl^- channel of the electric organ of Torpedo was predicted to consist of a protein of 805 amino acids containing 13 putative transmembrane domains. An important and structurally different Cl^- channel is the type operated by the GABA-A receptor; it is enhanced by the anaesthetic isoflurane, and inhibited by caffeine, and allegedly mediates the anticonvulsant action of benzodiazepines and barbiturates. A hypothetical Cl^- channel is the cystic fibrosis transmembrane conductance regulator in the apical membrane of secretory epithelia, the function of which is defective in cystic fibrosis.

The *Na^+/H^+* antiporter exchanges Na^+ for H^+ and vice versa, requiring no energy, and is inhibited by amiloride; it appears to be a protein of 815 amino acids with 12 putative transmembrane domains, also containing amino acid residues that can bind H^+ and presumably represent its pH sensor. The *Cl^-/HCO_3^- exchanger* performs the exchange of Cl^- for HCO_3^-, and is inhibited by disulfonic stilbenes such as DIDS, while some types are Na^+-dependent; the exchanger of the red cell membrane appears to be a transmembrane protein with a longitudinal transport domain, and a water-soluble domain located in the cytoplasm. The *Na^+ $K^+/2\,Cl^-$ cotransport mechanism* performs electroneutral transport of the cations Na^+ and K^+ and 2 anions Cl^-; it is present in astrocytes but not in neurones; it is inhibited by furosemide and bumetanide, and its stimulation by adrenergic agonists seems to be mediated by elevation of cytosol Ca^{++} or by cAMP, while it is also subject to cAMP-protein kinase dependent regulation (Noda *et al.* 1984, Tempel *et al.* 1987, Tanabe *et al.* 1987, Jentsch *et al.* 1990, Berger *et al.* 1993, Padan and Schuldiner 1993, Falke *et al.* 1985).

The Measurement of Intracellular Space

Changes of cell volume have conventionally been considered in conjunction with complementary changes of extracellular space. In brain tissue in situ, expansion of the intracellular compartment has been deduced from the decrease of the extracellular space, which can be measured by the various methods mentioned before.

The use of cells in culture has allowed the measurement of cell volume proper, by passing the suspension of cells through a Metricell flow cytometric system. Determination of cell volume is based upon the recording of electrical potential changes between electrodes in each of two chambers, which are interconnected by a window in the wall separating the chambers; as cells pass through the window, the electrical current passing through the window is impeded, while the recorded potential change is related to the volume of the passing particle. In this way the volume of C6 glioma cells has been measured to amount to 980 μm^3 (Chaussy *et al.* 1981).

Another method comprises the measurement of 3-0-methylglucose (3-MG) space of cells in a serum-free medium, which represents the volume of cell water (Latzkovits *et al.* 1993).

The advent of ^{31}P-NMR has recently allowed the measurement of cell volume in vivo, by means of the probe dimethylmethylphosphonate (DMMP), which has an intracellular NMR resonance shifted upfield from the extracellular (Lien *et al.* 1992).

The Maintenance of Cell Volume

Cell volume is subject to various changes, both physiological and pathological, such as those during growth and maturation, and on a shorter term those during excitation, spreading depression, hypoxia, and brain oedema.

The mechanism for maintenance of cell volume has conventionally been envisaged by the "pump and leak" hypothesis or double Gibbs-Donnan equilibrium (Tosteson and Hoffman 1960). The cell contains proteins, which behave as polyvalent anions ($Prot^{n-}$), resulting in a distribution of ions inside and outside the cell as reflected by a Gibbs-Donnan equilibrium:

$$[Na^+]_{in} + [K^+]_{in} = [Cl^-]_{in} + [Prot^{n-}]_{in}$$

$$[Na^+]_{out} + [K^+]_{out} = [Cl^-]_{out}$$

$$[K^+]_{in} \times [Cl^-]_{in} = [K^+]_{out} \times [Cl^-]_{out}$$

$$[Na^+]_{in} \times [Cl^-]_{in} = [Na^+]_{out} \times [Cl^-]_{out}$$

The impermeant intracellular proteins, moreover, exert an osmotic pressure which would lead to influx of water and cell swelling. This is prevented by outward pumping of Na^+ and Cl^-. By the efflux of Na^+ the cellular contents acquires a negative charge, which attracts K^+ inside the cell, and expells Cl^- from the cell (Macknight and Leaf 1978). The pump has been identified as the membrane Na^+ K^+-ATPase (Skou 1957); consequently, interference with its function should lead to cell swelling. The pathways for the efflux or influx of ions should currently be identified as the various ion channels, cotransport and countertransport (antiporter) systems.

When rat brain was subjected to hypernatraemia, water was lost from the tissue, but the loss was less than the amount predicted for ideal osmotic behaviour; this indicates the presence of mechanisms responsible for volume regulation. After 30 min of hypernatraemia, total tissue water decreased by 7%, and extracellular water decreased by 27%, whereas intracellular water did not change. Estimates of ion content indicated that extracellular Na^+, Cl^- and K^+ decreased, but the intracellular ions increased (Cserr *et al.* 1991).

In epithelial cells of the gall bladder as well as in red blood cells of the giant salamander Amphiuma, maintenance of cell volume after hyperosmolar shrinking by a process of regulatory volume increase involved the activation of the Na^+/H^+-antiporter and the Cl^-/HCO_3^--antiporter, which results in the uptake of Na^+ and Cl^- in exchange for extruded H^+ and HCO_3^-. In Ehrlich ascites tumour cells and renal epithelial cells, regulatory volume increase comprised the activation of Na^+/Cl^- and Na^+ $K^+/2$ Cl^- cotransport systems, inducing the uptake of Na^+, K^+, and Cl^-, together with activation of the Na^+ K^+ ATPase; the net result is uptake of KCl and water (Eveloff and Warnock 1987, Cala 1985).

In many tissues maintenance of cell volume during prolonged hypernatraemia generally not only involves shifts of inorganic ions, but also the accumulation of osmolytes; these are low-molecular weight organic solutes comprising mainly free amino acids including taurine, glutamate, glutamine, aspartate, glycine, β-alanine, γ-aminobutyrate (GABA), and substances such as myo-inositol, methylamines, and glycerophosphorylcholine (Trachtman 1992, Law 1994). However, it appears that not all these osmolytes are significant in brain cell volume regulation. In rat brain subjected to chronic hypernatraemia, the cerebral cortex showed large increases of amino acids, mainly taurine, glutamate and glutamine (Bedford and Leader 1993). When cultured rat brain cells were placed in hyposmotic media, neurones as well as astrocytes released taurine, glutamate and aspartate, while in addition neurones released GABA, and astrocytes liberated β-alanine; it could be calculated that in cultured astrocytes free amino acids contributed 54% to cell volume regulation versus inorganic ions 46% (Pasantes-Morales et $al.$ 1993). Another study on cultured astrocytes demonstrated the release during hyposmolarity mainly of taurine, and to some extent glutamate, aspartate and glycine, but not glutamine; the liberation of taurine was a consequence of swelling and unrelated to depolarization (Schousboe and Pasantes-Morales 1992). Myo-inositol appeared to be involved in cell volume regulation in hypernatraemia, but not in hyponatraemia (Trachtman et $al.$ 1991). Synaptosomes isolated from the brains of rats with hypernatraemia contained increased levels of taurine, due to an increment of the Na^+-specific taurine transport; however, glycine transport was unaltered (Trachtman et $al.$ 1992). As to the relevance of other osmolytes, it was demonstrated by a ^{31}P NMR study of C6 glioma cells that during exposure to a hyperosmolar medium there was a reduction of cell volume, but no change of the contents of glycerophosphorylcholine and glycerophosphorylethanolamine (Lien et $al.$ 1992). Hyperosmolarity not only exists in hypernatraemia, but also in diabetic hyperglycemia. Moreover, in diabetes polyols or polyalcohols, such as sorbitol and fructose, which are additional metabolites of sugar metabolism, may be involved in volume regulation. However, in rats subjected to anisosmolarity, sorbinil, which is an inhibitor of aldose and aldehyde reductase, had no effect on the size of water compartments under the various anisosmotic conditions, and it was concluded that the polyol sorbitol was not an essential cerebral osmolyte (Trachtman *et al.* 1991).

There are also hormonal influences on glial cell volume as measured by the 3-MG space; arginine-vasopressine resulted in an increase of 25%, whereas atriopeptin caused a 32% decrease of cell volume (Latzkovits *et al.* 1993). These findings may bear upon previous observations, such as the increase in brain water content, associated with a decrease of brain tissue sodium and potassium content, evoked in rats by intraventricular administration of vasopressin (Doczi *et al.* 1982). Moreover, intraventricular administration of atriopeptin appeared to prevent the water accumulation in rat brain elicited by systemic hyposmolar fluid loading, associated with a sodium loss from the neural tissue (Doczi *et al.* 1987).

In view of the significance of the Na^+/H^+-antiporter in cell volume regulation as well as in the regulation of intracellular pH, both functions may conceivably be coupled. The maintenance of cell volume in lymphocytes following hyperosmolar cell shrinkage involved the uptake of Na^+ via the Na^+/H^+-antiporter; this was associated with alkalinization of the cellular contents (Grinstein *et al.* 1985). In vivo measurement of cell volume by means of ^{31}P NMR and using DMMP as a probe, showed a 67% reduction of the volume of C6 glioma cells, which was associated with an increase of intracellular pH, and with an increase of the contents of ATP and CrP (Lien *et al.* 1992). Exposure of C6 glioma cells or astrocytes to an isotonic lactic acid solution caused cell swelling, provided that Na^+ was present in the medium; presumably the external H^+ ions were buffered by bicarbonate resulting in the formation of water and CO_2, the latter diffused into the cell and caused intracellular acidosis; the cellular carbonic anhydrase catalyzed the formation of H_2CO_3, which dissociated into H^+ and HCO_3^-; the H^+ ions were then extruded by the Na^+/H^+-antiporter in exchange for Na^+ entering the cell, and the HCO_3^- ions were exchanged by the Cl^-/HCO_3^--antiporter for Cl^- entering the cell, both accompanied by osmotically obliged water resulting in swelling (Staub *et al.* 1990).

The Abnormal Accumulation of Brain Water

Given the significance of brain tissue water as an essential constituent of the tissue, there are conditions in which brain water may accumulate and become a hazard. The accumulation of water may be located within the tissue, scattered among tissue elements as brain oedema, or contained within dilated ventricles in hydrocephalus; the fluid accumulation may also occur in unnatural cavities in the tissue designated as cystic lesions. In view of the possibilities of exchange between the various compartments, it is conceivable that the accumulation of water in one compartment may affect the other.

Brain Oedema

Cerebral oedema may best be defined as an abnormal increase of brain tissue water content, as the result of general or local pathology.

It is well known that clinically, brain oedema plays an important role in determining morbidity and mortality in brain tumours, cerebral ischaemia, and severe head injury. Other conditions, in which brain oedema is considered of great significance, are inflammatory lesions, including brain abscess and necrotizing encephalitis, and radionecrosis.

There are also systemic affections, associated with brain oedema, such as lead poisoning, e.g. by lead-containing paints (Clasen *et al.* 1984), organic tin compounds (such as Stalinon, which has been used in France for the treatment of furunculosis (Gruner 1958)), hexachlorophene (used as a disinfectant), vitamin A intoxication, water intoxication and posthaemodialysis syndrome, hypertensive encephalopathy, hyperthermia and Reye's syndrome.

Pathogenesis of Brain Oedema

The classification of brain oedema on the basis of pathogenesis (Klatzo 1967), into vasogenic and cytotoxic types, marked a significant advance in our understanding. However, several arguments warrant the refinement and extension of the classification into 4 basic types, which should include, either singly or in conjunction, all the various kinds of brain oedema.

Overview of basic oedema types:

Type	Pathogenesis	Oedema fluid	Localization	Causes	CSF formation
Vasogenic	barrier breakdown	water, Na^+, protein	extracellular	focal lesions	decreased
Cytotoxic	metabolic disturbance	water, Na^+	intracellular	hypoxia, poisons, ischaemia (early)	
Osmotic	osmotic gradient	water, (Na^+)	intra- and extracellular	water intoxication	increased
Hydrostatic	hydrostatic gradient	water, Na^+	extracellular	hydrocephalus, hypertension	

Vasogenic Brain Oedema

The presence of vasogenic brain oedema is an inescapable consequence of a breakdown of the blood-brain barrier (Klatzo *et al.* 1958), which results in leakage of plasma constituents into the parenchyma of the brain. Blood-brain barrier disruption with concomitant vasogenic oedema occurs in virtually all focal cerebral lesions, such as cerebral contusions, operative trauma, brain tumours, inflammatory lesions and haemorrhages, after radiation therapy, and in the later stage of cerebral ischaemia. Among the intoxications, lead poisoning especially provokes vasogenic oedema.

A familiar experimental model of vasogenic brain oedema, which has been used to study many of its aspects, is the oedema induced by a freezing injury to the cerebral cortex (Clasen *et al.* 1953); it has the advantage of reproducibility. Other experimental models of vasogenic oedema which illustrate its association with other lesions include: the inflammatory response to implantation of irritative substances, contusion by mechanical impact, implantation of tumours into the brain, ischaemia following occlusion of arteries and ionizing radiation.

Investigation of vasogenic oedema induced by the freezing injury has demonstrated that its evolution may be characterized by a stage of exudation, a stage of propagation and a final stage of resolution (Fig. 17).

In the *exudative* stage there is exudation of plasma proteins, water and plasma electrolytes. In the experimental model this can be monitored by the intravenous administration of Evans blue dye, which binds to plasma albumin and causes blue-staining of the exudate. Clinically, the disruption of the blood-brain barrier can be recognized by the exudation of X-ray contrast agents on the CT-scan, and of MRI-contrast agents on the

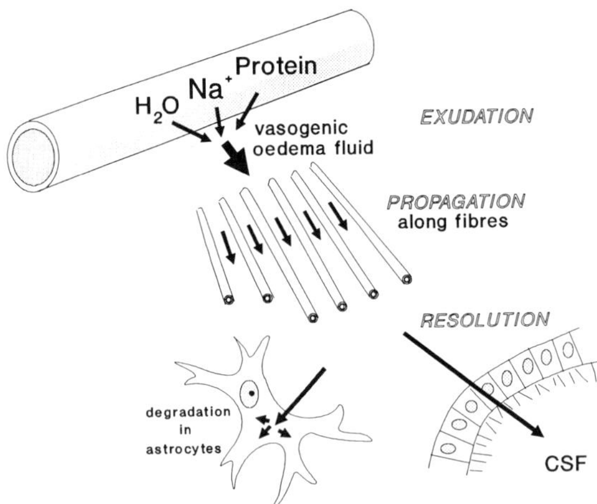

Fig. 17. Evolution of vasogenic cerebral oedema

MRI-scan. The exudate is extracellular and results in expansion of the extracellular space. Indeed electron microscopy has shown an increase of interstitial spaces in oedematous white matter amounting to 1000 nm, versus 60 nm in control white matter (Gonatas *et al.* 1963). Besides an increase of water content, the exudation of plasma constituents in brain tissue causes an increase of Na^+ content in the oedematous brain area, while K^+ content is reduced, usually by dilution in the swollen tissue, or occasionally by loss from the tissue.

The freezing injury model has allowed isolation of oedema fluid from the cat brain; analysis of the fluid has demonstrated a Na^+ content (143 meq/l) that more resembled that of plasma (146 meq/l) than that of CSF (158 meq/l); this is consistent with the alleged vasogenic origin (Go *et al.* 1976a, Patberg *et al.* 1977). The oedema fluid has an increased colloid-osmotic pressure due to the presence of plasma protein (23 mm Hg, corresponding to 3.98 g/100 ml of total protein) compared with 36 mm Hg in plasma (corresponding to 6.61 g/100 ml of total protein) (Go *et al.* 1985). This may be relevant in considerations on reabsorption of oedema fluid in the light of the Starling fluid flux equation.

The cryogenic injury model has also demonstrated the significance of the vascular bed in exudation. When the freezing lesion was immediately excised, the development of oedema was prevented, while excision at a later stage impeded further progress (Aarabi and Long 1979). Young animals tend to have less oedema than adults, which may be ascribed to a lower arterial blood pressure and a less developed vascular system in young animals (Streicher *et al.* 1965, Go *et al.* 1973a).

In the stage of *propagation*, spreading of the exudate takes place in the intercellular spaces of the tissue, and preferentially along fibre structures of the white matter, which are readily separated by the infiltrating exudate, whereas in grey matter interwoven cellular processes impede expansion of the intercellular spaces (Go *et al.* 1967). Clinically, the predilection of vasogenic oedema for white matter may be recognized on CT-scans as an area of low attenuation, or of signal hyperintensity on T_2-weighted MRI-scans, with a characteristic finger-like pattern of extension corresponding to the geometrical pattern of white matter. Therefore, the white matter may act as a trap, in which the exudate accumulates without a direct efflux route being available into surrounding grey matter structures, except possibly into the ventricle. As a consequence, the white matter compartment may rapidly swell to a considerable extent and become a space-occupying lesion. The exudate does not spread evenly into all white matter structures, however, as there are regions into which the oedema fluid penetrates less readily. These include the internal capsule, the optic radiation, the corpus callosum and the white matter structures of the lower brain stem. Therefore, the oedema rarely spreads from one hemisphere into the other across the corpus callosum, unless the latter is involved in the lesion itself (Go *et al.* 1967). The process of propagation of oedema fluid into the white matter is a process of convective fluid flow (bulk flow) through the extracellular space, with equal rates of movement for small- and large-molecular substances (Reulen *et al.* 1977).

Exudation and migration of oedema fluid are driven by the cerebral perfusion pressure, i.e. the capillary blood pressure minus the regional tissue pressure. The amount of vasogenic oedema has been shown to be correlated with the arterial blood pressure (Klatzo *et al.* 1967). However, another factor that seems to be significant, is cerebral vasomotor autoregulation. An intact autoregulation would respond to arterial blood pressure elevation with vasoconstriction, attenuating the propagation of arterial blood pressure into the capillary bed. When vasomotor autoregulation is disturbed, as may occur as a result of injury, arterial blood pressure may freely exert its influence upon exudation (Go *et al.* 1974, Go *et al.* 1976b).

The stage of *resolution* involves clearance of the exudate, by such mechanisms as: reabsorption into capillaries, drainage into the CSF, uptake and degradation by glial elements, or drainage to cervical lymph nodes, a pathway considered as an alternate route for the absorption of CSF (Bradbury *et al.* 1981). There have been observations suggesting the feasibility of reabsorption into capillaries, although reabsorption of the extravasated proteins tends to be restricted by the integrity of the blood-brain barrier in the white matter. Regarding the possibility of drainage into CSF, experiments in cats involving the infusion of radioactive serum albumin (RISA) with mock CSF into white matter have suggested that drainage into the ventricular CSF could take place only after saturation of the entire white matter compartment, which required three hours. The RISA efflux with CSF increased until a plateau was reached after seven hours; the efflux via this pathway then amounted to 38% of the quantity of RISA infused, while only 6% was retrieved in the blood and drainage to the cervical lymph nodes was less than 0.48% (Marmarou *et al.* 1984). Uptake and degradation by glia may also be relevant as a mechanism of resolution, since the exudate could be visualized immunohistochemically in astrocytes and microglial cells (Klatzo *et al.* 1980). High-performance liquid chromatography (HPLC) analysis of oedematous brain tissue demonstrated the presence of peptide fragments many hours after a freezing injury (Bodsch and Hossmann 1983).

The blood-brain barrier breakdown inherent in vasogenic oedema tends to jeopardize the efficacy of osmotherapy, which is used to reduce intracranial pressure by dehydrating the brain. Following administration of a hyperosmolar solution dehydration has been observed in brain regions with intact blood-brain barrier, but not in areas in which the blood-brain barrier was disrupted, and into which presumably the dehydrating agent has rapidly penetrated, abolishing the osmotic gradient required for dehydration (Beks and Kerckhoffs 1967). A rebound phenomenon, being the secondary rise of intracranial pressure which may even attain higher levels than before osmotherapy, seems to occur only in the presence of barrier breakdown; it presumably represents the resumption of intracranial pressure elevation due to progressing oedema formation after an interruption by the period of dehydration (Guisado *et al.* 1976).

Cytotoxic Brain Oedema

This type of oedema may be defined as cell swelling resulting from intracellular accumulation of fluid. The fluid is derived from the extracellular space, which consequently shrinks. The decrease of extracellular space has been documented by the rise of electrical impedance, such as in asphyxia (Van Harreveld 1966), in 6-amino-nicotinamide intoxication (Baethmann and Van Harreveld 1973), or following the intracerebral injection of ouabain (Gazendam *et al.* 1979c). Eventually the fluid taken up by the cells from the extracellular space must originate from the blood circulation, or from the CSF space which is in extensive diffusional contact with the tissue extracellular space.

Generally the cytotoxic oedemas may be classified into a group with evident disturbance of cellular energy metabolism, and those with impairment of other aspects of metabolism.

According to the hypothesis of the double Gibbs-Donnan equilibrium, energy deficit with consequent inadequate functioning of the Na^+K^+-ATPase must lead to cell swelling, as the influx of Na^+ and water is not pumped out. Therefore, cytotoxic oedema has been observed in such conditions as anoxia, ischaemia, decoupling of oxidative phosphorylation by dinitrophenol, intoxication with 6-amino-nicotinamide due to competitive inhibition of NAD enzymes, suppression of energy metabolism during deep hypothermia (15° C), intoxication with 3-nitropropionic acid resulting in irreversible inhibition of succinate dehydrogenase, inactivation of the Na^+K^+-pump by ouabain (Reulen and Baethmann 1967, Baethmann *et al.* 1968, Reulen *et al.* 1970b, Hamilton and Gould 1987, Gazendam *et al.* 1979b). Ultrastructural studies have revealed swelling of astrocytes and oligodendroglial cells and occasionally also of neurones (Bakay and Kobayashi 1971, Baethmann and Van Harreveld 1973, Towfighi and Gonatas 1973, Lowe 1978, Hamilton and Gould 1987). In anoxia and ischaemia, formation of lactic acid by anaerobic glycolysis may also be involved, resulting in intracellular acidosis and activation of the Na^+/H^+ antiporter, which tends to correct the acidosis by the efflux of H^+ ions in exchange for the influx of Na^+ with osmotically obliged water. Mediators that may induce cell swelling may also be released, allegedly by way of signal-transduction systems activating ion channels or ion exchange mechanisms.

Another group of cytotoxic oedemas comprise intoxications or diseases, in which the mechanism of the swelling has not been elucidated, such as the oedema following the ingestion of organic tin compounds, the use of hexachlorophene, cuprizone, the strongly epileptogenic agent methionine sulfoximine, isoniazid, cycloleucine, and in Reye's syndrome and hepatic encephalopathy (Gruner 1958, Aleu *et al.* 1963, Hirano *et al.* 1968, Lampert *et al.* 1973, Kesterson and Carlton 1971, Gutierrez and Norenberg 1977, Rizzuto and Gonatas 1974, Blakemore 1972, Greco *et al.* 1980, Partin *et al.* 1978, Gröflin and Thölen 1978). The cell swelling particularly affects astrocytes, but in many intoxications formation of large vacuoles has been observed in myelin sheaths. The vacuolation of astrocytes and myelin sheaths gives the tissue a spongy appearance, which has been described as status spongiosus or spongiform encephalopathy.

Even predominantly vasogenic types of oedema, such as cryogenic oedema, may often be accompanied by secondary cell swelling. It may be due to additional damage to cell membranes by the injury or by the action of factors that are produced in the injury, such as oxygen derived free radicals, e.g. resulting in a reduction of Na^+K^+ ATPase activity and retention of Na^+ and obliged water (Cohadon *et al.* 1984, Cohadon 1987).

Osmotic Brain Oedema

This is the result of water influx into the brain on account of hyperosmolarity of the brain with respect to plasma. The osmotic gradient may be due to water intoxication, infusion of fluids of incorrect composition, retention of water due to inappropriate antidiuretic hormone secretion or excessive natriuresis, which has been reported after subarachnoid haemorrhage. Since Na^+ is the prevailing cation, these conditions are associated with hyponatraemia. Osmotic brain oedema may develop during haemodialysis, when the blood urea level is lowered too rapidly (Szegedy 1966, Pappius *et al.* 1967). As the blood-brain barrier restricts the passage of urea, brain urea content cannot follow the rapid decline of blood urea level, and an increasing urea gradient develops between brain tissue and blood.

Integrity of the blood-brain barrier is not only required for the efficacy of osmotherapy but also for osmotic brain oedema to develop, as with a disruption of the barrier the change of plasma osmolarity is readily transmitted to the brain parenchyma, abolishing the osmotic gradient required for the development of oedema (Go *et al.* 1973b).

Analysis of oedema fluid from cats in which osmotic brain oedema had been induced by lowering plasma osmolarity, revealed the following composition: Na^+ 130 meq/l, K^+ 1.6 meq/l, compared to plasma Na^+ of 126 meq/l and plasma K^+ of 4.6 meq/l (Patberg *et al.* 1976). In the brains of rats subjected to plasma hyposmolarity (251 mOsm/l), ion-selective micro-electrodes measured the following interstitial electrolyte concentrations: a decreased Na^+ concentration of 124 mmol/l and Cl^- concentration of 106 mmol/l, but an unchanged K^+ concentration (Lundbaek *et al.* 1990). The changes of electrolyte content in oedema fluid are probably due to dilution and solvent drag in the presence of an increased flow of extracellular fluid towards the CSF. Under conditions of plasma hyposmolarity a consider-able increase of CSF formation rate has indeed been observed (Di Mattio *et al.* 1975), and this probably also accounts for the ephemeral character of osmotic brain oedema. The short duration of osmotic brain oedema may explain why in some early experiments no increase of water content was found two hours after water intoxication (Yannet 1939, Gerschenfeld *et al.* 1959).

Brain swelling following water intoxication in experimental animals was observed as early as 1919 by Weed and McKibben. In vitro incubation of brain slices in hyposmolar solutions resulted in swelling of the tissue, which could be localized to the non-sucrose space, allegedly the intra-cellular compartment (Pappius 1965). Osmotic cell swelling has been mea-sured in C_6 glioma cell suspensions using flow cytometry, with demonstra-tion of an increase of cell volume from a normal mean of 980 μm^3 to 1,469 μm^3 (Chaussy *et al.* 1981). Besides an increase of water content, in osmotic brain oedema generally a decline of the K^+, Cl^- and Na^+ contents has been reported (Van Harreveld *et al.* 1966, Gerschenfeld *et al.* 1959, Lundbaek *et al.* 1990). Electron-microscopy showed swelling of perivascu-lar glia in the cerebral cortex, and glial swelling along with enlargement of intercellular spaces in white matter (Luse and Harris 1960, Wasterlain and Torack 1968). In addition to cell swelling, there is also extracellular accu-mulation of fluid, which accounts for its drainage into CSF and the feasi-bility of its isolation by the insertion of needles into the tissue. Diffusion-weighted MR imaging of rat brain with oedema induced by hyponatraemia showed a reduction of the apparent diffusion coefficient for water by $\sim 8\%$ (Sevick *et al.* 1992).

Contrary to acute plasma hyposmolarity with inherent hyponatraemia, in which there is concomitant brain oedema, chronic hyponatraemia is no longer associated with elevated brain water content (Holliday *et al.* 1968). The regulatory process that normalizes water content involves the decrease of brain K^+ content (Rymer and Fishman 1973, Katzman and Pappius 1973), probably in conjunction with the intracellular reduction of organic osmolyte levels (Trachtman 1992). On the cellular level, loss of K^+ has been observed in several cell types as a mechanism for restoration of cell volume (regulatory volume decrease) (Grinstein *et al.* 1984). The cellular ion shifts are probably responsible for the symptoms of hyponatraemia, such as somnolence and epileptic seizures, or the phenomenon of pathoclisis, i.e. the manifestation of latent neurological disturbances (Espinas and Poser 1969, Goulon *et al.* 1971).

In the treatment of prolonged hyponatraemia by the administration of hypertonic saline, it is advisable not to exceed a rate of 0.5 mmol/l per hour or a total increment of plasma Na^+ of 25 mmol/l in 48 hours, lest the condition of central pontine myelinolysis is induced (Trachtman 1992).

Hydrostatic Brain Oedema

This type of oedema is actually a transudate or ultrafiltrate with a low protein content, which has entered the brain parenchyma as a result of a hydrostatic gradient. Hydrostatic oedema has been observed after experimental head injury, with hypertension and vasoparalysis (Schutta *et al.* 1968), or in experimentally induced hypertension with pronounced hypercapnic vasodilatation (Meinig *et al.* 1972), in which the elevated arterial pressure was transmitted into the capillary bed, unattenuated by autoregulatory vasoconstriction, and therefore capable of promoting increased transcapillary fluid filtration. The blood-brain barrier is intact in these brain areas showing elevated water content, as testified by the absence of Evans blue staining of the tissue.

Clinically, the most familiar example of hydrostatic oedema is the periventricular oedema in hydrocephalus, which appears as periventricular hypodensities on CT-scans, and in experimental hydrocephalus is based upon enlargement of intercellular spaces as visualized in electronmicrographs (Weller and Wisniewski 1969).

Brain Oedema in the Clinical Context

Important clinical conditions such as brain tumours, cerebral ischaemia, and head injury are almost always associated with brain oedema, which greatly contributes to morbidity and mortality.

Peritumoural Brain Oedema

Brain tumours are among the lesions that are often associated with surrounding brain oedema. Peritumoural brain oedema has been extensively studied after implantation of tumours in experimental animals, and has proved to be of the vasogenic type, with blood-brain barrier disruption, and localization of the oedema in the white matter. Clinically, the vasogenic nature of peritumoural brain oedema is evident from its preferential location in the white matter as shown by CT and MRI scans. Measurement of tissue impedance during operation has also demonstrated its extra-cellular location (Go *et al.* 1972b). The defective blood-brain barrier is mainly based upon a pathologically altered capillary endothelium, showing fenestrations, separation of tight junctions, and other abnormalities such as the presence of tubular bodies and an increased number of vesicles in the cytoplasm, and absence or irregular thickening of the basal lamina (Long 1970, Hirano and Matsui 1975, Lohle *et al.* 1992).

The mechanism of peritumoural brain oedema formation is related to the type of tumour as classified into intra-axial tumours (gliomas), extra-axial tumours (meningiomas and neurinomas), and metastatic tumours. As gliomas arise from the brain tissue itself and tend to infiltrate the sur-rounding tissue, there is no definite border separating the tumour from the surrounding tissue and restricting the flow of oedema fluid into the sur-rounding tissue; in the glioma the exudate especially originates in the marginal regions in which the blood-brain barrier is disrupted, as shown by contrast studies. However, not all gliomas form a solid mass of tumour; a histologic study of serial stereotaxic biopsies has demonstrated that low-grade gliomas may consist of isolated neoplastic cells scattered within the brain parenchyma rather than a central mass of tumour (Daumas-Duport *et al.* 1987). Extra-axial tumours arise outside the brain; these tumours are separated by several layers from the cerebral white matter in which oedema fluid tends to accumulate. These layers are the arachnoid mater, the sub-arachnoid space, the pia mater, and the cerebral cortex, all of which tend to impede to some degree the spread of oedema fluid from the tumour. With meningiomas and metastases, the oedema fluid originates from the tumour, since contrast studies demonstrate that the blood-brain barrier is not disrupted in the surrounding brain. As has been demonstrated in meningiomas, the amount of peritumoural oedema appeared to depend not only on the size and histological type of the tumour, but also on the integrity of the separating layers (Go *et al.* 1988a). Although metastases are usually well demarcated from surrounding brain, they are intra-axially located and not enveloped by layers which may impede the spread of oedema fluid from the tumour into the surrounding brain. In oedema surrounding metastases, the rate of formation of oedema fluid could be calculated from the spread of contrast agent on CT-scans (Ito *et al.* 1986, 1988). By using the spread of contrast agent on CT-scans, the rate of oedema fluid formation was also measured in meningiomas, and it proved to correlate with the amount and extent of peritumoural oedema (Go *et al.* 1993a).

The space occupying character of the tumour and of accompanying oedema may raise intracranial pressure, initially in the vicinity of the tumour, compromising regional tissue perfusion, but eventually in a global way, causing more widespread ischaemia. On the other hand, metabolites produced by the tumour may cause hyperaemia and increase of local tissue blood flow. The recent technique of proton magnetic resonance spectroscopy allows the study of various proton containing metabolites that occur in adequate concentration in the tissue, such as phosphocholine (CHOL), (phospho)creatine (CREAT), N-acetylaspartate (NAA), and lactate (LAC) (Go 1991). Areas of peritumoural oedema generally showed no increase of the CHOL/CREAT ratio, no decrease of the NAA/CREAT ratio, but there was an increase of the LAC/CREAT ratio, often to a lesser extent than in the margin of the tumour, although increased lactate in peritumoural oedema has been reported to exceed that in the tumour itself (Ott *et al.* 1993). Since these areas of peritumoural oedema do not contain tumour cells which might be responsible for the tumour-specific prevalence of glycolysis, the elevation of LAC may rather indicate hypoxia/ischaemia. Measurements of tissue oxygen tension have demonstrated low values in the tumour and in peritumoural oedematous areas, which markedly improved after operative decompression and therefore could be attributed to decreased perfusion (Kayama *et al.* 1991, Cruickshank and Rampling 1994).

When massive peritumoural oedema and absence of contrast enhancement obscure the exact site of a glioma on CT- or MRI scans, localization of the tumour for biopsy may be accomplished by MRSI on the basis of the increase of CHOL and LAC, and the NAA void (Go *et al.* 1994a). Oedematous areas which still exhibit NAA on the MRSI may be assumed to contain viable neurones, resection of which may conceivably increase the functional deficit in functionally critical areas.

In proton MRS the proton containing metabolites that occur in adequate concentration, appear as resonance peaks of marked height in the proton magnetic resonance spectrum. The substance (or a specific proton containing group it contains) is characterized by its place on the abscissa of the spectrum, which denotes the specific chemical shift of resonance frequency it exhibits on the basis of the specific molecular environment of the proton delivering the signal. Signals of adequate size may be obtained from 1 ml of tissue volume. Consequently unit volumes of tissue (voxels) of 1 cm^3 may be chosen to make up the total volume of brain to be studied, and in magnetic resonance spectroscopic imaging (MRSI) reconstructed into two-dimensional matrices representing the spatial distribution of a certain metabolite in the total volume studied. CHOL appears to be abundant in gliomas as a constituent of membrane components to be incorporated in the growing cells of the tumour. The elevation of CHOL in gliomas tends to occur in the marginal rather than in the central parts of the tumour. CREAT occurs in all living cells, subserving energy metabolism as creatine phosphate, and is often used as a reference to express the relative concentrations of the other metabolites. NAA is a component of neurones, the function of which is still poorly understood. Its disappearance in tumours presumably indicates that the normal neuronal population in the lesion has been replaced by tumour cells. LAC also tends to be elevated

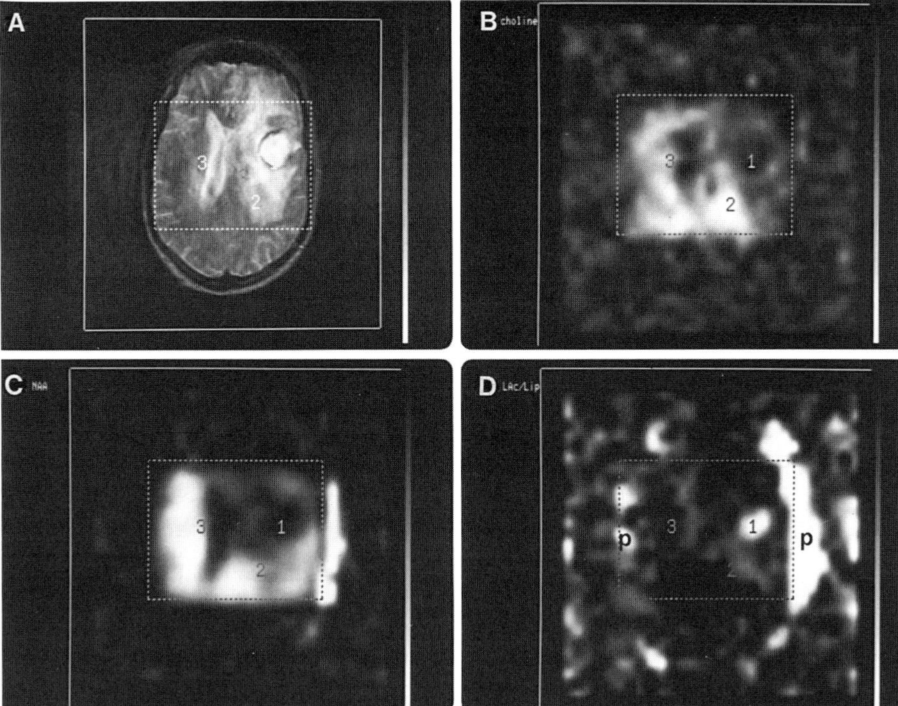

Fig. 18. Proton MR spectroscopic imaging of left parietal malignant astrocytoma: (A) is a T_2-weighted MRI showing anatomical relations and the area (box) depicted by the metabolite maps. (B) Choline map showing elevated CHOL, especially in the oedematous area *(2)* presumably infiltrated by proliferating tumour. (C) NAA map showing the tumour *(1)* and the lateral ventricles (between *3* and tumour), but not the oedematous area *(2)* being devoid of NAA. (D) Lactate/lipid map showing strong lactate signal in the tumour *(1)* and some lactate in the area of oedema *(2)*; the strong signals (*p*) at the periphery derive from subcutaneous fat

in tumours, presumably on the basis of the predominance of glycolysis, although another cause may be impaired perfusion due to elevated regional tissue pressure. LAC elevation occurs with the high-grade gliomas, in particular, and tends to be located in the core of the tumour rather than in its margin, possibly suggesting necrosis (Fig. 18).

Glucocorticosteroids have been shown to reduce both the symptoms and signs in brain tumour patients, as well as the peritumoural oedema. Calculations on the basis of the spread of contrast agent on CT-scans have demonstrated a decrease in the rate of oedema fluid formation by steroids, both in meningiomas and other tumours (Ito *et al.* 1986).

Ischaemic Brain Oedema

Brain oedema in ischaemia tends to have a dual nature: initially of the cytotoxic type, at later stages there is additional vasogenic oedema by blood-brain barrier breakdown.

With the onset of ischaemia very soon swelling of the tissue develops due to uptake of water (cytotoxic oedema), with concomitant elevation of total tissue Na^+ and decrease of total tissue K^+. Studies of interstitial ion activities in rat brain cortex by means of ion-sensitive microelectrodes have demonstrated that in cardiac arrest, for example, the extracellular K^+ concentration slowly increased in the first two min, and then abruptly rose to a plateau at around 80 mM within seconds; the cortical electrical activity ceased long before the surge in K^+ concentration took place (Hansen 1978). Simultaneously, Na^+ and Cl^- concentrations fell from around 140–110 to 70 mM, and there was concomitant shrinking of the extracellular space to about half of its normal size, reflecting the intracellular water shift.

A Na^+/K^+-ATPase failure due to the energy deficit can explain only part of the K^+ shift, as it can be calculated that the K^+ efflux would otherwise proceed much more slowly. An additional factor may be the opening of K^+ channels in response to the ischaemic changes (Hansen 1987). The activation of K^+ channels is considered to be mediated by elevation of cytosolic Ca^{++}, which has entered from the extracellular space (Krnjevic et al. 1978, Harris et al. 1981, Harris and Symon 1984). The influx of Na^+ may not be only a consequence of Na^+/K^+ pump failure, for other mechanisms that may contribute to the Na^+ shift are the Na^+/H^+ antiporter exchanging Na^+ uptake for H^+ extrusion to alleviate the intracellular acidosis, and activation of Na^+ channels by glutamate (NMDA) receptors (Mac Dermott et al. 1986) in response to elevated extracellular glutamate levels in ischaemia. Other cationic changes include elevation of tissue Ca^{++} and reduction of tissue Mg^{++} content.

Very soon after the onset of ischaemia there is a decrease of the apparent diffusion coefficient of water, which can be visualized as a significant change of the signal in the diffusion-weighted image (Moseley et al. 1990). The decrease in the ADC of water is generally ascribed to the shift of water into the intracellular compartment where diffusion is relatively more restricted. It occurs even before increase of T_2 (visible as hyperintensity on the T_2-weighted images) develops, indicating net water accumulation. After killing of the animal the ADC in the ischaemic area equals that in the rest of the brain, contrary to the anisotropy which changed neither during ischaemia, nor postmortem (Van Gelderen et al. 1994).

There is initially no exudation of proteins or of tracers to indicate blood-brain barrier breakdown; the oedema is merely of the cytotoxic type, which is related to the resistance of the blood-brain barrier to the energy deficit in anoxia. The secondary occurrence of barrier disruption after a period of latency has been referred to as a maturation phenomenon (Ito *et al.* 1976, Studygroup on Brain Edema in Stroke 1977). The latency period before barrier breakdown tends to be shorter the more severe the ischaemia. On CT-scans, ischaemic cytotoxic oedema specifically affects both grey and white matter, contrary to the vasogenic oedema at a later stage, which preferentially occupies the white matter. The blood-brain barrier disruption may be verified in animal experiments by the exudation of Evans blue or of horseradish peroxidase in ultrastructural studies (Westergaard *et al.* 1976, Go *et al.* 1984a), and clinically by the appearance of a radioactive focus on the isotope brain scan or of contrast enhancement on the CT-scan, four to seven days after the insult. In animal experiments the vasogenic oedema has been shown to increase, if the circulation is restored after prolonged ischaemia (Ito *et al.* 1979).

The effect of glucocorticosteroids on cerebral ischaemia proved to be controversial, at best (Studygroup on Brain Edema in Stroke 1977). Decrease of ischaemic oedema has only been achieved in the context of a reduction of the effects of cerebral ischaemia by protective measures or drugs, such as hypothermia, hypoglycaemia (Go *et al.* 1988b), or barbiturates (Safar *et al.* 1978), and drugs abolishing the causes of ischaemia, such as calcium antagonists (nimodipine) in vasospasm.

Traumatic Brain Oedema

Head injuries occur in various types and of variable severity. On one hand there is the type resulting from a more or less locally focused mechanical impact on the head, occasionally complicated by penetration of the skull and local laceration of the underlying brain. On the other hand there is the closed type, usually resulting from traffic accidents or falls, in which a large decelerating force is globally transferred to the cranial contents. The consequences of impact and tissue inertia may be a multitude of lesions, including neuronal damage, vasculare rupture resulting in subarachnoid, subdural and intracerebral haemorrhages, impairment of vasomotor autoregulatory mechanisms making the brain susceptible to hypoxia and hypotension, blood-brain barrier breakdown with consequent vasogenic oedema, and widespread shear-induced rupture of nerve fibres, called diffuse axonal injury.

Accordingly, several experimental models of head injury have been devised. A familiar model is the fluid percussion injury, in which the force of a swinging pendulum is transmitted to the brain of the animal by way of a column of fluid which is in immediate contact with the brain. The model rather represents injury to the brain stem, in which the maximum site of strain proved to be located (Thibault *et al.* 1992). The direct impact models include blows delivered by a special gun or a piston to the skull, which rather produce local laceration of the tissue underlying the site of impact. Diffuse axonal injury has been inflicted in monkeys by decelerating forces acting in the lateral direction upon the head, which even do not require direct impact (Gennarelli *et al.* 1982).

In head-injured patients, intracranial pressure elevation has been found to be correlated with mortality; among the patients with an intracranial pressure exceeding 20 mm Hg only 36% had a good outcome or moderate disability, versus 80% of the patients with normal intracranial pressure (Narayan *et al.* 1981). Intracranial pressure elevation following head trauma may be caused by brain oedema, next to haemorrhage and possibly also vascular factors (Marmarou *et al.* 1987). Regarding vascular engorgement, however, studies of cerebral blood volume and cerebral blood flow by means of dynamic stable Xenon-enhanced CT-scanning, have demonstrated decreased cerebral volume, as well as ischaemic flow values in head-injured patients with raised intracranial pressure.

In animal experiments, local laceration of the brain by direct impact is invariably associated with blood-brain barrier disruption and consequent vasogenic oedema as demonstrated by extravasation of Evans blue and increase of tissue water content soon after the impact (Tornheim and McLaurin 1984, Shapira *et al.* 1993). In human head injury, the presence of brain oedema has been corroborated by the increased water content, measured in white matter biopsies from both diffuse as well as mass lesions (Galbraith *et al.* 1984). MR measurement of water diffusion demonstrated that in the rat spinal cord, the tissue anisotropy which is normally evident from a greater apparent diffusion coefficient along the fibre tracts than tranverse to it, has diappeared after experimental injury (Ford *et al.* 1994).

However, blood-brain barrier disruption, which has been observed so frequently and early after experimental head injury, proved to be less conspicuous in human cases. Remarkable was the paucity (5.7% among 70 patients) of contrast enhancement on the CT-scans of head-injured patients (Mauser *et al.* 1984). Moreover, MR-contrast enhancement studies using Gadolinium showed no evidence of blood-brain barrier disruption one to 4 days after the injury; enhancement was found only in patients who were studied 6 or more days after the injury (Lang *et al.* 1991).

The secondary occurrence of blood-brain barrier impairment after head injury in humans has therefore been considered akin to the situation in cerebral ischaemia. Indeed, evidence of cerebral ischaemia has been amply found after head injury. In autopsies of 151 patients who had died from head injury, ischaemic damage has been found in 91%, 27% of which was severe, and 43% moderately severe (Graham *et al.* 1978). A consistent finding after head injury is a raised CSF lactate level, which proved to correlate with the degree of injury, with a poor outcome, and with elevation of intracranial pressure (Sood *et al.* 1980, De Salles *et al.* 1986). Predisposing to ischaemic damage are, on one hand, the attenuated cerebrovascular responses to hypoxaemia, and even more to arterial hypotension, as have been found in experimental animals after head trauma (Unterberg *et al.* 1988, Andersen *et al.* 1988, Ishige 1987, 1988), while on the other hand there is an increase of cerebral energy consumption soon after the injury, as animal experiments have demonstrated (Nelson *et al.* 1966, Duckrow *et al.* 1981).

Histological studies of contused brain after experimental injury, such as in the rat, showed swelling of astrocytes (cytotoxic oedema). Swelling of perivascular astrocytes has been related to compression of the microvascular lumen; moreover, other causes of microvascular obstruction were intra- and extravascular clotting (Hekmatpanah and Hekmatpanah 1985). In biopsies taken from head-injured patients during surgery, astrocytic swelling was observed from 3 hours to 5 days after injury, to an extent that it may account for compression of the vascular lumen. Initially, endothelial morphology was grossly normal; but from 2 days on the capillary endothelial cells in the contused areas showed irregular profiles due to the appearance of folds and processes on their luminal aspect. No disruption of endothelial tight junctions was observed. In the white matter astrocytic swelling was less pronounced than in the cortex, and occasionally there was marked accumulation of interstitial fluid in grossly disrupted tissue (Bullock *et al.* 1991).

The findings with diffusion-weighted MRI are controversial in experimentally induced head injury. Decrease of ADC has been reported as well as increase, which may reflect the controversy that exists regarding the intra- or extracellular nature of the oedema.

Glucocorticosteroids, even in doses higher than conventionally used to treat peritumoural oedema, have been shown to be ineffective in influencing mortality after head injury (Braakman *et al.* 1983). Assuming that their mechanism of action should be directed at the formation of vasogenic brain oedema, this is to be expected if the type of oedema in head injury is not predominantly vasogenic. Nimodipine, the calcium channel blocker that proved so effective in the treatment of vasospasm induced by subarachnoid heamorrhage, did not achieve a significant increase in the percentage of head-injured patients exhibiting a favourable outcome, although a trend toward a beneficial effect was found in a subgroup with traumatic subarachnoid haemorrhage (The European Studygroup on Nimodipine in Severe Head Injury 1994).

Hydrocephalus

In hydrocephalus the fluid accumulation is located in the CSF compartment, as a surplus resulting from CSF production in excess of CSF absorption. Rarely an abnormal increase of CSF formation is the cause of hydrocephalus; since ventriculocisternal perfusion first enabled us to measure CSF dynamics, abnormally increased CSF formation has only been measured in choroid plexus papilloma, 1.43 ml/min in one case (Eisenberg *et al.* 1974b), and in another case, 1.05 ml/min was found before, and 0.20 ml/min after removal of the tumour (Milhorat *et al.* 1976). Recently a case has been described with a 4-fold increase of CSF formation rate and no evidence of tumour or hypertrophy of the choroid plexus (Casey and Vries 1989).

Usually hydrocephalus is the result of an obstruction of CSF outflow. In obstructive hydrocephalus, which prior to the era of shunting was the only type amenable to treatment by draining the ventricles to a cistern, the obstruction is located within the ventricular system, such as in congenital atresia of the exits of the fourth ventricle (the Dandy-Walker syndrome), descent of the cerebellar tonsils (Arnold-Chiari malformation), tumours or cysts compressing the ventricles or the aqueduct, and stenosis of the Sylvian aqueduct.

In communicating hydrocephalus the obstruction is located outside the ventricular system, by factors such as fibrosis, formation of adhesions in the subarachnoid spaces following meningitis or subarachnoid haemorrhage, and aplasia of the arachnoid granulations (Winkelman and Fay 1930, Torvik *et al.* 1978).

Measurement of CSF dynamics in patients with hydrocephalus has revealed in one category of patients a deficit of CSF absorption based upon an elevated opening pressure, but normal outflow conductance, whereas in another category there was a normal opening pressure but a decreased opening conductance (Lorenzo *et al.* 1970). In a later study a third category was recognized with normal opening pressure and normal absorption at lower CSF pressures, but severely reduced outflow conductance at higher CSF pressures (Lorenzo *et al.* 1974). The CSF formation rate in patients with hydrocephalus was slightly lower (0.30 ml/min) than in children without hydrocephalus (Cutler *et al.* 1968) and in adults (0.40 ml/min) (Rubin *et al.* 1966).

There are patients in whom dilatation of the ventricular system, and often of peripheral CSF spaces as well, is a manifestation of a discrepancy between cranial volume and brain volume, due to a loss of brain tissue by other causes. These include Alzheimer, multi-infarct and severe posttraumatic dementias. The ventricular dilatation in these cases is designated as *ex vacuo hydrocephalus*, and is not thought to be associated with raised intracranial pressure. Therefore it should be differentiated from the syndrome of normal pressure hydrocephalus, although in the latter instance prolonged recording may reveal elevated pressures (Hakim and Adams 1965, Symon and Dorsch 1975).

As an illustration of the development of normal pressure hydrocephalus, an experiment was carried out in rabbits in which following the intracisternal injection of kaolin, there was a ten-fold elevation of intraventricular pressure in the first two days, which returned to normal values in the following five days. The pressure rise was associated with ventricular enlargement, which largely persisted after the pressure returned to normal levels (Edvinsson and West 1971). In rabbits with kaolin-induced hydrocephalus, CSF production appeared to be reduced to almost 50% of normal (Lindvall and Owman 1984). In cats with kaolin-induced hydrocephalus the development of the normal pressure type has been observed in relation to dilatation of the central canal of the spinal cord. After injection of Evans blue into the ventricular CSF there was blue-staining of the walls of the spinal central canal and the outer surface of the sacral cord, indicating that the dye had penetrated through slits in the dorsal columns of the lumbar cord (Eisenberg *et al.* 1974a, Nakamura *et al.* 1983). It is assumed that the CSF is then absorbed from the spinal subarachnoid space. The pressure measured in the central canal remained at a reasonably low level of 8 cm H_2O, when 22–43 $\mu l/min$ of fluid was infused into the ventricular system. The operation of this efflux mechanism may well explain the normal pressure stage of kaolin-induced hydrocephalus. Fluid infusions exceeding the maximum efflux capacity of 168 $\mu l/min$ provoked a rapid rise of pressure. The importance of the efflux pathway was demonstrated by ligation of the lumbar cord, whereupon the absorption rate of 47 $\mu l/min$ declined to zero; recording of intraventricular pressure revealed the development of plateau waves, eventually followed by death of the animal (Wald and Hochwald 1977). The role of spinal central canal dilatation in human hydrocephalus is probably negligible, since it has not been observed on sagittal MRI-scans of patients with communicating hydrocephalus.

In general, re-establishment of drainage of CSF in hydrocephalus, to account for the cases of spontaneous arrest of its clinical evolution, is assumed to proceed either by restoration of normal CSF pathways (Johnston *et al.* 1984), or because transventricular fluid absorption has become operative as an alternative pathway, involving the same mechanisms as those in the resolution of oedema fluid.

Cystic Lesions

Water collections may occur in cysts; these are unnatural cavities within the brain parenchyma, in which the tissue is replaced by fluid.

There exist a multitude of cystic lesions, for which the following classification may be useful: (I) Cysts containing CSF-like fluid; (II) Cysts with a lining of non-neural epithelium; (III) Cysts accompanying gliomas and other tumours; (IV) Cysts of infectious origin (Go *et al.* 1993b). The cysts with a lining of non-neural epithelium (II) have contents which are clearly the product of secretion (viz. colloid cysts, Rathke's cleft cysts), or of desquamation of the cyst wall (epidermoid and dermoid cysts, cysts accompanying craniopharyngiomas), while cysts of infectious origin (IV) such as brain abscesses or hydatid cysts have contents which in the former are the result of the inflammatory process, and in the latter are the secretory product of the parasite. Therefore, only the cysts containing CSF-like fluid (I), and those accompanying tumours (III), are relevant to the dynamics of brain tissue water accumulation, also pertaining to the question why the fluid persists and is not reabsorbed in the light of transcapillary fluid exchange.

The cysts containing CSF-like fluid comprise: (A) Ex vacuo type of cysts; (B) Cysts with fluid secreting walls and CSF-like content. Radiologically, they appear on CT-scans with the same attenuation value as that of CSF. On MR-scans they exhibit long T_1 and T_2 relaxation times, and like CSF, they are hypointense on T_1-weighted images, while on T_2-weighted images they present with a high signal intensity. Since there are no inflammatory changes with blood-brain barrier impairment in the surrounding tissue, there is no enhancement upon intravenous administration of contrast agents.

Ex vacuo Type Cysts

To understand their pathogenesis it is helpful to reflect upon the course of events after an injury to the tissue. Disruptions of tissue continuity like those resulting from surgical resection or cerebral haemorrhage, are initially filled with extracellular fluid (or CSF) when the acute phase of oedema and heamorrhage has subsided. Then the cavity tends to collapse and obliterate, with the fluid within the cavity being resolved by reabsorption and drainage to CSF spaces. For the process of reabsorption the Starling fluid flux equation applies, as discussed before. A cavity will persist, however, when the loss of tissue is too extensive to be accommodated by the elasticity of the surrounding brain. Typical examples of such ex vacuo types of cyst, i.e. cysts resulting from shortage of brain tissue are posttraumatic leptomeningeal cysts, ex vacuo cysts remaining after the resection of tumours; cysts resulting from extensive infarctions; and porencephalic cysts. Posttraumatic leptomeningeal cysts are in fact pockets of the subarachnoid space, which are formed by adhesions following trauma. There is other evidence of the ex vacuo condition, such as dilatation and retraction of adjacent ventricles (Taveras and Ransohoff 1953). These features of the ex vacuo situation are shared by the cavities remaining from extensive resections and infarctions. The porencephalic cysts have been defined as congenital cavities which frequently, but not always, exhibit communication with the ventricular system or subarachnoid spaces (Heschl 1859). They actually constitute an amalgam of more or less extensive congenital defects, which may be manifestations of developmental derangements (also called schizencephalies), or the results of brain damage due to vascular occlusion and haemorrhage (destructive encephaloclastic porencephaly) (Yakovlev 1946). In view of a shortage of tissue being the cause of ex vacuo cysts, there is no need to reduce intracranial pressure. Moreover, communication with normal CSF spaces allows ex vacuo cystic lesions to empty their contents into these spaces when they are compressed by surrounding brain during movements of the head. In terms of craniospinal pressure/volume relations this implies that unlike incompressible solid tumours these lesions do not reduce *compliance*.

It is therefore important to establish the presence of communication with physiological CSF spaces. Radioisotope scanning may be used to demonstrate the appearance of radioactivity in the cyst after intrathecal injection of a radioactive marker; currently CT-scanning is preferred following intrathecal injection of an X-ray contrast agent. A non-invasive method of assessing communication between a cyst and CSF spaces has been proposed using an interferographic MR-technique which is based on the RARE-fast imaging sequence. Essentially, the method averages CSF flow over an ECG cycle and therefore measures net flow rather than ECG-dependent flow variations, with a sensitivity below 1 mm/sec. This makes these slow currents visible in physiological CSF spaces and in other spaces with which they communicate (Hennig *et al.* 1990).

Cysts with Fluid Secreting Walls and CSF-Like Content

These comprise the *arachnoid cysts* and *neuroepithelial cysts*. Arachnoid cysts contain a fluid which resembles CSF. Nevertheless, there is no extensive communication with physiological CSF spaces. During operation it has been observed that the cyst is separated from adjacent subarachnoid spaces and cisterns by translucent walls, and after its emptying no fluid is seen entering the cyst from surrounding cisterns. Also, bleeding within the cyst does not progress into a subarachnoid haemorrhage, but rather develops into a subdural haematoma. Pneumoencephalography, radioisotope cisternography and CT-cisternography with intrathecal contrast agents generally demonstrate retarded filling from adjacent subarachnoid spaces. Other features indicate the existence of a mechanism that maintains or increases its fluid volume, such as expansion, indentation and displacement of adjoining (developing) brain structures (eventually resulting in "temporal lobe agenesis"), and recurrence after mere evacuation or after failure of a previously installed drainage system. Various suggestions have been made as to the nature of this mechanism, such as an open communication with the subarachnoid space at an early stage of development, allowing inflow of fluid and sequestration at a later stage by closure of the opening (Starkman 1958). This mechanism would not explain long-term maintenance or expansion of cyst volume. Valvular mechanisms have also been suggested, e.g. by way of a single small opening serving both as an entrance and an exit of fluid, presumably driven by the CSF pulse pressure. But it is difficult to envision how the CSF pulse pressure can act as a driving force and result in fluid accumulation, when the latter may cause elevation of intracranial pressure exceeding the driving force. Another mechanism comprises secretion of fluid by the cyst walls. By their possession of several characteristics, such as desmosomal junctions, vimentin-positive cytoplasmic tonofilaments, interdigitating cytoplasmic processes, large cytoplasmic vacuoles and pinocytotic vesicles, and an underlying basal lamina, the cells lining arachnoid cysts have been recognized as being similar to those of the outer layer of the arachnoid mater, designated as the subdural neurothelium (Go *et al.* 1978, Rascol and Izard 1969). Furthermore, subdural neurothelium has been recognized as constituents of arachnoid granulations. Like meningiomas and arachnoid granulations, which may be considered to be derived from subdural neurothelium, the cellular lining of arachnoid cysts appears to possess progesterone rather than estrogen receptors (Verhagen *et al.* 1994). It may be surmised that the mechanism of fluid secretion involves $Na^+K^{+-}ATPase$. Using the K-NPPase reaction (a reaction that is based upon the conversion of K-nitrophenylphosphate (K-NPP) by $Na^+K^+ATPase$ into a reaction product that is visible by electron microscopy), enzyme ultracytochemistry has shown the presence of $Na^+K^+ATPase$ in the luminal plasma membrane of the cells lining arachnoid cysts (Fig. 19), as well as those covering arachnoid granulations (Go *et al.* 1984b, 1986). In addition, ion-exchange and cotransport mechanisms in the cell membrane may be involved, with the $Na^+K^+ATPase$ providing the driving force of the transport. Similar to the process of CSF secretion by the choroid plexus, it may be envisaged that the $Na^+K^+ATPase$ of the cyst wall transports Na^+ from the cell contents into the cyst lumen, with the Na^+ then attracting osmotically obliged water. Such a biochemical mechanism of fluid secretion is inherently independent of pressure and may well account for elevation of intracranial pressure. As to the formation of arachnoid cysts, it is conceivable that, (—unlike arachnoid villi or granulations, transporting CSF from the subarachnoid space into the lumen of a venous vessel—), arachnoid cysts lack the blood circulation as the drainage pathway, and therefore

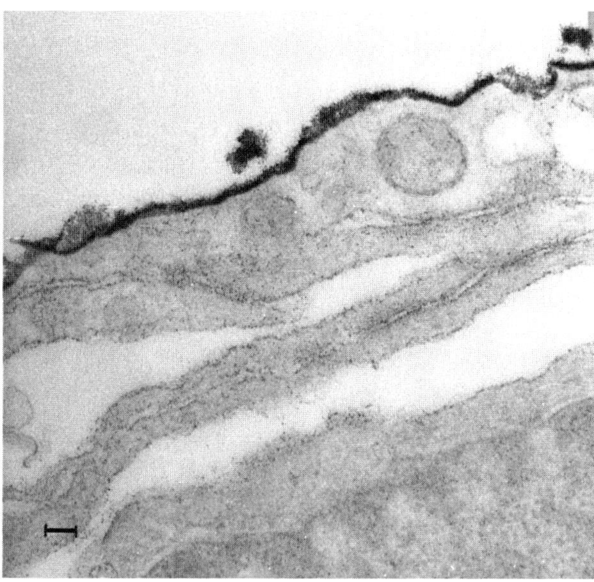

Fig. 19. Ultracytochemical demonstration of the enzyme Na^+K^+ ATPase on the basis of the K-nitrophenylphosphatase reaction in the wall of an arachnoid cyst. The dark (electron dense) reaction product is localized at the luminal membrane of lining neurothelial cells of the cyst wall. Section unstained in order not to obscure the reaction product. Scale bar: 0.1 μm

the transported fluid accumulates in the cyst cavity in the same way as epidermoid cysts are formed by accumulation of desquamated keratin. The situation may arise as a developmental defect of the leptomeninges, in the sense that rudiments of arachnoid villi are developing without the establishment of a connection to draining veins.

Neuroepithelial cysts (also called *ependymal cysts*) contain fluid similar to CSF, and unlike arachnoid cysts they are located intra-axially (from the cerebral convexity to deep within the brain parenchyma). They possess a lining that consists of ependyma or choroid plexus (Inoue *et al.* 1985). From the resemblance of their fluid contents to CSF it may be assumed that the mechanism of secretion is similar to that in arachnoid cysts.

By virtue of their contents of CSF-like fluid, the cysts with CSF-secreting walls display the same features on CT- and MR-scans as the ex-vacuo type of cysts, the only difference being the lack of communication with surrounding CSF spaces in cisternographic studies. Because of their lack of communication they have no way of emptying their contents upon compression, and they tend to behave like real space occupying lesions which may well reduce cranial compliance.

Cysts Associated with Gliomas and Other Tumours

Cysts occur in 20%–55% of brain tumours, and typically contain a yellow-coloured proteinaceous fluid, which is not separated from the tissue by a special cellular lining. In the light of the Starling fluid flux equation for transcapillary fluid exchange the high protein content (exerting an increased colloid osmotic pressure) tends to counteract reabsorption of fluid, which may account for their persistence in the tissue in spite of the absence of a special lining.

With respect to the mechanism of their formation, tumour cyst fluid has been regarded as the product of necrosis, and has been reported to contain various endogenous cerebral proteins, such as glial fibrillary acidic protein, S-100 protein, enolase, and thymidine kinase (Szymas *et al.* 1986, Persson *et al.* 1985). However, analysis of cyst fluid proteins has demonstrated that more than 92% of total cyst fluid protein appears to consist of plasma protein fractions. This implies that the majority of the cyst fluid proteins must derive from plasma, while the remainder (less than 8%) may constitute endogenous brain proteins. This is not consistent with the assumption of necrosis being the origin of the cyst contents, since endogenous proteins would then have prevailed. Analysis of cyst fluid proteins has also demonstrated that the concentration of the various plasma protein fractions within the tumour cyst fluid, when expressed as ratios of their plasma concentrations, appeared to be elevated by as much as 50-fold with respect to their concentration in normal CSF, which indicates increased barrier permeability. Blood-brain barrier disruption is common in gliomatous tumours, particularly in those of malignant grade, as may be inferred from the degree and extent of contrast exudation on CT- or MR-scans. It is also inherent in the formation of vasogenic brain oedema, frequently associated with the tumours. Histology and electron microscopy of tumour cyst walls show gradual transition of the spongy appearance of oedematous tissue to the contents of the cyst lumen (Fig. 20), while at other places the cyst wall shows a distinct cellular lining. On CT- and MR-scans the cyst walls tend to show areas, in which delineation from the surrounding oedematous tissue is vague, probably reflecting the gradual liquefaction of oedematous tissue into cyst contents (Fig. 21). There are also areas of the cyst wall which are sharply delineated on the scans, probably representing those sides of the cyst, which impinge upon the tissue by expansive growth, and histologically probably corresponding to areas exhibiting a distinct cellular lining (Lohle *et al.* 1992). With longstanding oedema some balance may be assumed to exist between the rates of oedema formation and oedema resolution, as otherwise the pressure/volume relations would soon be severely deranged, with elevation of intracranial pressure and coning. It may be surmised that cyst formation indi-

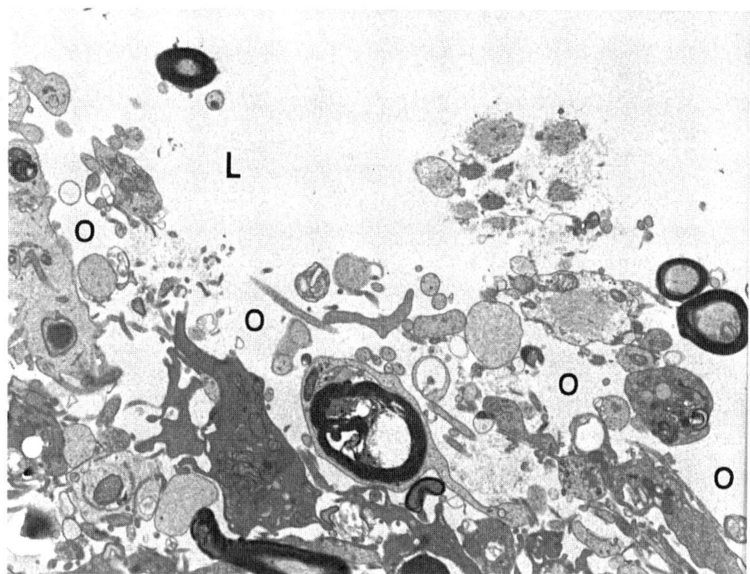

Fig. 20. Electron micrograph of the wall of a cyst, which was associated with a glioblastoma. There is a gradual transition of the oedematous tissue with enlarged intercellular spaces *(O)* into the cyst lumen *(L)*

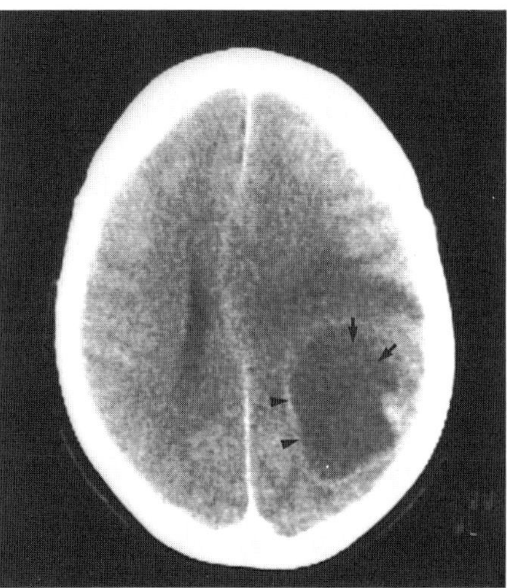

Fig. 21. CT-scan of cyst associated with a malignant astrocytoma; vaguely delineated area of cyst wall (arrows) is probably the site where oedematous tissue liquifies into cyst contents; other areas of cyst wall are well defined (arrow heads)

cates a possible deficiency of the resolution mechanism. Another relevant factor may be the geometry of cysts, which by their globular shape imply an unfavourable surface/volume ratio, as resolution may be assumed to proceed across the surface into the surrounding tissue. Also, ischaemic/ hypoxic factors may account for the gradual liquefaction of tissue in the areas flooded by oedema fluid, as in these areas the density of feeding vessels is greatly reduced, and by the increased distance to blood vessels these areas may experience inadequate supply of nutrients and oxygen. In this light the finding of low tissue oxygen pressures, measured with *in situ* oxygen electrodes in brain tumours and peritumoural oedema, may be significant. With proton MR spectroscopy, brain tumours, areas of peritumoural oedema, and associated cysts, in particular, have been found to contain increased lactate, which is indeed consistent with the existence of ischaemia, presumably due to decreased perfusion pressure as a result of regionally increased tissue pressure (Go *et al.* 1994b).

On account of their proteinaceous fluid content, tumour-associated cysts exhibit prolonged T_1 and T_2 values that are less than those of CSF, contrary to cysts containing CSF-like fluid. Consequently, they have a hypointense appearance on T_1-weighted, but a reasonable brightness on T_2-weighted MR-images (Go *et al.* 1983). The associated blood-brain barrier impairment also characterizes them by a rim of enhancement on intravenous contrast administration. Tumour-associated cysts are among those that show rapid expansion.

Acknowledgement

I am indebted to Prof. W. G. Perdok (Department of Chemistry) for his invaluable comments regarding the structural aspects of the water molecule, and to Prof. A. Okken (Section of Neonatology) for his comments on fluid balance in the infant.

References

1. Aarabi B, Long DM (1979) Dynamics of cerebral edema. The role of an intact vascular bed in the production and propagation of vasogenic brain edema. J Neurosurg 51: 779–784
2. Aleu FP, Katzman R, Terry RD (1963) Fine structure and electrolyte analysis of cerebral edema induced by alkyltin intoxication. J Neuropath Exp Neurol 22: 403–413
3. Alksne JF, Lovings ET (1972) Functional ultrastructure of the arachnoid villus. Arch Neurol 27: 371–377
4. Alksne JF, White LE (1965) Electron microscopic study of the effect of increased intracranial pressure on the arachnoid villus. J Neurosurg 22: 481–488

5. Amenta F, Cavalotti C, Collier WL, Ferrante F, Napoleone P (1989) ^{3}H-muscimol binding sites within the rat choroid plexus: pharmacological characterization and autoradiographic localization. Pharmacol Res 21: 369–373
6. Ames A III, Sakanoue M, Endo S (1964) Na, K, Ca, Mg and Cl concentrations in choroid plexus fluid and cisternal fluid compared with plasma ultrafiltrate. J Neurophysiol 27: 672–681
7. Andersen BJ, Unterberg AW, Clarke GD, Marmarou A (1988) Effect of posttraumatic hypoventilation on cerebral energy metabolism. J Neurosurg 68: 601–607
8. Andersson B, Westbye O (1970) Synergistic action of sodium and angiotensin on brain mechanisms controlling fluid balance. Life Sci 9: 601–608
9. Andres KH (1967) Zur Feinstruktur der Arachnoidalzotten bei Mammalia. Z Zellforsch 82: 92–109
10. Ariëns-Kappers CU (1929) The evolution of the nervous system in invertebrates, vertebrates and man. de Erven, Bohn, Haarlem
11. Back A (1993) Liquid water and the origin of life. Orig Life Evol Biosph 23: 3–10
12. Baethmann A, Reulen HJ, Brendel W (1968) Die Wirkung des Antimetaboliten 6-Aminonicotinamid (6-ANA) auf Wasser- und Elektrolytgehalt des Rattenhirns und ihre Hemmung durch Nicotinsäure. Zschr Ges Exp Med 146: 226–240
13. Baethmann A, Van Harreveld A (1973) Water and electrolyte distribution in gray matter rendered edematous with a metabolic inhibitor. J Neuropath Exp Neurol 32: 408–423
14. Bakay L, Kobayashi T (1971) Cerebral isotope uptake in acute experimental hypercapnic hypoxia. Exp Neurol 32: 303–312
15. Baldissera S, Menani JW, Sotero dos Santos LF, Favaretto ALV, Gutkowska J, Turrin MQA, McCann SM, Antunes-Rodriguez J (1989) Role of the hypothalamus in the control of atrial natriuretic peptide release. Proc Natl Acad Sci USA 86: 9621–9625
16. Banks WA, Kastin AJ, Fischman AJ, Coy DH, Strauss SL (1986) Carrier-mediated transport of enkephalins and N-Tyr-MIF-1 across blood-brain barrier. Am J Physiol (London) 251: E477–482
17. Bedford JJ, Leader JP (1993) Response of tissues of the rat to anisosmolarity in vivo. Am J Physiol 264: R1164–R1179
18. Beks JWF, Kerckhoffs HPM (1972) Studies on the water content of cerebral tissues and intracranial pressure in vasogenic brain oedema. In: Brock M, Dietz H (eds) Intracranial pressure. Springer, Berlin Heidelberg New York Tokyo, pp 119–126
19. Berendsen HJC (1975) Specific interactions of water with biopolymers. In: Franks F (ed) Water, a comprehensive treatise, 5. Water in disperse systems. Plenum, New York, pp 293–330
20. Berendsen HJC, Edzes HT (1973) The observation and general interpretation of sodium magnetic resonance in biological material. Ann NY Acad Sci 204: 459–489
21. Berger HA, Travis SM, Welsh MJ (1993) Regulation of the cystic fibrosis

transmembrane conductance regulator Cl$^-$ channel by specific protein kinases and protein phosphatases. J Biol Chem 268: 2037–2047

22. Bering EA (1958) Problems of the dynamics of the cerebrospinal fluid with particular reference to the formation of cerebrospinal fluid and its relationship to cerebral metabolism. Clin Neurosurg 5: 77–98

23. Betz AL, Firth JA, Goldstein GW (1980) Polarity of the blood-brain barrier: distribution of enzymes between the luminal and antiluminal membranes of brain capillary endothelial cells. Brain Res 192: 17–28

24. Betz AL (1983a) Sodium transport in capillaries isolated from rat brain. J Neurochem 41: 1150–1157

25. Betz AL (1983b) Sodium transport from blood to brain: inhibition by furosemide and amiloride. J Neurochem 41: 1158–1164

26. Blakemore WF (1972) Observations on oligodendrocyte degeneration, the resolution of status spongiosus and remyelination in cuprizone intoxication in mice. J Neurocytol 1: 413–426

27. Bodsch W, Hossmann KA (1983) ^{125}I-antibody autoradiography and peptide fragments of albumin in cerebral edema. J Neurochem 41: 239–243

28. Braakman R, Schouten HJA, Blaauw-van Dishoeck M, Minderhoud M (1983) Megadose steroids in severe head injury. Results of a prospective double-blind clinical trial. J Neurosurg 58: 326–330

29. Bradbury MWB, Cserr HF, Westrop RJ (1981) Drainage of cerebral interstitial fluid into deep cervical lymph of the rabbit. Am J Physiol 240: F329–F336

30. Brightman MW, Hori M, Rapoport SI, Reese TS, Westergaard E (1973) Osmotic opening of tight junctions in cerebral endothelium. J Comp Neurol 152: 317–326

31. Brody MJ, Alpers RH, O'Neill TP, Porter JP (1986) 1. Central neural control of the cardiovascular system. In: Zanchetti A, Tarazi RC (eds) Pathophysiology of hypertension, Handbook of hypertension, vol 8. Elsevier, Amsterdam, pp 1–25

32. Bullock R, Maxwell WL, Graham DI, Teasdale GM, Adams JH (1991) Glial swelling following human cerebral contusion: an ultrastructural study. J Neurol Neurosurg Psychiatry 54: 427–434

33. Burstein D (1988) On the in vivo detection of intracellular water and sodium by nuclear magnetic resonance with shift reagents. Biophys J 54: 191–192

34. Burstyn PGR (1978) Sodium and water metabolism under the influence of prolactin, aldosterone, and antidiuretic hormone. J Physiol 275: 39–50

35. Cala PM (1985) Volume regulation by amphiuma red blood cells: strategies for identifying alkali metal/H$^+$ transport. Fed Proc 44: 2500–2507

36. Canessa CM, Horisberger JD, Rossier BC (1993) Epithelial sodium channel related to proteins involved in neurodegeneration. Nature 361: 467–470

37. Carey ME, Vela AR (1974) Effect of systemic arterial hypotension on the rate of cerebrospinal fluid formation in dogs. J Neurosurg 41: 350–355

38. Casey KF, Vries JK (1989) Cerebral fluid overproduction in the absence of tumor or villous hypertrophy of the choroid plexus. Childs Nerv Syst 5: 332–334

39. Chabrier PE, Roubert P, Braquet P (1987) Specific binding of atrial natriuretic factor in brain microvessels. Proc Natl Acad Sci USA 84: 2078–2081

40. Chaplin ER, Free RG, Goldstein GW (1981) Inhibition by steroids of the uptake of potassium by capillaries isolated from rat brain. Biochem Pharmacol 30: 241–245

41. Chaussy L, Baethmann A, Lubitz W (1981) Electrical sizing of nerve and glia cells in the study of cell volume regulation. In: Cervos-Navarro J, Fritschka E (eds) Cerebral microcirculation and metabolism. Raven, New York, pp 29–40

42. Clasen RA, Brown DVL, Leavitt S, Hass GM (1953) The production by liquid nitrogen of acute closed cerebral lesions. Surg Gynecol Obstet 96: 605–616

43. Clasen RA, Pandolfi S, Hoeppner TJ, Clasen JR (1984) Treatment of experimental acute lead encephalopathy. In: Go KG, Baethmann A (eds) Recent progress in the study and therapy of brain edema. Plenum, New York, pp 633–642

44. Cohadon F, Rigoulet M, Averet N (1984) Alterations of membrane-bound enzymes in vasogenic edema. In: Go KG, Baethmann A (eds) Recent progress in the study and therapy of brain edema. Plenum, New York, pp 223–231

45. Cohadon F (1987) Physiopathologie des oedèmes cérébraux. Rev Neurol 143: 3–20

46. Coulter DM (1989) Postnatal fluid and electrolyte changes and clinical implications. In: Brace RA, Ross MG, Robillard JE (eds) Fetal and neonatal body fluids: the scientific basis for clinical practice. Perinatal, Ithaca, pp 319–367

47. Crockard A, Ianotti F, Hunstock AT, Smith RD, Harris RJ, Symon L (1980) Cerebral blood flow and edema following carotid occlusion in the gerbil. Stroke 11: 494–498

48. Crone C (1963) The permeability of capillaries in various organs as determined by use of the indicator diffusion method. Acta Physiol Scand 58: 292–305

49. Crook RB, Farber MB, Prusiner SB (1984) Hormones and neurotransmitters control cyclic AMP metabolism in choroid plexus epithelial cells. J Neurochem 42: 340–350

50. Crook RB, Farber MB, Prusiner SB (1986) H_2 histamine receptors on the epithelial cells of choroid plexus. J Neurochem 46: 489–493

51. Cruickshank GC, Rampling R (1994) Peri-tumoural hypoxia in human brain: peroperative measurement of the tissue oxygen tension around malignant brain tumours. Acta Neurochir (Wien) [Suppl] 60: 375–377

52. Cserr HF, Cooper DN, Milhorat TH (1976) Production, circulation, and absorption of brain interstitial fluid. In: Pappius HM, Feindel W (eds) Dynamics of brain edema. Springer, Berlin Heidelberg New York, pp 95–97

53. Cserr HF, De Pasquale M, Nicholson C, Patlak CS, Pettigrew KD, Rice ME (1991) Extracellular volume decreases while cell volume is maintained by ion

uptake in rat brain during acute hypernatremia. J Physiol (London) 442: 277–295

54. Cushing H (1914) Studies on the cerebrospinal fluid. I. Introduction. J Med Res 31: 1–19

55. Cutler RWP, Page L, Galicich J, Watters GV (1968) Formation and absorption of cerebrospinal fluid in man. Brain 91: 707–720

56. Dandy WE, Blackfan KD (1914) Internal hydrocephalus. An experimental clinical and pathological study. Am J Dis Child 8: 406–482

57. Dani JW, Chernjavsky A, Smith SJ (1992) Neuronal activity triggers calcium waves in hippocampal astrocyte networks. Neuron 8: 429–440

58. Daumas-Duport C, Monsaigneon V, Blond S, Munari C, Musolino A, Chodkiewicz JP, Missir O (1987) Serial stereotactic biopsies and CT scan in gliomas: correlative study in 100 astrocytomas, oligo-astrocytomas and oligodendrogliomas. J Neurooncol 4: 317–328

59. D'Avella D, Baroni A, Mingrino S, Scanarini M (1980) An electron microscope study of human arachnoid villi. Surg Neurol 14: 41–47

60. Davson H, Luck CP (1957) The effect of acetazolamide on the chemical composition of the aqueous humour and cerebrospinal fluid of some mammalian species and on the rate of turnover of ^{24}Na in these fluids. J Physiol (London) 137: 279–293

61. Davson H, Spaziani E (1962) Effect of hypothermia on certain aspects of the cerebrospinal fluid. Exp Neurol 6: 118–128

62. Davson H, Pollay M (1963) Influence of various drugs on the transport of ^{131}I and PAH across the cerebrospinal fluid—blood barrier. J Physiol (London) 167: 239–246

63. De Bold AJ (1986) Atrial natriuretic factor: an overview. Fed Proc 45: 2081–2085

64. De Rougemont J, Ames A III, Nesbett FB, Hofmann HF (1960) Fluid formed by choroid plexus. J Neurophysiol 23: 485–495

65. De Salles AAF, Kontos HA, Becker DP, Yang MS, Ward JD, Moulton R, Gruemer HD, Lutz H, Maset AL, Jenkins L, Marmarou A, Muizelaar (1986) Prognostic significance of ventricular CSF lactate acidosis in severe head injury. J Neurosurg 65: 615–624

66. De Souza SW, Dobbing J (1971) Cerebral edema in developing brain. I. Normal water and cation content in developing rat brain and postmortem changes. Exp Neurol 32: 431–438

67. Diamond JM, Bossert WH (1967) Standing gradient osmotic flow. A mechanism for coupling of water and solute transport in epithelia. J Gen Physiol 50: 2061–2083

68. Di Mattio J, Hochwald GM, Malhan C, Wald A (1975) Effects of changes in serum osmolarity on bulk flow of fluid into cerebral ventricles and on brain water content. Pflügers Arch 359: 253–264

69. Diringer M, Ladenson PW, Stern BJ, Schleimer J, Hanley DF (1988) Plasma atrial natriuretic factor and subarachnoid hemorrhage. Stroke 19: 1119–1124

70. Doczi T, Szerdahelyi P, Gulya K, Kiss J (1982) Brain water accumulation after the central administration of vasopressin. Neurosurgery 11: 402–407

71. Doczi T, Joo F, Szerdahelyi P, Bodosi M (1987) Regulation of brain water and electrolyte contents: the possible involvement of central atrial natriuretic factor. Neurosurgery 21: 454–458
72. Domer FR (1969) The effect of furosemide on cerebrospinal fluid formation and potassium movement. Exp Neurol 24: 54–64
73. Duckrow RB, La Manna JC, Rosenthal M, Levasseur JE, Patterson JL (1981) Oxidative metabolic activity of cerebral cortex after fluid percussion head injury in the cat. J Neurosurg 54: 607–614
74. Edvinsson L, West KA (1971) Relation between intracranial pressure and ventricular size at various stages of experimental hydrocephalus. Acta Neurol Scand 47: 451–457
75. Eisenberg HM, McLennan JE, Welch K (1974a) Ventricular perfusion in cats with kaolin-induced hydrocephalus. J Neurosurg 41: 20–28
76. Eisenberg HM, McComb JG, Lorenzo AV (1974b) Cerebrospinal fluid overproduction and hydrocephalus associated with choroid plexus papilloma. J Neurosurg 40: 381–385
77. Eisenberg HM, Suddith RL (1979) Cerebral vessels have the capacity to transport sodium and potassium. Science 206: 1083–1085
78. Engel J (1991) Domains in proteins and proteoglycans of the extracellular matrix with functions in assembly and cellular activities. Int J Biol Macromol 13: 147–151
79. Epstein MH, Feldman AM, Brusilow SW (1977) Cerebrospinal fluid production: stimulation by cholera toxin. Science 196: 1012–1013
80. Espinas OE, Poser CM (1969) Blood hyperosmolality and neurologic deficit. Arch Neurol 20: 182–186
81. Eveloff JL, Warnock DG (1987) Activation of ion transport systems during cell volume regulation. Am J Physiol 252: F1–F10
82. Faber WM (1937) The nasal mucosa and the subarachnoid space. Am J Anat 62: 121–148
83. Falke JJ, Kanes KJ, Chan SI (1985) The minimal structure containing the band 3 anion transport site. A ^{35}Cl NMR study. J Biol Chem 260: 13294–13303
84. Faraci FM, Kinzenbaw D, Heistad DD (1994) Effect of endogenous vasopressin on blood flow to choroid plexus during hypoxia and intracranial hypertension. Am J Physiol 266: H393–H398
85. Feinberg DA, Mark AS (1987) Human brain motion and cerebrospinal fluid circulation demonstrated with MR velocity imaging. Radiology 103: 793–799
86. Felgenhauer K, Schliep G, Rapic N (1976) Evaluation of the blood-CSF barrier by protein gradients and the humoral immune response within the central nervous system. J Neurol Sci 30: 113–128
87. Fenstermacher JD, Li CL, Levin VA (1970) Extracellular space of the cerebral cortex of normothermic and hypothermic cats. Exp Neurol 27: 101–114
88. Flamm ES, Ransohoff J, Wuchinich D, Broadwin A (1978) Preliminary experience with ultrasonic aspiration in neurosurgery. Neurosurgery 2: 240–245

89. Ford JC, Hackney DB, Alsop DC, Jara H, Joseph PM, Hand CM, Black P (1994) MRI characterization of diffusion coefficients in a rat spinal cord injury model. Magn Reson Med 31: 488–494

90. Friis-Hansen B (1961) Body water compartments in children: changes during growth and related changes in body composition. Pediatrics 28: 169–181

91. Fullerton GD, Potter JL, Dornbluth NC (1982) NMR relaxation of protons in tissues and other macromolecular water solutions. Magn Reson Imag 1: 39–55

92. Furuse M, Gonda T, Kuchiwaki H, Hirai N, Inao S, Kageyama N (1984) Thermal analysis on the state of free and bound water in normal and edematous brains. In: Go KG, Baethmann A (eds) Recent progress in the study and therapy of brain edema. Plenum, New York, pp 293–298

93. Galambos R (1971) The glia-neuronal interaction: some observations. J Psychiatr Res 8: 219–224

94. Galbraith S, Cardoso E, Patterson J, Marmarou A (1984) The water content of white matter after head injury in man. In: Go KG, Baethmann A (eds) Recent progress in the study and therapy of brain edema. Plenum, New York, pp 323–330

95. Gazendam J, Go KG, Van Zanten AK (1979a) Composition of isolated edema fluid in cold-induced edema. J Neurosurg 51: 70–77

96. Gazendam J, Go KG, Van Zanten AK (1979b) The effect of intracerebral ouabain administration on the composition of edema fluid isolated from cats with cold-induced brain edema. Brain Res 175: 279–298

97. Gazendam J, Go KG, Van der Meer J, Zuiderveen F (1979c) Changes of electrical impedance in edematous cat brain during hypoxia and after intracerebral ouabain injections. Exp Neurol 55: 78–87

98. Gazendam J, Houthoff HJ, Huitema S, Go KG (1984a) Cerebral edema formation and blood-brain barrier impairment by intraventricular collagenase infusion. In: Go KG, Baethmann A (eds) Recent progress in the study and therapy of brain edema. Plenum, New York, pp 159–173

99. Gennarelli TA, Thibault LE, Adams JH, Graham DI, Thompson CJ, Marcincin RP (1982) Diffuse axonal injury and traumatic coma in the primate. Ann Neurol 12: 564–574

100. Gerschenfeld HM, Wald F, Zadunaisky JA, de Robertis EDP (1959) Function of astroglia in the water-ion metabolism of the central nervous system. Neurology 9: 412–425

101. Ghandour MS, Langley OK, Zhu XL, Waheed A, Sly WS (1992) Carbonic anhydrase IV in brain capillary endothelial cells: a marker associated with the blood-brain barrier. Proc Nat Acad Sci USA 89: 6823–6827

102. Go KG, Ebels EJ, Beks JWF, ter Weeme CA (1967) The spreading of cerebral edema from a cold injury in cats. Psychiat Neurol Neurochir (Amsterdam) 70: 403–411

103. Go KG, van Woudenberg F, de Lange WE, Sluiter WJ (1972a) The influence of saline-loading on cold-induced cerebral oedema in the rat. J Neurol Sci 16: 209–214

104. Go KG, Van der Veen PH, Ebels EJ, Van Woudenberg F (1972b) A study of

electrical impedance of oedematous cerebral tissue during operations. Acta Neurochir (Wien) 27: 113–124

105. Go KG, Ebels EJ, Van Woudenberg F, Geerlings T (1973a) The development of oedema in the immature brain. Psychiat Neurol Neurochir (Amsterdam) 76: 427–437

106. Go KG, de Lange WE, Sluiter WJ, van Woudenberg F, Ebels EJ, Blaauw EH (1973b) The influence of salt-free solutions on cold-induced cerebral oedema. A chemical and morphological study in the rat. J Neurol Sci 18: 323–333

107. Go KG, Zijlstra WG, Flanderijn H, Zuiderveen F (1974) Circulatory factors influencing exudation in cold-induced cerebral edema. Exp Neurol 42: 332–338

108. Go KG, Edzes HT (1975) Water in brain edema. Observations by the pulsed nuclear magnetic resonance technique. Arch Neurol 32: 464–465

109. Go KG, Pratt JJ (1975) The dependence of the blood to brain passage of radioactive sodium on blood pressure and temperature. Brain Res 93: 329–336

110. Go KG, Patberg WR, Teelken AW, Gazendam J (1976a) The Starling hypothesis of capillary fluid exchange in relation to brain edema. In: Pappius HM, Feindel W (eds) Dynamics of brain edema. Springer, Berlin Heidelberg New York, pp 63–67

111. Go KG, Zuiderveen F, Kuipers-de Jager TI (1976b) Responses of cortical vein wedge pressure, ventricular fluid pressure and brain tissue pressure to elevation of arterial blood pressure under conditions of hyperventilation and freezing injury to the brain. In: Beks JWF, Bosch DA, Brock M (eds) Intracranial pressure III. Springer, Berlin Heidelberg New York, pp 5–9

112. Go KG, Houthoff HJ, Blaauw EH, Stokroos I, Blaauw G (1978) Morphology and origin of arachnoid cysts. Scanning and transmission electron microscopy of three cases. Acta Neuropathol (Berl) 44: 57–62

113. Go KG, Gazendam J, Van Zanten AK (1979b) Influence of hypoxia on the composition of isolated edema fluid in cold-induced brain edema. J Neurosurg 51: 78–84

114. Go KG, Koster-Otte L, Pratt JJ (1979a) Brain sodium uptake after choroid plexectomy. Brain Res 170: 325–331

115. Go KG, Lammertsma AA, Paans AMJ, Vaalburg W, Woldring M (1981) Extraction of water labeled with oxygen-15 during single capillary transit. Influence of blood pressure, osmolarity and blood-brain barrier damage. Arch Neurol 38: 581–584

116. Go KG, van Dijk P, Luiten AL, Brouwer-van Herwijnen AA, van der Leeuw IJCL, Kamman RL, Vencken LM, Wilmink J, Berendsen HJC (1983) Interpretation of nuclear magnetic resonance tomograms of the brain. J Neurosurg 59: 574–584

117. Go KG, Houthoff HJ, Huitema S, Spatz M (1984a) Protein tracer permeability of the blood-brain barrier after transient cerebral ischemia in gerbils. In: Go KG, Baetmann A (eds) Recent progress in the study and therapy of brain edema. Plenum, New York, pp 539–550

118. Go KG, Houthoff HJ, Blaauw EH, Havinga P, Hartsuiker J (1984b) Arachnoid cysts of the Sylvian fissure. Evidence of fluid secretion. J Neurosurg 60: 803–813

119. Go KG, Houthoff HJ, Hartsuiker J, Van der Molen-Woldendorp D, Zuiderveen F, Teelken AW (1985) Exudation of plasma protein fractions in vasogenic brain edema. In: Inaba Y, Klatzo I, Spatz M (eds) Brain edema. Springer, Berlin Heidelberg New York Tokyo, pp 76–87

120. Go KG, Houthoff HJ, Hartsuiker J, Blaauw EH, Havinga P (1986) Fluid secretion in arachnoid cysts as a clue to cerebrospinal fluid absorption at the arachnoid granulation. J Neurosurg 65: 642–648

121. Go KG, Wilmink JT, Molenaar WM (1988a) Peritumoral brain edema associated with meningiomas. Neurosurgery 23: 175–179

122. Go KG, Prenen GHM, Korf J (1988b) Protective effect of fasting upon cerebral hypoxic-ischemic injury. Metab Brain Dis 3: 257–264

123. Go KG (1988c) Physical and biochemical methods for analysis of fluid compartments. In: Boulton AA, Baker GB, Waltz W (eds) Neuromethods. The neuronal microenvironment, vol 9. The Humana Press, Clifton, pp 127–185

124. Go KG (1991) Cerebral pathophysiology. An integral approach with some emphasis on clinical implications. Elsevier, Amsterdam

125. Go KG, Kamman RL, Wilmink JT, Mooyaart EL (1993a) A study on peritumoural brain oedema around meningiomas by CT and MRI scanning. Acta Neurochir (Wien) 125: 41–46

126. Go KG, Hew JM, Kamman RL, Molenaar WM, Pruim J, Blaauw EH (1993b) Cystic lesions of the brain. A classification based on pathogenesis, with consideration of histological and radiological features. Eur J Radiol 17: 69–84

127. Go KG, Keuter EJW, Kamman RL, Pruim J, Metzemaekers JDM, Staal MJ, Paans AMJ, Vaalburg W (1994a) Contribution of magnetic resonance spectroscopic imaging and L-[1-^{11}C]tyrosine positron emission tomography to localization of cerebral gliomas for biopsy. Neurosurgery 34: 994–1002

128. Go KG, Kamman RL, Mooyaart EL, Heesters MAAM, Pruim J, Vaalburg W, Paans AMJ (1995) Localised proton spectroscopy and spectroscopic imaging in cerebral gliomas, with comparison to positron emission tomography. Neuroradiology 37: 198–206

129. Goldstein GW, Betz L (1983) Recent advances in understanding brain capillary functions. Ann Neurol 14: 389–395

130. Gomez DG, Potts DG (1977) Effects of pressure on the arachnoid villus. Exp Eye Res 25: 117–125

131. Gonatas NK, Zimmerman HM, Levine S (1963) Ultrastructure of inflammation with edema in the rat brain. Am J Pathol 42: 455–469

132. Goodfriend TL, Elliot ME, Atlas SA (1984) Actions of synthetic atrial natriuretic factor on bovine adrenal glomerulosa. Life Sci 35: 1675–1682

133. Goulon M, Babinet P, Raphael JC, Grosbuis S, Gajdos P (1971) Les manifestations neurologiques des hyponatrémies. Rev Neurol 125: 219–237

134. Graham DI, Adams JH, Doyle (1978) Ischaemic brain damage in fatal non-missile head injuries. J Neurol Sci 39: 213–234

135. Grant R, Condon B, Lawrence A, Hadley DM, Patterson J, Bone I, Teasdale GM (1988) Is cranial CSF volume under hormonal influence? An MR study. J Comp Ass Tomogr 12: 36–39
136. Graves J, Himwich HE (1955) Age and the water content of rabbit brain parts. Am J Physiol 180: 205–208
137. Greco CM, Powell HC, Garrett RS, Lampert PW (1980) Cycloleucine encephalopathy. Neuropathol Appl Neurobiol 6: 349–360
138. Grinstein S, Rothstein A, Sarkadi B, Gelfand EW (1984) Responses of lymphocytes to anisotonic media: volume regulating behavior. Am J Physiol 246: C204–C215
139. Grinstein S, Goetz JD, Cohen S, Furuya W, Rothstein A, Gelfand EW (1985) Mechanisms of regulatory volume increase in osmotically shrunken lymphocytes. Molec Physiol 8: 185–198
140. Gröflin UB, Thölen H (1978) Cerebral edema in the rat with galactosamine induced severe hepatitis. Experientia 34: 1501
141. Gruner JE (1958) Lésions du névraxe secondaires à l'ingestion d'éthyl-étain (Stalinon). Rev Neurol 98: 109–116
142. Guisado R, Arieff AJ, Massry SG (1976) Effects of glycerol administration on experimental brain edema. Neurology 26: 69–75
143. Gutierrez JA, Norenberg MD (1977) Ultrastructural study of methionine sulfoximine-induced Alzheimer type II astrocytosis. Am J Path 86: 285–300
144. Hakim S, Adams RD (1965) The special clinical problem of symptomatic hydrocephalus with normal cerebrospinal fluid pressure. Observations on cerebrospinal fluid hydrodynamics. J Neurol Sci 2: 307–327
145. Hallaq HA, Haupert GT (1989) Positive inotropic effects of the endogenous Na^+K^+-transporting ATPase inhibitor from the hypothalamus. Proc Natl Acad Sci USA 86: 10080–10084
146. Hamilton BF, Gould DH (1987) Nature and distribution of brain lesions in rats intoxicated with 3-nitropropionic acid: a type of hypoxic (energy deficient) brain damage. Acta Neuropathol 72: 286–297
147. Hansen AJ (1978) The extracellular potassium concentration in brain cortex following ischemia in hypo- and hyperglycemic rats. Acta Physiol Scand 102: 324–329
148. Hansen AJ (1987) Disturbed ion gradients in brain anoxia. NIPS 2: 54–57
149. Hansson E, Rönnbäck L (1991) Receptor regulation of the glutamate, GABA and taurine high-affinity uptake into astrocytes in primary culture. Brain Res 548: 215–221
150. Harris HW, Paredes A, Zeidel ML (1993) The molecular structure of the antidiuretic hormone elicited water channel. Pediatr Nephrol 7: 680–684
151. Harris RJ, Symon L, Branston NM, Bayhan M (1981) Changes in extracellular calcium activity in cerebral ischemia. J Cereb Blood Flow Metab 1: 203–210
152. Harris RJ, Symon L (1984) Extracellular pH, potassium and calcium activities in progressive ischaemia of rat cortex. J Cereb Blood Flow Metab 4: 178–186
153. Harrison HE, Darrow DC, Yannet H (1936) The total electrolyte content of

animals and its probable relation to the distribution of body water. J Biol Chem 113: 515–529

154. Haupert GT, Sancho JM (1979) Sodium transport inhibitor from bovine hypothalamus. Proc Nat Acad Sci USA 76: 4658–4660

155. Heisey SR, Held D, Pappenheimer JR (1962) Bulk flow and diffusion in the cerebrospinal fluid system of the goat. Am J Physiol 203: 775–781

156. Hekmatpanah J, Hekmatpanah CR (1985) Microvascular alterations following cerebral contusion in rats. J Neurosurg 62: 888–897

157. Henderson LJ (1913) The fitness of the environment. MacMillan, New York

158. Hennig J, Ott D, Adam T, Friedburg H (1990) Measurement of CSF flow using an interferographic MR technique based on the RARE-fast imaging sequence. Magn Reson Imag 8: 541–556

159. Hertz L (1978) An intense potassium uptake into astrocytes, its further enhancement by high concentrations of potassium, and its possible involvement in potassium homeostasis at the cellular level. Brain Res 145: 202–208

160. Heschl R (1859) Gehirndefekt und Hydrocephalus. Vierteljahrschrift Praktische Heilkunde 61: 59–74

161. Hilal SK, Maudsley AA, Ra JB, Simon HE, Roschmann P, Wittekoek S, Cho ZH, Mun SK (1985) In vivo NMR imaging of sodium-23 in the human head. J Comp Ass Tomogr 9: 1–7

162. Hirano A, Zimmerman HM, Levine S (1968) Intramyelinic and extracellular spaces in triethyltin intoxication. J Neuropath Exp Neurol 27: 571–580

163. Hirano A, Matsui T (1975) Vascular structures in brain tumors. Human Pathol 6: 611–621

164. Hiratsuka H, Tabata H, Tsuruoka S, Aoyagi M, Okada K, Inaba Y (1982) Evaluation of periventricular hypodensity in experimental hydrocephalus by metrizamide CT ventriculography. J Neurosurg 56: 235–240

165. Hochwald GM, Wald A, Di Mattio J, Malhan C (1974) The effect of serum osmolarity on cerebrospinal fluid volume flow. Life Sci 15: 1309–1316

166. Holliday MA, Kalayci MN, Harrah J (1968) Factors that limit brain volume changes in response to acute and sustained hyper- and hyponatremia. J Clin Invest 47: 1916–1928

167. Hopkins LN, Bakay L, Kinkel WR, Grand W (1977) Demonstration of transventricular CSF absorption by computerized tomography. Acta Neurochir (Wien) 39: 151–157

168. Hounsfield GN, Ambrose J (1973) Computerized transverse axial scanning (tomography). I. Description of system. II. Clinical application. Br J Radiol 46: 1016–1047

169. Houthoff HJ, Go KG, Gerrits PO (1982) The mechanisms of blood-brain barrier impairment by hyperosmolar perfusion. Acta Neuropathol 56: 99–112

170. Inoue T, Kuromatsu C, Iwata Y, Matsushima T (1985) Symptomatic choroidal epithelial cyst in the fourth ventricle. Surg Neurol 24: 57–62

171. Ishige N, Pitts LH, Pogliani L, Hashimoto T, Nishimura MC, Bartkowski HM, James TL (1987) Effect of hypoxia on traumatic brain injury in rats.

Part 2: Changes in high energy phosphate metabolism. Neurosurgery 20: 854–858

172. Ishige N, Pitts LH, Berry I, Nishimura MC, James TL (1988) The effects of hypovolemic hypotension on high-energy phosphate metabolism of traumatized brain in rats. J Neurosurg 68: 129–136

173. Isales CM, Bollag WB, Kiernan LC, Barrett PG (1989) Effect of ANP on sustained aldosterone secretion stimulated by angiotensin II. Am J Physiol 256: C89–C95

174. Ito U, Go KG, Walker JT, Spatz M, Klatzo I (1976) Experimental cerebral ischemia in Mongolian gerbils. Behavior of the blood-brain barrier. Acta Neuropathol 34: 1–6

175. Ito U, Ohno K, Nakamura R, Suganuma F, Inaba Y (1979) Brain edema during ischemia and after restoration of blood flow. Measurement of water, sodium, potassium content and plasma protein permeability. Stroke 10: 542–547

176. Ito U, Reulen HJ, Huber P (1986) Spatial and quantitative distribution of human peritumoural ooedema in computerised tomography. Acta Neurochir (Wien) 81: 53–60

177. Ito U, Reulen HJ, Tomita H, Ikeda J, Saito J, Maehara T (1988) Formation and propagation of brain oedema fluid around human brain metastases. A CT study. Acta Neurochir (Wien) 90: 35–41

178. Jackson RL, Busch SJ, Cardin AD (1991) Glycosaminoglycans: molecular properties, protein intercations, and role in physiological processes. Physiol Rev 71: 481–539

179. Jaffe LF (1993) Classes and mechanisms of calcium waves. Cell Calcium 14: 736–745

180. Javaheri S, Wagner KR (1992) Bumetanide decreases canine cerebrospinal fluid production. In vivo evidence for NaCl cotransport in the central nervous system. J Clin Invest 92: 2257–2261

181. Jayatilaka ADP (1965) An electronmicroscopic study of sheep arachnoid granulations. J Anat 99: 635–649

182. Jentsch TJ, Steinmeyer K, Schwarz G (1990) Primary structure of Torpedo marmorata chloride channel isolated by expression cloning in Xenopus oocytes. Nature 348: 510–514

183. Johnston IH, Howman-Giles R, Whittle IR (1984) The arrest of treated hydrocephalus in children. A radionuclide study. J Neurosurg 61: 752–756

184. Kamman RL, Go KG, Muskiet FAJ, Stomp GP, Van Dijk P, Berendsen HJC (1984) Proton spin relaxation studies of fatty tissue and cerebral white matter. Magn Reson Med 2: 211–220

185. Katzman R, Hussey F (1970) A simple constant-infusion manometric test for measurement of CSF absorption. I. Rationale and method. Neurology 20: 534–544

186. Katzman R, Pappius HM (1973) Brain electrolytes and fluid metabolism. Williams and Wilkins, Baltimore

187. Kayama T, Yoshimoto T, Fujimoto S, Sakurai Y (1991) Intratumoral oxygen pressure in malignant brain tumor. J Neurosurg 74: 55–59

188. Kesterson JW, Carlton WW (1971) Histopathologic and enzyme histochemical observations of the cuprizone-induced brain edema. Exp Molec Path 15: 82–96
189. Kita T, Kida O, Kato J, Nakamura S, Eto T, Minamino N, Kangawa K, Matsuo H, Tanaka K (1989) Natriuretic and hypotensive effects of brain natriuretic peptide (BNP) in spontaneously hypertensive rats. Life Sci 44: 1541–1545
190. Kiwit JCW, Schröders C, Wambach G (1988) Untersuchung des Plasma-ANP-Spiegels und seiner Beziehung zum Elektrolyt- und Wasserhaushalt bei neurochirurgischen Intensivpatienten. Z Kardiol 77: 119–123
191. Klatzo I, Piraux A, Laskowski EJ (1958) The relationship between edema, blood-brain barrier and tissue elements in a local brain injury. J Neuropath Exp Neurol 17: 548–564
192. Klatzo I (1967) Neuropathological aspects of brain edema. J Neuropath Exp Neurol 26: 1–14
193. Klatzo I, Wisniewski H, Steinwall O, Streicher E (1967) Dynamics of cold-injury edema. In: Klatzo I, Seitelberger F (eds) Brain edema. Springer, Berlin Göttingen Heidelberg New York, pp 554–563
194. Klatzo I, Chui E, Fujiwara K, Spatz M (1980) Resolution of vasogenic brain edema. Adv Neurol 28: 359–373
195. Klein HC (1992) Over de preventie van ischemische hersenschade. Thesis. University of Groningen, Groningen
196. Korf J (1989) Lactography: a novel technique to monitor brain energy metabolism in physiology and pathology. Neurosci Res Comm 4: 129–138
197. Krisch B, Leonhardt H (1978a) The functional and structural border of the neurohemal region of the median eminence. Cell Tiss Res 192: 327–339
198. Krnjevic K, Puil E, Werman R (1978) Significance of 2,4-dinitrophenol action on spinal motoneurones. J Physiol (London) 275: 225–229
199. Lampert P, O'Brien JO, Garrett R (1973) Hexachlorophene encephalopathy. Acta Neuropathol 23: 326–333
200. Lang DA, Hadley DM, Teasdale GM, MacPherson P, Teasadale E (1991) Gadolinium DTPA enhanced magnetic resonance imaging in acute head injury. Acta Neurochir (Wien) 109: 5–11
201. Latzkovits L, Cserr HF, Park JT, Patlak CS, Pettigrew KD, Rimanoczy A (1993) Effects of arginine vasopressine and atriopeptin on glial cell volume measured as 3-MG space. Am J Physiol 264: C603–C608
202. Law RO (1994) Regulation of mammalian brain cell volume. J Exp Zool 268: 90–96
203. Le Beux YJ, Willemot J (1978) Actin-like filaments in the endothelial cells of adult rat brain capillaries. Exp Neurol 58: 446–454
204. Le Bihan D, Breton E, Lallemand D, Grenier P, Cabanis E, Laval-Jeantet M (1986) MR imaging of intravoxel incoherent motions: application to diffusion and perfusion in neurologic disorders. Radiology 161: 401–407
205. Le Bihan D, Breton E, Lallemand D, Aubin ML, Vignaud J, Laval-Jeantet M (1988) Separation of diffusion and perfusion in intravoxel incoherent motion MR imaging. Radiology 168: 497–505

206. Lien YH, Zhou HZ, Job C, Barry JA, Gillies RJ (1992) In vivo ^{31}P NMR study of early cellular responses to hyperosmotic shock in cultured glioma cells. Biochimie 74: 931–939
207. Lindvall M, Owman C (1984) Sympathetic nervous control of cerebrospinal fluid production in experimental obstructive hydrocephalus. Exp Neurol 84: 606–615
208. Lindvall M, Gustafson A, Hedner P, Owman C (1985) Stimulation of cyclic adenosine 3',5'-monophosphate formation in rabbit choroid plexus by beta-receptor agonist and vasoactive intestinal polypeptide. Neurosci Lett 54: 153–157
209. Lindvall-Axelsson M, Mathew C, Nilsson C, Owman C (1988) Effect of 5-hydroxytryptamine on the rate of cerebrospinal fluid production in rabbit. Exp Neurol 99: 362–368
210. Lohle PNM, Verhagen ITHJ, Teelken AW, Blaauw EH, Go KG (1992) The pathogenesis of cerebral gliomatous cysts. Neurosurgery 30: 180–185
211. Long DM (1970) Capillary ultrastructure and the blood-brain barrier in human malignant brain tumors. J Neurosurg 32: 127–144
212. Lorenzo AV, Page LK, Watters GV (1970) Relationship between cerebrospinal fluid formation, absorption and pressure in human hydrocephalus. Brain 93: 679–692
213. Lorenzo AV, Bresnan MJ, Barlow CF (1974) Cerebrospinal fluid absorption deficit in normal pressure hydrocephalus. Arch Neurol 30: 387–393
214. Lorenzo AV (1974) Amino acid transport mechanisms of the cerebrospinal fluid. Fed Proc 33: 2079–2085
215. Lorenzo AV, Winston KR, Welch K, Adler JR, Granholm L (1983) Evidence of prolactin receptors in the choroid plexus and a possible role in water balance in neonatal brain. Z Kinderchir 38 [Suppl II]: 68–70
216. Lorenzo AV, Taratuska A, Halperin JA (1989) Suppression of cerebrospinal fluid (CSF) production by a Na^+/K^+ pump inhibitor extracted from human cerebrospinal fluid. Z Kinderchir 44 [Suppl I]: 24–26
217. Love JA, Fridén H, Ekstedt J (1984) Effect of corticosteroids at the level of the arachnoid villi. In: Go KG, Baethmann A (eds) Recent progress in the study and therapy of brain edema. Plenum, New York, pp 589–595
218. Lowe DA (1978) Morphological changes in the cat cerebral cortex produced by superfusion of ouabain. Brain Res 148: 347–363
219. Lundbaek JA, Tonnesen T, Laursen H, Hansen AJ (1990) Brain interstitial composition during acute hyponatremia. Acta Neurochir (Wien) [Suppl] 51: 17–18
220. Luse SA, Harris B (1960) Electronmicroscopy of the brain in experimental edema. J Neurosurg 17: 439–446
221. Mac Dermott AB, Mayer ML, Westbrook GL, Smith SJ, Barker JL (1986) NMDA-receptor activation increases cytoplasmic calcium concentration in cultured spinal cord neurones. Nature 321: 519–522
222. Macknight ADC, Leaf A (1978) Regulation of cellular volume. In: Andreoli TE, Hoffman F, Fanestil DD (eds) Physiology of membrane disorders. Plenum, New York, pp 315–334

223. Madara JL, Moore R, Carlson S (1987) Alteration of intestinal tight junction structure and permeability by cytoskeletal contraction. Am J Physiol 253: C854–C861

224. Majewska MD, Harrison NL, Schwartz RD, Barker JL, Paul SM (1986) Steroid hormone metabolites are barbiturate-like modulators of the GABA receptor. Science 232: 1004–1007

225. Manery JF, Hastings AB (1939) The distribution of electrolytes in mammalian tissues. J Biol Chem 127: 657–676

226. Maren TH, Broder LE (1970) The role of carbonic anhydrase in anion secretion into cerebrospinal fluid. J Pharmacol Exp Ther 172: 192–202

227. Marmarou A, Tanaka K, Shulman K (1982) An improved gravimetric measure of cerebral edema. J Neurosurg 56: 246–253

228. Marmarou A, Nakamura T, Tanaka K, Hochwald GM (1984) The time course and distribution of water in the resolution phase of infusion edema. In: Go KG, Baethmann A (eds) Recent progress in the study and therapy of brain edema. Plenum, New York, pp 37–44

229. Marmarou A, Maset AL, Ward JD, Choi S, Brooks D, Lutz HA, Moulton RJ, Muizelaar JP, De Salles A, Young HF (1987) Contribution of CSF and vascular factors to elevation of ICP in severely head-injured patients. J Neurosurg 66: 883–890

230. Martins A, Ramirez A, Doyle TF (1975) Comparison of radioiodinated serum albumin and blue dextran as indicators to measure rate of formation of cerebrospinal fluid. Exp Neurol 47: 249–256

231. Masserman JH (1934) Cerebrospinal hydrodynamics. IV. Clinical experimental studies. Arch Neurol Psychiat (Chicago) 32: 226–234

232. Mauser HW, Van Nieuwenhuisen O, Veiga-Pires JA (1984) Is contrast enhanced CT indicated in acute head injury? Neuroradiology 26: 31–32

233. Mayman CI (1972) Inhibitory effect of dexamethasone on sodium-potassium activated adenosine triphosphatase of choroid plexus in cat and rabbit. Fed Proc 31: 591

234. Meinig G, Reulen HJ, Hadjidimos A, Siemon C, Bartko D, Schürmann K (1972) Induction of filtration edema by extreme reduction of cerebrovascular resistance associated with hypertension. Eur Neurol 8: 97–103

235. Messert B, Wannamaker BB, Dudley AW (1972) Reevaluation of the size of the lateral ventricles of the brain. Neurology 22: 941–951

236. Milhorat TH, Hammock MK, Fenstermacher JD, Rall DP, Levin VA (1971) Cerebrospinal fluid production by the choroid plexus and brain. Science 173: 330–332

237. Milhorat TH, Hammock MK, Chien T, Davis DA (1976) Normal rate of cerebrospinal fluid formation five years after bilateral choroid plexectomy. J Neurosurg 44: 735–739

238. Miner LC, Reed DJ (1972) Composition of fluid obtained from choroid plexus tissue isolated in a chamber in situ. J Physiol (London) 227: 127–139

239. Moseley ME, Cohen Y, Mintorovitch J, Chileuitt L, Shimizu H, Kucharczyk J, Wendland MF, Weinstein PR (1990) Early detection of regional cerebral

ischemia in cats: comparison of diffusion- and T_2-weighted MRI and spectroscopy. Magn Reson Med 14: 330–346

240. Nakamura S, Camins MB, Hochwald GM (1983) Pressure-absorption responses to the infusion of fluid into the spinal cord central canal of kaolin-hydrocephalic cats. J Neurosurg 58: 198–203

241. Narayan RK, Greenberg RP, Miller DJ, Enas GG, Choi SC, Kishore PRS, Selhorst JB, Lutz HA, Becker DP (1981) Improved confidence of outcome prediction in sever head injury. A comparative analysis of the clinical examination, multimodality evoked potentials, CT scanning, and intracranial pressure. J Neurosurg 54: 751–762

242. Nelson SR, Lowry OH, Passonneau JV (1966) Changes in energy reserves in mouse brain associated with compressive head injury. In: Caveness WF, Walker AE (eds) Head injury. Conference Proceedings. Lippincott, Philadelphia, pp 444–447

243. Nelson SR, Mantz ML, Maxwell JA (1971) Use of specific gravity in the measurement of cerebral edema. J Appl Physiol 30: 268–271

244. Nicholson C, Rice ME (1988) Use of ion-selective microelectrodes and voltammetric microsensors to study brain cell microenvironment. In: Boulton AA, Baker GB, Walz W (eds) Neuromethods 9. The neural microenvironment. Humana, Clifton, pp 247–361

245. Nilsson C, Lindvall-Axelsson M, Owman C (1991) Simultaneous and continuous measurement of choroid plexus flow and cerebrospinal fluid production: effects of vasoactive intestinal polypeptide. J Cereb Blood Flow Metab 11: 861–867

246. Nilsson C, Stahlberg F, Thomsen C, Henriksen O, Herning M, Owman C (1992) Circadian variation in human cerebrospinal fluid production measured by magnetic resonance imaging. Am J Physiol 262: R20–R24

247. Noda M, Shimizu S, Tanabe T, Takai T, Kayano T, Ikeda T, Takahashi H, Nakayama H, Kanaoka Y, Minamino N, Kangawa K, Matsuo H, Raftery MA, Hirose T, Inayama S, Hayashide H, Miyata T, Numa S (1984) Primary structure of electrophorus electricus sodium channel deduced from cDNA sequence. Nature 312: 121–127

248. Oldendorf WH, Davson H (1967) Brain extracellular space and the sink action of cerebrospinal fluid. Arch Neurol 17: 196–205

249. Oppelt WW, Maren TH, Owens ES, Rall DP (1963) Effects of acid-base alterations on cerebrospinal fluid production. Proc Soc Expl Biol Med 144: 86–89

250. Organ LW, Tasker RR, Moody F (1968) Brain tumor localization using an electrical impedance technique. J Neurosurg 28: 35–44

251. Orkand RK, Nicholls JG, Kuffler SW (1966) Effect of nerve impulses on the membrane potential of glial cells in the central nervous system of amphibia. J Neurophysiol 29: 788–806

252. Ott D, Hennig J, Ernst T (1993) Human brain tumors: assessment with in vivo proton MR spectroscopy. Radiology 186: 745–752

253. Padan E, Schuldiner S (1993) Na^+/H^+ antiporters, molecular devices that couple the Na^+ and H^+ circulation in cells. J Bioenerget Biomembr 25: 647–669

254. Pappius HM (1965) The distribution of water in brain tissue swollen in vitro and in vivo. Biology of neuroglia. Progr Brain Res 15: 135–154
255. Pappius HM, Oh JH, Dossetor JB (1967) The effects of rapid hemodialysis on brain tissues and cerebrospinal fluid of dogs. Can J Physiol (London) Pharmacol 45: 129–147
256. Partin JS, Mc Adams AJ, Partin JC, Schubert WK, Mc Laurin RL (1978) Brain ultrastructure in Reye's disease. II Acute injury and recovery processes in three children. J Neuropath Exp Neurol 37: 796–819
257. Pasantes-Morales H, Alavez S, Sanchez Olea R, Moran J (1993) Contribution of organic and inorganic osmolytes to volume regulation in rat brain cells in culture. Neurochem Res 18: 445–452
258. Patberg WR, Go KG, Teelken AW (1977) Isolation of edema fluid in cold-induced cerebral edema for the study of colloid-osmotic pressure, lactate dehydrogenase activity, and electrolytes. Exp Neurol 54: 141–147
259. Penning L, Front D (1975) Brain scintigraphy, a neuroradiological approach. Excerpta Medica, Amsterdam
260. Persson L, Boethius J, Gronowitz JS, Kallander C, Lindgren L (1985) Thymidine kinase in brain-tumor cyst. J Neurosurg 63: 568–572
261. Phillips PA, Kelly LM, Abrahams JM, Grzonka Z, Paxinos G, Mendelsohn FA, Johnston CI (1988) Vasopressin receptors in rat brain and kidney: studies using a radio-iodinated V_1 receptor antagonist. J Hypertens [Suppl] 6: 550–553
262. Pollay M, Stevens A, Estrada E, Kaplan R (1972) Extracorporeal perfusion of choroid plexus. J Appl Physiol 32: 612–617
263. Popp R, Hoyer J, Meyer J, Galla HJ, Gogelein H (1992) Stretch-activated non-selective cation channels in the antiluminal membrane of porcine cerebral capillaries. J Physiol (London) 454: 435–449
264. Potts DG, Gomez DG (1974) Arachnoid villi and granulations. In: Lundberg N *et al* (eds) Intracranial pressure II. Springer, Berlin Heidelberg New York, pp 42–45
265. Raichle ME, Eichling JO, Straatman MG, Welch MJ, Larson KB, Ter Pogossian MM (1976) Blood-brain barrier permeability of ^{11}C-labeled alcohols and [13]O-labeled water. Am J Physiol 230: 543–552
266. Raichle ME, Grubb RL (1978) Regulation of brain water permeability by centrally-released vasopressin. Brain Res 143: 191–194
267. Rall DP (1968) Transport through the ependymal lining. Progr Brain Res 29: 159–172
268. Rapoport SI: Blood-brain barrier in physiology and medicine. Raven, New York
269. Rascol MM, Izard JY (1969) Ultrastructure des granulations de Pacchioni de la méninge humaine chez l'adulte. J Microsc 8: 1017–1030
270. Reed DJ (1969) The effect of furosemide on cerebrospinal fluid flow in rabbits. Arch Int Pharmacodyn Ther 178: 324–330
271. Renkin EM (1959) Transport of potassium-42 from blood to tissue in isolated mammalian skeletal muscles. Am J Physiol 197: 1205–1210
272. Reulen HJ, Baethmann A (1967) Das Dinitrophenol-Ödem. Klin Wschr 45: 149–154

273. Reulen HJ, Hase U, Fenske A, Samii M, Schürmann K (1970a) Extrazellulärraum und Ionenverteilung in grauer und weißer Substanz des Hundehirns. Acta Neurochir (Wien) 22: 305–325
274. Reulen HJ, Steude U, Brendel W, Hilber C, Prusiner S (1970b) Energetische Störung des Kationentransports als Ursache des intrazellulären Hirnödems. Acta Neurochir (Wien) 22: 129–166
275. Reulen HJ, Graham R, Spatz M, Klatzo I (1977) Role of pressure gradients and bulk flow in dynamics of vasogenic brain edema. J Neurosurg 46: 24–35
276. Ripellino JA, Margolis RU, Margolis RK (1989) Immunoelectron microscopic localization of hyaluronic acid-binding region and link with protein epitopes in brain. J Cell Biol 108: 1899–1907
277. Rizzuto N, Gonatas NK (1974) Ultrastructural study of effect of methionine sulfoximine on developing and adult rat cerebral cortex. J Neuropath Exp Neurol 33: 237–250
278. Robinson BW (1962) Localization of intracerebral electrodes. Exp Neurol 6: 201–223
279. Rosenberg CA, Kyner WT, Estrada E (1980) Bulk flow of brain interstitial fluid under normal and hyperosmolar conditions. Am J Physiol 238: F42–F49
280. Ross CA, Mac Cumber MW, Glatt CE, Snyder SH (1989) Brain phospholipase C isozymes: differential mRNA localizations by in situ hybridization. Proc Nat Acad Sci USA 86: 2923–2927
281. Rubin RC, Henderson ES, Ommaya AK, Walker MD, Rall DP (1966) The production of cerebrospinal fluid in man and its modification by acetazolamide. J Neurosurg 25: 430–436
282. Rymer MM, Fishman RA (1973) Protective adaptation of brain to water intoxication. Arch Neurol 28: 49–54
283. Saavedra JM, Israel A, Kurihara M, Fuchs E (1986) Decreased number and affinity of rat atrial natriuretic peptide (6–32) binding sites in the subfornical organ of spontaneously hypertensive rats. Circ Res 58: 389–392
284. Saavedra JM (1988) Alteration in atrial natriuretic peptide receptors in rat brain nuclei during hypertension and dehydration. Can J Physiol Pharmacol 66: 288–294
285. Safar P, Bleyaert A, Nemoto EM, Moossy J, Snyder JV (1978) Resuscitation after global brain ischemia-anoxia. Care Med 6: 215–217
286. Saper CB, Standaert DG, Currie MG, Schwartz D, Geller DM, Needleham P (1985) Atriopeptin-immunoreactive neurons in the brain: presence in cardiovascular regulatory areas. Science 227: 1047–1049
287. Schousboe A, Svenneby G, Hertz L (1977) Uptake and metabolism of glutamate in astrocytes cultured from dissociated mouse brain hemispheres. J Neurochem 29: 999–1005
288. Schousboe A, Pasantes-Morales H (1992) Role of taurine in neural cell volume regulation. Can J Physiol Pharmacol 70 [Suppl]: S356–361
289. Schutta HS, Kassell NF, Langfitt TW (1968) Brain swelling produced by injury and aggravated by arterial hypertension. A light and electronmicroscopic study. Brain 91: 281–294
290. Schwartz WB, Bennett W, Curelop S, Bartter FC (1957) A syndrome of renal

sodium loss and hyponatremia probably resulting from inappropriate secretion of antidiuretic hormone. Am J Med 23: 529–542

291. Sevick RI, Kanda F, Mintorovitch J, Arieff AI, Kucharczyk J, Tsuruda JS, Norman D, Mosely ME (1992) Cytotoxic brain edema: assessment with diffusion weighted MR imaging. Radiology 185: 687–690

292. Shapira Y, Setton D, Artru AA, Shohami E (1993) Blood-brain barrier permeability, cerebral edema, and neurologic function after closed head injury in rats. Anesth Analg 77: 141–148

293. Shulman K, Yarnell P, Ransohoff J (1964) Dural sinus pressure in normal and hydrocephalic dogs. Arch Neurol 10: 575–580

294. Simpson JB, Routtenberg A (1973) Subfornical organ: site of drinking elicitation by angiotensin. Science 181: 1172–1175

295. Skeggs LT, Lentz KE, Gould AM, Hochstrasser H, Kahn JR (1967) Biochemistry and kinetics of the renin angiotensin system. Fed Proc 26: 42–47

296. Skou JC (1957) The influence of some cations on an adenosine triphosphatase from peripheral nerves. Biochim Biophys Acta 23: 394–401

297. Snodgrass SR, Lorenzo AV (1972) Temperature and cerebrospinal fluid production rate. Am J Physiol 222: 1524–1527

298. Snyder GL, Girault JA, Chen JY, Czernik AJ, Kebabian JW, Nathanson JA, Greengard P (1992) Phosphorylation of DARPP-32 and protein phosphatase inhibitor-1 in rat choroid plexus: regulation by factors other than dopamine. J Neurosci 12: 3071–3083

299. Sood SC, Gulati SC, Kumar M, Kak VK (1980) Cerebral metabolism following brain injury. II. Lactic acid changes. Acta Neurochir (Wien) 53: 47–51

300. Spector R (1977) Vitamin homeostasis in the central nervous system. N Engl J Med 296: 1393–1398

301. Spector R (1980b) Thymidine transport in the central nervous system. J Neurochem 35: 1092–1098

302. Speth RC, Harik SI (1985) Angiotensin II receptor binding sites in brain microvessels. Proc Natl Acad Sci USA 82: 6340–6343

303. Staub F, Baethmann A, Peters J, Kempski O (1990) Effects of lactacidosis on volume and viability of glial cells. Acta Neurochir (Wien) [Suppl] 51: 3–6

304. Starkman SP, Brown TC, Linell EA (1958) Cerebral arachnoid cysts. J Neuropath Exp Neurol 17: 484–500

305. Steardo L, Nathanson JA (1987) Brain barrier tissues: end organs for atriopeptins. Science 235: 470–473

306. Stewart-Wallace AM (1939) A biochemical study of cerebral tissue and of the changes in cerebral oedema. Brain 62: 426–438

307. Strecker EP, Kelley JET, Merz T, James AE (1974) Transventricular albumin absorption in communicating hydrocephalus. Semiquantitative analysis of periventricular extracellular space utilizing autoradiography. Arch Psychiatr Nervenkr 218: 369–377

308. Streicher E, Wisniewski H, Klatzo I (1965) Resistance of immature brain to experimental cerebral edema. Neurology 15: 833–836

309. Stricker EM, Verbalis JG (1988) Hormones and behavior: the biology of thrist and sodium appetite. Am Scientist 76: 261–267
310. Studygroup on Brain Edema in Stroke (1977) brain edema in stroke. Report of Joint Committee for Stroke Resources. Stroke 8: 512–540
311. Sykova E, Jendelova P, Svoboda J, Chvatal A (1992) Extracellular K^+, pH and volume changes in spinal cord of adult rats and during postnatal development. Can J Physiol Pharmacol 70 [Suppl]: S301–309
312. Symon L, Dorsch NWC (1975) Use of long-term intracranial pressure measurement to assess hydrocephalic patients prior to shunt surgery. J Neurosurg 42: 258–273
313. Szegedy L (1966) The influence of hemodialysis treatment on the injuries of the central nervous system in uremia. Acta Neurol Scand 42: 105–117
314. Szentágothai J (1970) Glomerular synapses, complex synaptic arrangements, and their operational significance. In: Evolution of brain and behavior. The neurosciences. Second Study Program. Rockefeller University Press, New York, pp 427–443
315. Szymas J, Morkowski S, Tokarz F (1986) Determination of the glial acidic protein in human cerebrospinal fluid and in cyst fluid of brain tumors. Acta Neurochir (Wien) 83: 144–150
316. Takagi H, Shapiro K, Marmarou A, Wisoff H (1981) Microgravimetric analysis of human brain tissue. J Neurosurg 54: 797–801
317. Tanabe T, Takeshima H, Mikami A, Flockerzi V, Takahashi H, Kangawa K, Kojima M, Matsuo H, Hirose T, Numa S (1987) Primary structure of the receptor for calcium channel blockers from skeletal muscle. Nature 328: 313–318
318. Taveras JM, Ransohoff J (1953) Leptomeningeal cysts of the brain following trauma with erosion of the skull. A study of seven cases treated by surgery. J Neurosurg 10: 233–241
319. Tempel BL, Papazian DM, Schwarz TL, Jan YN, Jan LY (1987) Sequence of a probable potassium channel component encoded at Shaker locus of Drosophila. Science 237: 770–775
320. The European Studygroup on Nimodipine in Severe Head Injury (1994) A multicentral trial of the efficacy of nimodipine on outcome after severe head injury. J Neurosurg 80: 797–804
321. Thibault LE, Meaney DF, Anderson BJ, Marmarou A (1992) Biomechanical aspects of a fluid percussion model of brain injury. J Neurotrauma 9: 311–322
322. Torack RM, Alcala H, Gado M (1976) Water, specific gravity and histology as determinants of diagnostic computerized cranial tomogtaphy (CCT). In: Pappius M, Feindel W (eds) Dynamics of brain edema. Springer, Berlin Heidelberg New York, pp 271–277
323. Tornheim PA, McLaurin RL (1984) Effects of mechanical impact to the skull on tissue density of the cerebral cortex. In: Go KG, Baethmann A (eds) Recent progress in the study and therapy of brain edema. Plenum, New York, pp 81–92
324. Torvik A, Bhatia R, Murthy VS (1978) Transitory block of the arachnoid

granulations following subarachnoid haemorrhage. Acta Neurochir (Wien) 41: 137–146
325. Tosteson DC, Hoffman JF (1960) Regulation of cell volume by active cation transport in high and low potassium sheep red cells. J Gen Physiol 44: 169–194
326. Towfighi J, Gonatas NK (1973) Effect of intracerebral injection of ouabain in adult and developing rats. Lab Invest 28: 170–180
327. Townsend JB, Ziedonis DM, Bryan RM, Brennan RW, Page RB (1984) Choroid plexus blood flow: evidence for dopaminergic influence. Brain Res 290: 165–169
328. Trachtenberg MC, Pollen DA (1970) Neuroglia: biophysical properties and physiologic function. Science 167: 1248–1252
329. Trachtman H, Futterweit S, Hammer E, Siegel TW, Oates P (1991) The role of polyols in cerebral cell volume regulation in hypernatremic and hyponatremic states. Life Sci 49: 677–688
330. Trachtman H (1992) Cell volume regulation: a review of cerebral adaptative mechanisms and implications for clinical treatment of osmolal disturbances. Pediatr Nephrol 6: 104–112
331. Trachtman H, Futterweit S, Del Pizzo R (1992) Taurine and osmoregulation. IV. cerebral taurine transport is increased in rats with hypernatremic dehydration. Pediatr Res 32: 118–124
332. Tripathi RC (1977) The functional morphology of the outflow systems of ocular and cerebrospinal fluid. Exp Eye Res 25: 65–116
333. Tschirgi RD, Frost RW, Taylor JL (1954) Inhibition of cerebrospinal fluid formation by a carbonic anhydrase inhibitor 2-acetylamino-1,3,4-thiadazole-5-sulfonamide (Diamox). Proc Soc Exp Biol Med 87: 373–376
334. Turski PA, Perman WH, Houston L, Winkler SS (1988) Clinical and experimental sodium magnetic resonance imaging. Radiol Clin North Am 26: 861–871
335. Unterberg AW, Andersen BJ, Clarke GD, Marmarou A (1988) Cerebral energy metabolism following fluid-percussion brain injury in cats. J Neurosurg 68: 594–600
336. Upton ML, Weller RO (1985) The morphology of cerebrospinal fluid drainage pathways in human arachnoid granulations. J Neurosurg 63: 867–875
337. Van Bree JBMM, De Boer AG, Danhof M, Ginsel LA, Breimer DD (1988) Characterization of an "in vitro" blood-brain barrier: effects of molecular size and lipophilicity on cerebrovascular endothelial transport rates of drugs. J Pharmacol Exp Ther 247: 1233–1239
338. Van Gelder NM (1983) Metabolic interactions between neurons and astroglia: glutamin synthetase, carbonic anhydrase, and water balance. In: Jasper HH, Van Gelder NM (eds) Basic mechanisms of neuronal hyperexcitability. Liss, New York, pp 5–29
339. Van Gelderen P, de Vleeschouwer MHM, DesPres D, Pekar J, Van Zijl PCM, Moonen CTW (1994) Water diffusion and acute stroke. Magn Reson Med 31: 154–163
340. Van Harreveld A (1966) Brain tissue electrolytes. Butterworths, London

341. Verhagen A, Go KG, Visser GM, Blankenstein MA, Vaalburg W (1994) Presence of progesterone receptors in arachnoid granulations and in the lining of arachnoid cysts. Its relevance to expression of progesterone receptors in meningiomas. Br J Neurosurg

342. Verney EB (1947) Antidiuretic hormone and the factors which determine its release. Proc Roy Soc (London) B135: 25–201

343. Vigne P, Champigny G, Marsault R, Barbry P, Frélin C, Lazdunski M (1989) A new type of amiloride-sensitive cationic channel in endothelial cells of brain microvessels. J Biol Chem 264: 7663–7668

344. Wald A, Hochwald GM (1977) An animal model for the production of intracranial pressure plateau waves. Ann Neurol 1: 486–488

345. Wasterlain CG, Torack RM (1968) Cerebral edema in water intoxication. Arch Neurol 19: 79–87

346. Weed LH (1914) Studies on cerebrospinal fluid, vol II. The theory of drainage of cerebrospinal fluid, with an analysis of the methods of investigation. J Med Res 31: 21–49

347. Weinberger MH (1988) Hypertension: the sodium connection. Clin Physiol Biochem 6: 130–135

348. Weiss MH, Wertman N (1978) Modulation of CSF production by alterations in cerebral perfusion pressure. Arch Neurol 35: 527–529

349. Welch K, Friedman V (1960) The cerebrospinal fluid valves. Brain 83: 454–469

350. Welch K, Pollay M (1963) The spinal arachnoid villi of the monkeys Cercopithecus aethiops sabaceus and Macacus irus. Anat Rec 145: 43–48

351. Weller RO, Wisniewski H (1969) Histological and ultrastructural changes with experimental hydrocephalus in adult rabbits. Brain 92: 819–828

352. Westergaard E (1975) Enhanced vesicular transport of exogenous peroxidase across cerebral vessels, induced by serotonin. Acta Neuropathol 32: 27–42

353. Westergaard E, Go KG, Klatzo I, Spatz M (1976) Increased permeability of cerebral vessels to horse radish peroxidase induced by ischemia in Mongolian gerbils. Acta Neuropathol 35: 307–325

354. Wijdicks EFM, Vermeulen M, Van Brummelen P, Den Boer NC, Van Gijn J (1987) Digoxin-like immunoreactive substance in patients with aneurysmal subarachnoid haemorrhage. B M J 294: 729–732

355. Winkelman NW, Fay T (1930) The Pacchionian system. Histologic amd pathologic changes with particular reference to the idiopathic and symptomatic convulsive states. Arch Neurol Psychiat 23: 44–64

356. Wolff SD, Balaban RS (1989) Magnetization transfer contrast (MTC) and tissue water proton relaxation in vivo. Magn Reson Med 10: 135–144

357. Wolfenden R (1983) Waterlogged molecules. Science 222: 1087–1093

358. Wolpow ER, Schaumburg HH (1972) Structure of the human arachnoid granulation. J Neurosurg 37: 724–727

359. Woollam DHM, Millen JW (1958) Observations on the production and circulation of the cerebrospinal fluid. In: Wolstenholme GEW, O'Connor CM (eds) Ciba Foundation Symposium on Production, Circulation and Absorption of the Cerebrospinal Fluid. Little and Brown, Boston, pp 124–146

360. Wright EM (1972) Mechanisms of ion transport across the choroid plexus. J Physiol (London) 226: 545–571
361. Yakovlev PI, Wadsworth RC (1946) Schizencephalies. A study of the congenital clefts in the cerebral mantle. I. Clefts with fused lips. J Neuropathol Exp Neurol 5: 116–129
362. Yannet H (1939) Changes in the brain resulting from depletion of extracellular electrolytes. Am J Physiol 128: 683–689
363. Zlokovic BV, Segal MB, Davson H, Lipovac MN, Hyman S, Mc Comb JG (1990) Circulating neuroactive peptides and the blood-brain barrier and blood-cerebrospinal fluid barriers. Endocrin Exp 24: 9–17
364. Zucker RS, Lando L (1986) Mechanism of transmitter release: voltage hypothesis and calcium hypothesis. Science 231: 574–578

B. Technical Standards

Transfacial Approaches to the Skull Base

D. Uttley

Department of Neurosurgery, Atkinson Morley's Hospital, Wimbledon,
London (U.K.)

With 8 Figures

Contents

Transfacial Approaches to the Clivus

Introduction

Until very recently the skull base and adjacent stuctures were only accessible as a result of severe and sustained brain retraction, which inevitably lead to increased postoperative neurovascular complications, often of a serious and permanent nature. It is a measure of the success of skull base surgery that many of these obstacles to a better outcome have been overcome by means of novel applications of operative techniques, some new, but, more often than not, extant already in the repertoire of disciplines not overtly concerned in transclival penetration. The major spur to progress has been the evolution of team-work, without which much of this work would never have come to fruition. The conjunction of multiple disciplines to form teams, each bringing complementary expertise to bear on the tasks in hand, has created a tremendous impetus to the development of the complex techniques that are often necessary to achieve optimal exposure of the conditions involving the skull base. It is true to say that there are no areas of the brain's surface that are denied surgical access, thanks to these recent innovations. The revolution in radiological imaging techniques has been an enormous boon to students of this region. The combination of computerised transverse axial scanning (CT), and magnetic resonance imaging (MRI) has transformed our perceptions of tumour pathology and its consequences. Improved diagnosis has resulted in better patient management, and the imaging techniques are invaluable in charting postoperative progress, both in the immediate phase, and in the long term. The new angiographic MRI sequences have largely supplanted invasive angiography in studying the vascular relationships of skull base tumours, except where fine detail is still required, or embolisation is being considered, and, of course, in those cases where ballon occlusion may be necessary.

Anaesthetic advances have contributed to improved operating conditions, and increased use of intraoperative monitoring has led to safer surgery by sparing brain, nerves, and blood vessels from operative damage. On the surgical front there have been important technical strides. Equipment such as the ultrasonic aspirator and the laser are in everyday use as operative aids of great value, and a new type of instrumentation has been adapted or invented to cope with operating at the considerable depths that exist between the surface of the face and the clivus.

All these developments have been seized upon with gratitude by surgeons, who have drawn the various strands together to extend and broaden the scope of surgery. The operative approaches to be discussed in this chapter would not have been initiated, let alone flourished, without them.

The clivus has been not only a natural barrier between the base of the brain and the nasopharynx, but has been regarded as a psychological barrier as well, albeit from a specialist surgical standpoint until very recently. It is the purpose of this chapter to describe how these barriers have fallen, and what lies beyond them to generate such interest and enthusiasm in the skull base surgical fraternity.

Anatomy of the Clivus

The clivus (Lat. = a slope) is a composite bony structure formed from the basilar part of the occipital bone and the posterior part of the body of the sphenoid bone which articulate by a cartilaginous epiphysis until the age of 25 years when ossification takes place. It presents a broad inclined intracranial surface, extending from the base of the posterior clinoid processes above down to the anterior margin of the foramen magnum below. This aspect is slightly concave from side to side, in its lower reaches CSF separates its dural surface from the medulla oblongata with the vertebral arteries interposed between them, and at a higher level, this intimate relationship is continued as the pons and basilar artery. A groove on each side of the clivus laterally is occupied by the inferior petrosal sinus, which begins above at the apex of the petrous temporal bone where it drains the posterior end of the cavernous sinus. The sinus in its descending course moves backwards and slightly laterally along the petro-occipital suture to leave the skull through the jugular foramen. There are two layers of dura covering the intracranial portion of the clivus in which run a profusion of venous channels, called the plexus of basilar sinuses (among other things!), which interconnect the right and left inferior petrosal sinuses, they tend to be concentrated in the upper third of the clivus and become less numerous as the foramen magnum is reached. Deep to the dura the anterior margin of the foramen magnum gives attachment to ligaments passing to the axis: the membrana tectoria is fused with the dura, in front of this lies the vertical fibres of the cruciate ligament, and anterior to this are the apical and the pair of alar ligaments joined to the odontoid process.

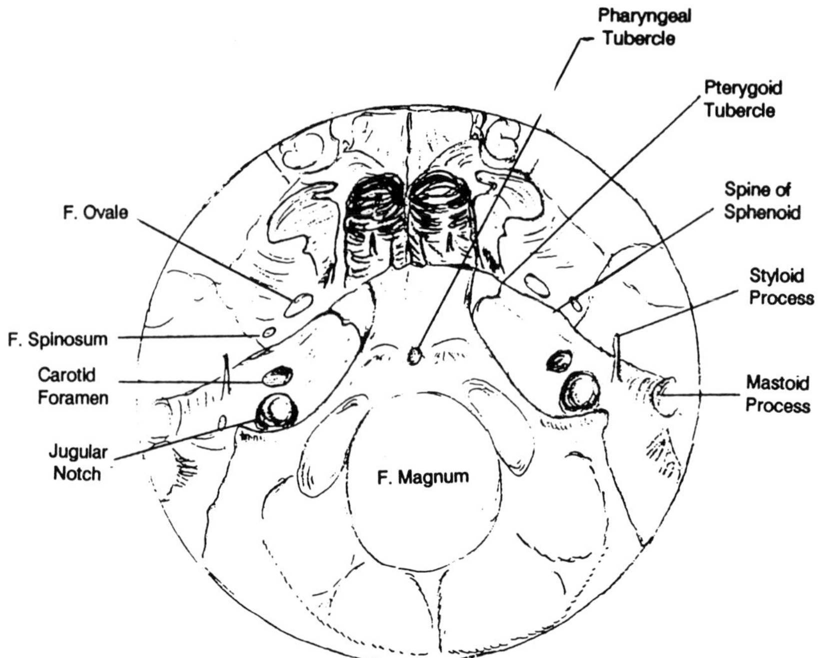

Fig. 1. Inferior aspect of dried skull showing clivus in centre and important lateral
landmarks

The anterior margin of the foramen magnum is thin and in the sagittal
plane expands as it ascends to the region of the sella, producing a wedge-
shaped appearance, resembling a slice of pie; compact bone on each surface
of this encloses a central mass of cancellous bone. Just over 1 centimetre
above the margin of the foramen magnum, and in the midline is situated a
small raised area in the bone: the pharyngeal tubercle, anterior to which
the bone forms the roof of the nasopharynx, the mucous membrane of
which is attached to the periosteum. In front of the tubercle two raised
lines radiate laterally, convex forwards, furnishing attachments for the
prevertebral fascia and the pharyngobasilar fascia (Fig. 1). Posterior to
these ridges lie the insertions of the longus capitis muscles on either side
of the midline, with the rectus capitis anterior situated behind and lateral
to them.

Functional Anatomy

No structures of significance pierce the clivus. The fault lines on either side
limit its lateral extension. These are formed by the apices of the petrous
temporal bones above, and the occipital tubercles below. The upper

boundary is the sphenoid sinus, and the lower the anterior margin of the foramen magnum. A line drawn though the tips of the mastoid processes divides the latter into an anterior third and a posterior two thirds, and divides the occipital condyles in the opposite proportions. A further line may be drawn from the mastoid tips extending anteriorly from the original line at 45° as far as the pterygoid tubercles, posteriorly the jugular and carotid foramina lie within this line, and the foramen spinosum and foramen ovale more anteriorly are situated just outside it; these represent the absolute lateral limits to a transclival approach to the brain stem, but dissection may proceed up to, and even beyond, these boundaries in the presence of soft tumour infiltrating the skull base. A recent study was undertaken to try to define more clearly the midline anatomic relationships as they are likely to be encountered in standard transoral and transpalatal operations. The appropriate measurements were made in 15 human cadavers. Landmarks approximating the the midline of the skull base and the upper cervical spinal canal were defined to assist the surgeon's orientation, but only the former will be noted here (Table 1). Taking structures as they are found from below upwards; the mean distance in the axial plane between the vertebral arteries as they enter the dura is 2.18 cm, between the hypoglossal foramina: 2.64 cm, the jugular foramina: 4.32 cm, the inferior petrosal sinuses (midway between their exit from the cavernous sinuses and their entrance into the jugular bulbs): 2.94 cm, the medial aspects of the internal auditory foramina: 4.89 cm, the dural exits of the VI cranial nerves: 2.18 cm, the medial borders of Meckel's caves: 3.03 cm,

Table 1. *Intracranial Axial Measurements*

Structures	Mean distance (cm)
VA-VA	2.18
XII-XII	2.64
JF-JF	4.32
IPS-IPS	2.94
IAC-IAC	4.89
VI-VI	2.18
V-V	3.03
CA-CA	1.55

Distance between similar structures on intracranial surface of the clivus. *VA* vertebral arteries as they enter dura, *XII* hypoglossal foramen, *JF* jugular foramen, *IPS* inferior petrosal sinus, *IAC* internal auditory meatus, *VI* dural exit of VI cranial nerve, *V* medial aspect of Meckel's cave, *CA* medial loop cavernous carotid artery. Details in text. (After Rock *et al.* 1993).

and the inner aspects of the medial loops of the carotid arteries in the cavernous sinuses: 1.55 cm (Rock *et al.* 1993). Serious damage to vital structures may occur if due consideration is not given to these important measurements during the planning stages of the surgical process.

Surgical Pathology

Pathology relating to the clivus is fortunately rare, which is a compelling reason for those involved in its management to be experts in the surgical access to the region, and in dealing with the disorders found there. The pathology is best considered in terms of the "surgical sieve", and it is important to note that all the conditions to be mentioned are situated extradurally until the tumour category is reached, when for the first time intradural lesions are mentioned. This brief overview of clival pathology highlights the most common of the unusual clinical conditions found in the region.

Developmental

These problems are usually situated at the craniocervical junction and can rarely be considered in isolation. Clival exposure is obviously necessary to deal with anomalies of the foramen magnum and the arch of the atlas. These are due to the complexity of the embryological formation of the region. Multiple related problems are common. In addition to these multiple bony abnormalities there may be associated failures of development in the nervous system itself (List 1941). Thus the neurological picture may not be resolved by attempts to decompress the bony deformities or segmentation anomalies alone, or by attempts to stabilise subluxation in the presence of coexisting damage to the nervous system, which by definition is irreversible. The most common lesion in this group is primary basilar invagination occurring as a consequence of multiple complex developmental failures, often associated with other bony abnormalities such as the Klippel-Feil syndrome, where distortion of the clivus and the craniocervical junction produces effects on the brain stem and its vascular supply leading to neurological symptoms and signs. This disorder may be associated with abnormalities of the neuraxis such as Chiari malformations, syringobulbia or syringomyelia (Hurwitz *et al.* 1966, List 1941, Spillane *et al.* 1957).

Metabolic Causes

Secondary basilar impression occurs as a sequel to secondary softening of bone due to a diversity of metabolic causes. All of them have the same effect and culminate in invagination of the skull base by the anterior margin of the foramen magnum which is subjected to same infolding process that also affects the rest of the clivus. This disturbance in the sagittal plane leads to contraction of the axial distances as noted in the section on functional anatomy and renders the various structures more vulnerable to surgical damage if this is not borne in mind. Some of the conditions leading to this include Hurlers syndrome, achondroplasia, rickets, infections, osteomalacia, osteoporosis, hyperparathyroidism and Paget's disease. Despite the considerable deformities that may occur at the craniocervical junction in these conditions the junction is usually stable and so the correction of the deformity can be undertaken by anterior decompression with a reasonable prospect of success.

Trauma

This is very rare in the clivus and obviously anything in this context that disturbs its structural integrity is likely to be fatal. Again it is difficult to consider this structure in isolation; it has to be taken in conjunction with the atlas and axis. Craniocervical dislocation is usually fatal due to damage to the spinal cord and/or avulsion of the vertebral arteries as they enter the dura (Bohlman 1979). These injuries require considerable force to produce their results, and are commonly the sequel to high velocity impacts associated with road traffic accidents (Huelke *et al.* 1981).

Inflammatory Conditions

Some of the earliest reports on the approach to the clivus were concerned with the need to relieve accumulations of purulent material caused by bacterial infections, which included tuberculosis (Fang *et al.* 1962). Acute inflammatory diseases leading to atlanto-axial dislocation are most common in children; and Greenberg noted the fact that 77% of published cases of non-traumatic occipito-atlanto-axial dislocation occurred in children under 13 years of age (Greenberg 1968). The most prominent of the chronic inflammatory conditions is rheumatoid arthritis. When it occurs at the craniocervical junction it may be associated with the twin dangers of a mass lesion on the one hand occurring in conjunction with instability on the other, to create a spectrum of neurological damage, which, not uncommonly, may lead to fatal consequences. It is said that 50% of people die within a year of developing a rheumatoid myelopathy (Marks *et al.* 1981, Meijers *et al.* 1984) and death may occur as a sudden event (Redlund-Johnell 1984). The need for anterior surgery in this situation has been highlighted by Crockard and his colleagues in a very extensive series of cases, who conclude from their experience that the most suitable treatment for irreducible subluxation of the craniocervical junction is the combination of anterior decompression with posterior stabilisation (Crockard *et al.* 1990).

Tumours

Tumours situated in and around the skull base are rare: only 1% of all intracranial tumours are found in this locality. Because of the rich diversity of tissues in and around the skull base many very unusual tumours may be encountered. In many cases the clivus is the principal structure involved, and the majority are usually extradural. If there are considerable extensions laterally on either side then clearly anterior surgery alone is probably inadequate to deal with them and some form of combined operation is likely to be necessary. Although the pathology is very variable the tumours share considerable affinities in terms of their behaviour. They are usually of low malignancy and therefore non-metastasising, but they are locally invasive and resistent to radiotherapy. These similarities lead to a degree of uniformity in management. Some typical examples of the pathology found here are chordomas (Laws 1985), chondrosarcomas (Stapleton *et al.* 1993), giant-cell tumours (Watkins *et al.* 1992), invasive pituitary adenomas (Cook *et al.* 1994) (Table 2), and even softened ligaments in the craniocervical junction may behave, in the elderly, as a benign space occupying lesion (Crockard *et al.* 1991). Again these are all extradural tumours but an anterior approach may be considered suitable for surgery upon intradural lesions such as meningiomas (most frequently), neurofibromas, epidermoids, congenital cysts, and also in dealing with intrinsic brain stem space occupying lesions with exophytic components erupting onto the anterior surface of the brain stem, or major cystic abnormalities presenting on the clival aspect of the brain stem. These may very well lend themselves to an approach through the clivus (Uttley *et al.* 1989).

Vascular Lesions

Naturally these are all intradural, and take the form of aneurysms occurring on the distal extremities of the vertebral arteries, the vertebrobasilar

Table 2. *Histology of Skull Base Tumours*

Chordomas	15%
Chondrosarcomas	15%
Pituitary adenomas (invasive)	15%
Squamous cell carcinomas	10%

Most frequent tumour types in author's series of 46 clival tumours.

junction, and the trunk and termination of the basilar artery. An anterior approach is a logical step in view of the anatomical relationships of these lesions, lying, as they do, between the brain stem and the dural surface of the clivus. As long as they lie within 1.5 cm of the midline, it is usually possible to deal with them more satisfactorily from an anterior approach, in view of the difficulties inherent in postero-lateral access (Archer *et al.* 1987, Uttley *et al.* 1993).

Clinical Presentations

The complex relationships of the clivus are responsible for a diverse range of neurological findings that are of considerable fascination to the clinical neurologist. All the cranial nerves fall within the ambit of clival pathology, together with the pons, brain stem, and upper cervical spinal cord, as well as the major vascular stuctures lying in front of them. At first sight the combinations may appear endless, but in fact there is a fairly standard sequence of involvment as far as the tumour categories are concerned: about half the patients present with cranial nerve palsies, a third have headache or neck pain, a third have visual disturbances, another third present with airway obstruction, and a quarter with bulbar palsy (Table 3). In the developmental group there may be obvious external deformities, such as varieties of dwarfism, or the cervical deformity of the Klippel-Feil syndrome. The rheumatoid sufferers should manifest the typical joint deformities of that condition. Children who complain of neck pain and have a wry neck after an acute infective illness should be suspected of having an incipient occipito-atlanto-axial dislocation. Few trauma cases survive, and this may be just as well for them and their relatives as the degree of neurological deficit may not be compatible with an independent existence. Finally the vascular cases present with a typical history of subarachnoid haemorrhage in the main, but rare giant aneurysms may masquerade as tumours, and behave as space-occupying lesions.

Table 3. *Clinical Presentation: Tumours*

Cranial nerve palsies	50%
Headache and/or neck pain	33%
Visual disturbances	33%
Airway obstruction	33%
Bulbar palsy	25%

Frequency of clinical features in author's series of 50 operations for clival tumours.

Investigations

1. Plain x-Rays

These have a suffered a decline in popularity since the advent of sophisticated scanning techniques. Standard views of the skull in the sagittal and PA planes have never been particularly useful in demonstrating the clivus. If it was thought necessary to visualise this region then pluridirectional tomography was considered to be essential for the purpose. Bony erosion by, or ectopic calcification in tumours could be seen, but there would be little help forthcoming as to the exact operative approach that should be adopted in any given circumstances. Of greater value is the role of plain x-rays in the determination of stability at the occipito-atlanto-axial joints, where thin slice tomography may show degrees of subluxation, and reveal the various types of fracture that may occur in the region locally. When views in flexion and extension are employed (with caution!) much useful information may be gleaned as to the extent and level of the dislocation. A number of eponymous lines have been formulated slicing across and through the foramen magnum. The distances, angles, and ratios they define may be used as guides to measure the existence of significant discrepancies from normal values.

2. Angiography

Here again there has been a recent sea change in the indications for this investigation. No longer, with pneumoencephalography, is it the automatic choice for the examination of the posterior fossa in cases of tumour. There are still major, and so far unchallenged, areas in which vertebral angiograms are of fundamental importance and the main application is in the delineation of the detailed anatomy of aneurysms and arteriovenous malformations in the posterior fossa. These abnormalities may not be easy to recognise on the usual lateral and PA views, so oblique views may be necessary to demonstrate their presence, and subtraction techniques to illuminate the neighbouring vessels. Angiography for tumour pathology is important to assess the contribution made to the vascular supply by internal and external vessels respectively, to see if vessels are displaced, distorted, or occluded, and to determine whether embolisation has a part to play in the preoperative preparation of the patient. Lastly, useful information relating to the patency of the venous sinuses may be gained, particularly in identifying the dominant sigmoid sinus.

3. Computerised Tomography (CT)

The first of the modern scanning techniques to become available has had a profound influence on the way pathology is regarded by the present generation of surgeons. The boundaries, nature, and consistency of the tumour can be predicted, and in addition the secondary pathological chacteristics, such as the degree of vasogenic oedaema, necrosis, and its invasive properties may be accurately assessed. Usually an informed opinion can be given as to the tumour type. The technique has a special place in skull base surgery, because it is here that thin-slice high resolution bone windows may determine the nature of the tumour and the actual approach to the lesion. The ability to process complex information permits the presentation of data in other forms, so that reformatting of the cranio-cervical junction in the sagittal plane is a routine component of the examination, and three-dimensional images in any plane may be generated; these, taken with views in flexion and extension, have led almost to the abandonment of plain tomograms in this region. The 3-D reformats also play a part in the improved precision with which facial osteotomies may be made. CT scans after the instillation of water-soluble contrast medium into the CSF by lateral cervical puncture make it possible to outline the CSF pathways in and around the skull base to show where obliteration and distortion have occurred.

4. Magnetic Resonance Imaging

This latest developement has marked a further major step in imaging. Its strength lies in being able to produce high quality images of soft tissues, separating them into normal and abnormal components, and revealing borders of great clarity. Signal voids indicate flow in vessels, which enables decisions to be made regarding displacment and compression of vascular elements that it may be vital to preserve during the course of surgery. Taken one step further the angiographic sequences that are now available help to rationalise operative planning, and render surgery safer, though the detail is not adequate at present to identify small tumour vessels with absolute certainty.

5. Evoked Potentials

Visual, brain-stem auditory, and somatosensory evoked potentials (VEP, BAEP, and SSEP) may all in their different ways make valuable contributions to the acquisition of relevant information in the preoperative phase, though their role in this process is currently less critical than that of the imaging techniques.

General Operative Considerations

As many of the points regarding preoperative assessment, positioning, anaesthesia, and post operative management are common to all the transfacial approaches, it is appropriate to combine them in this section.

1. Preoperative Preparation

Intensive sterilisation of the nasal pathways or oral cavity prior to surgery is probably unnecessary. It has been recommended that an accurate picture of the bacterial flora in these cavities is obtained prior to surgery, and in addition it has been suggested that antibiotic cream should be applied to the nasal cavity for three or four days before the operation, and the mouth treated with mouth washes of appropriate disinfectants for the same time. These are counsels of perfection as they require some degree of patient supervision and it is both impractical and prohibitively expensive to have them in hospital for this length of time prior to surgery. The author's practice is to assume the normal commensal organisms are present in the posterior part of the nares or in the oral cavity and that special pre-operative application of topical antibiotics is superfluous, particularly when it is borne in mind that systemic prophylactic antibiotics are to be given during the course of the operation. In several hundred transnasal pituitary operations and over 60 maxillotomy procedures no evidence has accumulated to demonstrate that this practice has led to serious post-operative infections.

2. General Anaesthesia

An extremely detailed pre-operative assessment of the patient is made by the surgeon and the anaesthetist and it is during these final stages of preparation that detailed consent must be sought for the operation that is undertaken, so that the patient is fully aware of the risks and potential complications that may occur during the course of surgery. Due attention should be paid to rectifying preoperative medical problems. If these are of a chronic nature and already receiving medical attention, special care is necessary during the operation to make sure that failure to maintain treatment does not compromise the conduct of anaesthesia, or lead to deleterious drug interactions. Selection of anaesthetic agents is done with care to avoid those with a tendency to increase intracranial pressure or produce systemic hypotension. Ideally they should ensure haemodynamic stability and a decrease in cerebral metabolic demands. It is our practice to use large doses of a standard combination of neurosurgical anaesthetic agents from the beginning of the operation, because it is known that they are likely to be lengthy procedures, and then gradually to give smaller aliquots of drugs to maintain anaesthesia for the duration of the operation. Effective peri-operative monitoring is essential for the stability of the operation, while at the same time being alert to the possibility of sudden changes dictated by surgical emergencies and requirements, and having a rapid response time to them. Central venous and arterial lines are essential, and electronic monitoring of cerebral electrical function and evoked potentials are used where necessary. Orotracheal intubation is standard with the transfacial approaches, the tubing being anchored very firmly to prevent displacement, and usually on the left side of the oral cavity. After suitable neuromuscular blockade, mechanical hyperventilation is instituted to reduce cerebral vasodilatation and prevent increases in intracranial pressure which may be induced by the inhalational agents as well as the operative conditions. Adequate neuromuscular relaxants are required throughout the operation to maintain this steady state and prevent patient movement.

3. Control of Intracranial Pressure

During the anaesthetic preparations an indwelling catheter is placed in the bladder so that osmotic diuretics can be used safely. The one in everyday use and by far the quickest in action is a hypertonic solution of mannitol, with loop diuretics such as frusemide being used for more protracted purposes. These are normally only administered if an intradural exposure is required, otherwise they are of little value. A lumbar spinal drain is inserted during this stage of the operative preparation which permits continuous CSF drainage during the operation. This is an extremely useful facility, but again it is more useful if the intention is to open the dura, and a surgeon will normally request that the drain be opened shortly before this is undertaken in order to reduce the intracranial pressure. There are no fixed times for the drain to remain in place after surgery, but it is generally accepted that for cases where the dura has not been breached the drain could be removed within 48 hours, particularly if the draining CSF remains crystal clear. If the dura has been opened then it is more important that a waterproof seal is obtained and the drain is left in place longer. In this unit it is arbitrarily removed at 5 days after a short period of clamping, providing there is no evidence of CSF leakage during this phase.

There are dangers inherent in the use of lumbar drains: a profound fall in intracranial pressure may delay recovery of full conciousness after the anaesthetic and this may conceal the insidious accumulation of a postoperative clot or a pneumoencephalocoele, the latter may be avoided by draining against a gradient. The important lesson is to resort to frequent CT scans in the unresponsive patient, during the immediate postoperative phase when clinical progress may be difficult to assess.

4. Prophylactic Antibiotics

In recent years there has been growing evidence to suggest that these do have a part to play in combatting postoperative neurosurgical sepsis, particularly in major operations of this nature. The standard practice is to institute cover at the beginning of the operation with an intravenous injection of a cefalosporine (cefotaxime) with or without the addition of met-ronidazole. This antibiotic cover is maintained for the next three days before being discontinued, but only in the absence of overt infection.

5. Corticosteroids: Replacement

With large tumours involving the clivus there is a distinct possibility that pituitary function may be defective and most surgeons would recommend the exhibition of corticosteroids during the beginning of the operation and then maintainance for several days afterwards. If the patient is obviously deficient in pituitary hormones prior to surgery, then a wider range of replacements may need to be given than steroids alone. It is widely believed by the surgical fraternity that steroids protect the nervous system from operative damage, but there is little scientific evidence to support this. Indeed Hout prospectively examined the integrity of the hypothalamic-pituitary-adrenal axis in 88 consecutive patients with pituiary adenomas (Hout *et al.* 1983). In 83 patients in whom it was intact glucocorticoids were not given before, during, or after pituitary surgery, but they were closely monitored and their serum cortisol levels were measured in the early post-operative period and found to be satisfactory. Only two of the cases were suspected of adrenal insufficiency after surgery and they were treated accordingly. It therefore appears that even in the presence of a pituitary lesion the vast majority of patients will not require additional steroid cover, and its use in current practice may be to bolster surgical confidence rather than promote neurological protection.

6. Positioning

The patient is normally placed on the table in the supine position with the head and body tilted upwards at an angle of 20° to the lower extremities, to facilitate access, and also to reduce the intracranial venous load. For a very limited objective it may be advisable to use the Mayfield headrest and pins to stabilise the head, but in more major procedures where access to different areas is essential it is better to have the head supported on a horseshoe headrest, so that it can be moved as required during the opera-tion. Care should be taken during these lengthy procedures to pad depen-dent parts, and avoid contact with hard surfaces to spare pressure areas. Some form of thermal protection should be adopted to avoid dangerous levels of hypothermia developing during the operation.

7. Blood Pressure Control

This is continuously monitored by the arterial line and the operation is normally conducted with the pressure in the low-normal range of values. In younger patients with few adverse risk factors short periods of controlled hypotension may be very valuable to the surgeon during difficult technical manoeuvres. Reductions in blood pressure should be avoided wherever possible in the older patient where serious consequences may follow. In this type of surgery blood loss is usually substantial, and of a sudden may become torrential. Adequate reserves of blood for transfusion should be available, and should be used at an early stage in the operation to counteract the possibility of precipitate losses which could have profound hypovolaemic and hypotensive sequelae, leading to irreversible ischaemic changes in the nervous system. If large quantities of stored blood are transfused the possibility of a transfusional coagulopathy may exacerbate the bleeding problems, particularly in these lengthy and traumatic operations, with wide exposures. Even minor abnormalities may have disastrous consequences, in the shape of postoperative clots which are very damaging to the nervous system. A rapid and accurate diagnosis of the nature of the coagulopathy is essential to rectify it. Most commonly this would take the form of a dilutional thrombocytopaenia which will respond to platelet administration. The deficiency of clotting factors is the second most common cause of intraoperative coagulopathy. To counteract this may require fresh frozen plasma or more specialised haematological products, depending on an accurate laboratory diagnosis.

8. Post-Operative Nutrition

At the end of the major transfacial operations some means of instituting post-operative feeding has to be implemented. We choose to use a pharyngogastric tube which is inserted via a puncture pharyngostomy, through which fluids may be given on the first post-operative day, provided the patient is not suffering unduly from post-operative emesis. Aqueous oral fluids may be given as early as the second day in favourable circumstances, and may be gradually increased to constitute the major source of nutritional replacement at an early stage. With sutures in the oral cavity it is advisable for milk products to be withheld until the sutures have been removed at ten to fourteen days postoperatively. Careful measurement and observation of the fluid balance is essential from the outset, to make sure that adequate replenishment of fluid losses is given. Diabetes insipidus is always a potential threat if the pituitary gland has been disturbed by the presence of large tumours. Appropriate action needs to be taken in these circumstances. The clinical situation may also be adversely affected by inappropriate secretion of ADH, and every precaution should be exercised to avoid what is usually an easily rectified disorder.

9. Dural Closure

If the dura is opened intentionally or accidentally during the course of the procedure, the surgeon should be at great pains to ensure that a watertight seal is achieved before the conclusion of the operation. If the dura has been torn inadvertently the fact usually becomes obvious with the persistent appearance of diluted blood in one part of the operative field, often in places where bleeding is not expected, and careful search should be made for these defects, because they demand the same meticulous attention to closure as a formal dural incision. Failure to do so leads to a CSF fistula and a high risk of subsequent meningitis. It is always frustrating, and often futile, to try and close a clival dural defect by suture, as the margins may well have shrunk after coagulation or manipulation. Great difficulty may be experienced in the correct placement of sutures, which during tightening not infrequently cut out of the dura, leaving the remnants in a worse state for repair than they were originally. The solution to this problem is to place a layer of dural substitute inside (i.e. on the intracranial side of) the dura and another on the extracranial aspect, and bond the three layers together with human fibrin adhesive (Tisseel, Immuno, Vienna), so that the cross section rather resembles a sandwich, with the original dura featuring as its filling. After this has been done bone defects may be filled with multiple layers of oxidised cellulose, again held in place by human fibrin adhesive. Quite recently coral and hydroxylapatite preparations have been used to obliterate bone defects. Other materials are available and worthy of consideration. Biocompatible osteoconductive polymer (BOP, Diversified Tech International, subsidiary DTI s.a. Belgium) is another such product which would promote bone formation and ultimately create a solid barrier between the intracranial cavity and the pharynx. It is important to consider reconstruction of the clivus in cases where further surgery is not contemplated, for example following the treatment of aneurysms or the excision of benign tumours, because it is theoretically possible for such patients to undergo surgical emergencies where they are unable to explain what has happened to them in the past, and be subjected to an endonasal intubation where there may exist a potential for serious injury. In these cases it may be prudent for patients to carry some form of card to identify their susceptibility to these risks. As noted earlier in this section the lumbar drain is left in place for a minimum of 5 days if the dura has been opened, and longer if there is evidence of continued leakage. In the face of a recalcitrant fistula our policy is to re-explore the site and make further efforts to close the defect, hitherto always successful. The alternative is to insert a lumbo-peritoneal shunt to lower hydrostatic pressure and divert the CSF, to provide an opportunity for the defect to be sealed by the healing process.

10. Extubation

The crucial question which arises as the operation draws towards its conclusion is perhaps the most difficult one to be faced in the whole sequence of the management process, and revolves around the problem of extubation. Our anaesthetic colleagues have identified four factors which they feel are of prime importance in arriving at a decision. These are: excessive local haemorrhage, a greater degree of swelling in the airways than is customary with the type of operation, pre-existing or anticipated bulbar damage or lower cranial nerve IX to XII dysfunction, and finally whether there is likely to be depression of the patient's conscious level as a result of the procedure. If one or more of these criteria are noted extubation is delayed until a further asssessment is made on the day following surgery. In practical terms this means that aneurysm patients are extubated on the table, but occasionally amongst the tumour cases airway protection is needed, though we have never found it necessary for this to be prolonged for more than 24 hours, and we have yet to perform an immediate tracheostomy.

Surgical Approaches

The transfacial approaches to the skull base are few in number. As noted previously they are traditionally undertaken through the middle third of the face. Only one proceedure involves a facial incision, and thus may be categorised as an open operation. In most instances the incisions are concealed, either by working within the nasal cavity, or sublabially within the mouth. It must also be noted at the outset that some of the approaches are extremely restricted in terms of clival access, and confined to only a small portion of it. Only two methods expose the clivus to any reasonable degree, and only the method to be described last encompasses the whole of the clivus and the territory above and below it.

Transfacial Approach

This is the technique involving facial incisions which are usually neither mutilating nor severely damaging to underlying structures. Briefly the object of the exercise is to mobilise the maxilla medially and then rotate it laterally on a hinge formed by the flesh of the cheek and an osteotomy through the zygomatic arch.

In more detail the technique involves orotracheal intubation or even a tracheostomy if this is thought necessary. The patient is placed in a supine position with the head slightly elevated and lying on a horse-shoe head rest. A temporary tarsorrhaphy is first performed and then an incision is made extending from the vermilion of the upper lip vertically along the philtral crest on the side of the operation, around the posterior border of the

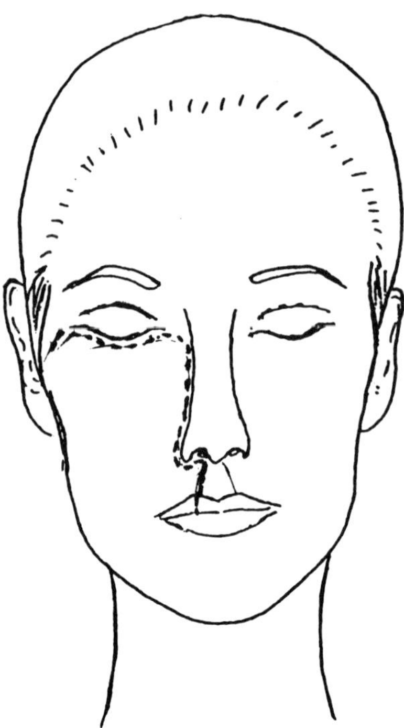

Fig. 2. Transfacial approach: skin incision (dotted line)

ipsilateral naris and upwards along the lateral aspect of the nose to the inner canthus, taking every precaution to preserve the latter. The incision then becomes horizontal passing laterally beneath the eye to the outer canthus, and comes to an end by curving slightly downwards over the zygomatic process (Fig. 2). A vertical incision is now made through the vestibular sulcus. Next a palatal flap extending from the retrotuberosity area on the side of the operation to the contralateral bicuspid area is elevated. Various bony landmarks are now accessible: including the upper part of the zygoma, the lower half of the orbital rim including the orbital floor (but taking care to preserve the lacrymal system), the piriform aperture from which the nasal mucosa has been reflected as far medially as possible, and the alveolar process in the paramedian area. A series of osteotomies are now undertaken (Fig. 3). Firstly a vertical cut is made at the level of the temporo-zygomatic junction. Another cut detaches the frontal process of the zygoma, and then a further osteotomy divides the floor of the orbit behind the orbital rim, and crosses to the highest point of the piriform aperture, again cautiously preserving the lacrymal system. On the orbital floor the infraorbital nerve has to be identified and marked, because it has to be divided. A vertical saw cut is then made in the alveolus between the central and lateral incisors which is continued posteriorly onto

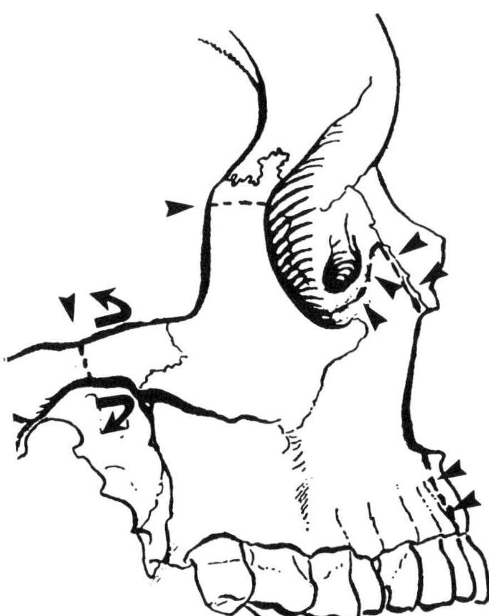

Fig. 3. Transfacial approach: osteotomy cuts (dotted lines), note hinge of bony
segment on root of zygoma (curved arrows)

the palate, in the sagittal plane, to its posterior border. The palatine artery
is now freed from its bony channel using an osteotome, thus preserving the
arterial pedicle of the palatal flap. Finally the pterigo-maxillary junction is
divided with an osteotome inserted medially. It is now possible to mobilise
the maxilla, which remains vascularised on the pedicle of the cheek, and
rotates around the hinge formed by the bisected temporal process of the
zygoma. The pedicle is kept in hot saline packs for the duration of the
procedure. If necessary the operation can be performed bilaterally leaving
only the central strut of the palate in position, though clearly this is an
over-elaborate option when simpler alternatives are available. The operation on one side exposes the ipsilateral pterygo-mandibular and retro-
maxillary areas, the rhinopharynx, the nasal fossa, the sphenoid sinus, the
ethmoids, the suborbital and subtemporal regions, and proceeding backwards to the clivus in the central skull base with access to all the foramina
and fissures through which neurovascular structures enter and leave the
skull. This technique was first described by Curioni (Curioni *et al.* 1984),
and Altemir who describes the method in relation to the removal of a large
angiofibroma with very little blood loss (Hernandez Altamir 1986). One of
the major drawbacks is the extensive packing required for the sphenoid
sinus, the nasal cavity and the maxillary sinus which has to be withdrawn
gradually over the next few days, and the re-suturing of the intraorbital
nerve. The osseus block is replaced and secured in position with wires or
minicompression plates which achieve a satisfactory cosmetic result.

Vascularisation of the flap is principally based on the facial and transverse facial arteries and the viability of the pedicle is well maintained even in situations where pre-operative embolisation has been undertaken, or where ligation of the external carotid artery, on a temporary or permanent basis, has been deemed necessary during the procedure. Although generally very satisfactory for retro-maxillary lesions including those adjacent to the clivus, it does not fulfill those ideal desiderata that would make it the operation of choice for a full anterior assault on the clivus. In current usage it is much more popular with ENT surgeons than with neurosurgeons, and in this respect accurately reflects their respective interests.

Facial Translocation

In this technique the maxillotomy described in the previous section is allied to mobilisation of the zygoma which increases the exposure of the skull base to facilitate better access to lesions arising from it (Arriaga *et al.* 1989, Janecka *et al.* 1990). The method involves a paranasal incision from the top of the philtral crest to the medial canthus which is divided, the incision then sweeps around the infaorbital conjunctiva and then severs the lateral canthus before it reappears on the surface to extend posteriorly across the temporal region to end at the upper attachment of the ear, where the incision is carried upwards in the coronal plane to the midline, the incision is extended in a downwards direction anterior to the tragus as far as the lower border of the ear, but may be taken down into the neck, when circumstances require an even greater exposure. Now the scalp flap may be turned anteriorly. The frontal branches of the facial nerve, the infraorbital nerve, and the nasolacrimal duct are identified, marked to allow for ultimate reconstuction, and then divided.

At this point the temporalis and masseter muscles are dissected away from their bony attachments to expose the mid portion of the facial skeleton. Next the cheek flap may be mobilised as far down as the palate; dissection should be deep to the masseteric fascia in an attempt to preserve facial nerve branches.

Osteotomies of the maxilla and the zygoma are performed at this stage, followed by removal of the posterior wall of the maxillary sinus and both pterygoid plates by means of horizontal osteotomies at the level of the hard palate and the skull. The temporalis muscle may be mobilised further inferiorly by a subperiosteal osteotomy and down-fracturing of the coronoid process of the mandible. At the end of the operation the bony osteotomies may be reassembled by the application of mini-plating systems. The nerves may be sutured at the conclusion of the operation, and good cosmetic results are claimed; the nasolacrimal duct is repaired over a stent which is removed after six weeks. Temporalis muscle may be used to obliterate "dead space", close defects, and protect dura when bone has been removed; its size and rich vascular supply makes it ideally suited to these roles. The soft tissue flaps are well vascularised, and heal well with minimal scarring. This complex procedure offers access to tumours of the anterior skull base that are extending laterally into the infratemporal fossa, and combines elements of both the anterior and lateral approaches to good effect.

Midfacial Degloving

This is another approach born out of the necessity to provide access to lesions lying in and around the skull base, and, like most of these techniques, it can be combined with transfrontal or temporal or palatal operations for the treatment of extensive lesions. The technique was first described in 1974 (Casson *et al.* 1974) and more recently in current practice by Price (Price 1986). General anaesthesia is maintained via orotracheal intubation, and the tube is firmly secured to prevent it becoming dislodged during the procedure. The patient is placed in a supine position with the head slightly elevated at about 30%, and supported by a horse-shoe head rest during the course of the operation. After the nasal application of cocaine paste, infiltration with local anaesthetic and a dilute solution of adrenaline to achieve local haemostasis is undertaken. The nose is injected first as if for a rhinoplasty, and then the buccogingival sulcus and the canine fossa are infiltrated next. Temporary tarsorrhaphies or some alternative corneal protection is provided bilaterally. Complete transfixion and intercartilaginous incisions separate the nasal tip from the dorsum. The incision is then extended around the piriform margin to complete a "circumvestibular" division, and then a sublabial incision usually extends across the midline to just above the first molars. The soft tissues of the nasal dorsum are then widely elevated in the subperiosteal plane. Now the tissues of the face may be elevated from the anterior maxilla: from its most lateral extension to the nasal bones medially, and then upwards to the intraorbital rim. The contents of the intraorbital foramen are to be protected as far as possible. The subperiosteal dissection is continued on each side of the midline as far as the piriform margins. Returning now to work through the nose, it is possible to release the remaining soft tissue attachments from the columella and anterior maxillary spine, and then the nasal and sublabial incisions are brought into communication. The upper lip along with the intact nasal columella and nasal tip including the alar cartilages may be now retracted over the nose to the level of the inferior orbital rim. At this point exposed bone may be removed to facilitate the excision of the surgical lesion. The ipsilateral antrum is entered first and the anterior maxillary bone rongeured away. The bone removal may continue up to the frontal process of the maxilla, and then osteotomies are carried out across the piriform margin superiorly and inferiorly to complete the medial maxillectomy. Ethmoidectomy and sphenoidectomy may be carried out under full vision at this stage, and the entire nasal septum is then accessible and may be released and deflected or resected up to the cribriform plate. If reqired these processes may be duplicated on the opposite side to improve access. Complete exposure of the naso-pharynx requires removal of the posterior wall of the maxillary antrum and the ascending process of the palatine bone. It should be noted that brisk bleeding may be experienced from the palatine arteries. The pterygoid muscles and plates, the posterior wall of the sphenoid sinus and the clivus form the posterior limits of resection. The cribriform plate and the adjacent portion of the floor of the anterior cranial fossa are the upper limits. The lateral limit of the dissection is the coronoid process of the mandible and the inferior boundary is the palate, although this too can be mobilised should the need arise. The major vascular supply of the flap includes facial, infraorbital and supratrochlear vessels, all of which are preserved in this procedure, with the result that ischaemic complications are exceptionally rare.

At the conclusion of the procedure a considerable amount of packing is required to obliterate the spaces. It has to be carefully applied so that it may be sequentially removed as the days go by. The nasal tip is carefully repositioned with a transfixion suture and a second suture placed at the base of the columella. The vestibular skin is then sutured to the piriform mucosal margin. The central frenulum of the sublabial incision is carefully approximated, and then a one layer closure of the oral membranes is completed.

Price described this operation as being of value for most ENT conditions involving the maxilla and its surroundings including chondromas, chordomas and chondrosarcomas, which presumably arise from the neighbourhood of the clivus (Price 1986). The operation has the merit of being suitable for large lesions because the potential for a bilateral approach to lesions much simplifies the surgery of this region, and is therefore in this respect superior to the more cumbersome transfacial approach. There are, of course, only minimal facial scars in what is an almost wholly "concealed" approach, but there may well be complaints of facial numbness in the distribution of the intraorbital nerves, although this tends to become less noticeable with time. Cosmetic problems may arise if too much of the anterior wall of the maxilla has been removed.

In a further article Price commented that the procedure was extremely useful in a wide variety of conditions and versatile in application, so that with bilateral medial maxillectomies and complete ethmoidectomy, there was ample access for dealing with lesions of the sphenoid sinus and clivus complex. A combination of this operation with other approaches may be used in very extensive lesions. It was noted that resection of the clivus was undertaken three times in their series, but the results were not analysed independently of the other lesions with which they dealt (Price *et al.* 1988).

Transsphenoidal Approach

In the early days of neurosurgery it was the case that surgical approaches were focused on the pituitary gland and only in the last 20 years or so that they have been extended to involve other structures. It is perhaps surprising that both the transsphenoidal and the transfrontal approaches to the pituitary fossa were being postulated at approximately the same time, and perhaps even more surprising to realise that this was almost a 100 years ago. It was Giodano who first suggested the transsphenoidal route after cadaveric dissections in 1897. This was an unacceptably mutilating operation in which the nose was split down the midline and the septum and turbinates were removed before access was gained to the sphenoid sinus and the region of the pituitary. Other propositions included reflecting the patient's nose laterally and them resecting the septum and turbinates, and the first successful operation of this nature was performed in 1907 (Schloffer 1907). These alarming procedures were rapidly discarded when more sophisticated alternatives appeared and Kaneval was one of the first to develop an infranasal transseptal approach, which was much preferable to the original methods, in that it preserved normal nasal function and facial appearance (Kanavel 1909). Cushing followed Halstead's suggestion (Halstead 1910), to adopt the sublabial transseptal approach, and used it between the years 1912–1925; he operated on a total of 231 patients using this approach with an operative mortality of 5.6% (Henderson 1939). Unfortunately his early enthusiasm for this method was dampened by several problems which included impaired visibility due to the considerable haemorrhage which occurred, and the lack of adequate magnification and illumination in the pre-microscope days. This led to portions of the tumour being left behind, and thus to an unacceptably high recurrence rate when compared to the transfrontal method, and, lastly, and perhaps most importantly, the degree of uncertainty regarding the exact nature and location of the pathology before modern imaging techniques became available. The historical evolution of pituitary surgery has been traced in an elegant review (Wellbourn 1986). In Edinburgh Norman Dott continued with this transseptal approach throughout his career (Rosegay 1981), and passed on the torch to Guiot (Guiot 1978), from whom Hardy adopted the method and introduced it into the canon of modern neurosurgery (Hardy *et al.* 1965), to the point where, in the last 20–30 years, it has superseded the transfrontal route. So much so that Guiot in 1978 did more than 90% of his pituitary operations by the transsphenoidal route (Guiot 1978), and Wilson six years later indicated that he only employed the transfrontal route in 1% of his pituitary operations (Wilson 1984). Clearly the success of the operation is predicated by the size of the sphenoid sinus. If this is commodious then the operation is much easier than in the presence of a small or absent sinus, when a good deal of bone dissection would need to be undertaken to approach the clivus. It is clear that only the small portion of the clivus that lies behind the sphenoid sinus and immediately inferior to it are likely to be accessible by this means. It is essential for an absolutely mid-sagittal plane to be followed during the operation to avoid damage to the important neurovascular structures which lie on either side of it in the skull base or cavernous sinus.

The sublabial technique is extensively used throughout the world. In its original form it was first proposed by Halstead (Halstead 1910) and then used subsequently by Cushing to complete his large series of cases (Henderson 1939). As a prelude to all the transnasal approaches the nasal mucous membranes are given a liberal application of cocaine paste, which helps to reduce vascularity, and produces long-lasting post-operative local analgesia. The technique consists of infiltrating the gingival margin above the upper incisors with a mixture of local anaesthetic and a $1:200,000$ solution of Adrenaline, and then dividing the margin in a horizontal plane parallel to the teeth and the floor of the nose. The mucosa is then dissected away from the nasal spine and floor of the nose and, as far as possible, from the nasal septum. The bony spine is then removed and the septum is either incised and deflected laterally or excised in its turn. It is now possible to place the self retaining speculum between the two layers of nasal mucosa and extend the dissection backwards and upwards to the region of the vomer. This structure almost always lies in the mid sagittal plane and is naturally a most important landmark. The actual direction of this nasal dissection can be monitored on the image intensifier to make sure that it always takes place in the direction of the sphenoid sinus. When the vomer is encountered, both it and the anterior wall of the sphenoid sinus can then be removed using bone forceps or a small osteotome to gain entry; following this the size of the window into the sinus may be increased using Kerrison punches. At this stage reference to a pre-operative CT scan in the transverse axial plane will suffice to demonstrate the position and number of the sphenoid septa; these should be removed together with the covering mucosa which normally harbours only comensal organisms. One can then either remove the anterior wall or the floor of the pituitary fossa and approach the gland, or excise the posterior wall of the sphenoid sinus which at this point is the uppermost portion of the clivus.

In 1909 Hirsch proposed the anterior endonasal transseptal approach which he used successfully for many years (Hirsch 1909). The problem with both this and the preceeding method is the amount of tedious dissection that is necessary at the beginning of the operation. The approaches are to a variable extent rendered difficult by significant septal deviation. In addition the sublabial method will produce the additional unacceptable complications of anaesthesia and possible discolouration of the upper front teeth.

In the course of the 1970s surgeons in various countries began to take account of the cardinal feature of the vomer, which was its almost invariable position in the midsagittal plane. This led to the development of the posterior endonasal approach (Griffith *et al.* 1987), which the author helped to pioneer. In this method septal deviation becomes irrelevant. The speculum can be placed in the most capacious of the nares, either left or right; it is then possible to identify the spine of the vomer which normally lies in the same vertical plane as the posterior end of the middle turbinate. This means that the speculum is placed in the nostril at approximately 45° to the floor of the nose, and with the help of the image intensifier a probe is placed through the mucosa, into what is considered to be the anterior aspect of the sphenoid sinus. Using the image intensifier, adjustments are made to the probe until this position is achieved. At this point the speculum is retracted several millimetres and then opened widely to fracture the cartilaginous septum from the vomer. This normally produces linear ischaemia in the septal mucosa in which an incision is made from above downwards in a vertical plane with a fine knife. The mucosa may then be dissected away from the junction of septum and vomer very easily so that the anterior aspect of the sphenoid sinus is visualised on one side, and then by dissecting on the opposite side of the vomer the mucosa is reflected away from the adjacent anterior surface of the sphenoid sinus. By insinuating the arms of the speculum between the two leaves of the nasal mucosa posteriorly and then distracting them, it is possible to expose the vomer and the anterior wall of the sphenoid sinus, looking rather like the keel of a boat. Bony dissection may be then made using either bone forceps or an osteotome through the anterior wall of the sphenoid sinus, and then the operation proceeds as did the sublabial procedure by stripping out the mucosa and the septa which divide the sphenoid sinus.

This simple technique is easy to teach: it avoids the complications to the teeth, and the nasal septum with its covering mucosa is retained intact (problem areas inherent in the sublabial approach), also it saves precious operating time. It is essentially a transsphenoidal approach and confines the operator to the posterior wall of the sphenoid sinus and the portion of the clivus immediately adjacent to it. The transsphenoidal approach is not suitable for lesions which are larger than the bony exposure, which extend laterally, or which are very vascular, because of the limitations imposed by the restricted access. On the other hand it must be admitted that it is by far the best way of dealing with pituitary microadenomas, and most of the macroadenomas which are situated in the sagittal plane. The operation will retain its established popularity for these conditions (Uttley 1994).

It is important when dealing with a clivus lesion or with a pituitary tumour or, indeed, pathology which straddles both regions, to ensure that there is no CSF leak following dural tear. This may happen in macro-adenomas which have thinned the capsule and where the arachnoid has been torn, or it may occur if the clival dura has been divided for the clipping of a terminal basilar aneurysm. This may be repaired in the manner already described and then the pituitary fossa and the sphenoid sinus should be packed. Various materials have been used including muscle from the thigh, or fat from the abdominal wall. It is superfluous to embark on a second operation because it is usually satisfactory to use some form of oxidised cellulose held in position with human fibrin adhesive.

At the conclusion of the operation the nasal mucosa is forced together by packing both nares with paraffin gauze ribbons, which have been soaked in an antibiotic suspension. These are left in place for 24 hours before they are removed. Patients are advised not to blow their nose for about a month following surgery by which time the mucosa will be thoroughly healed.

Transethmoidal Approach

First described by Chiari (Chiari 1912), this method is even more limited as a means of exposing the clivus than the transsphenoidal one and is really only suitable for removing strictly intrasellar lesions. In its customary form the pituitary fossa was viewed through the ethmoidectomy exposure, with the instruments being passed to the target via the nostril (James 1967). It had a short-lived vogue when hypophysectomy was being used as a treatment for the control of metastatic bone pain and diabetic retinopathy, but it has no part to play in the treatment of pituitary macroadenomas, or of adjoining clival disturbances. The eyelids on the side where the operation is to take place are sutured as a preliminary, and then a semicircular skin incision is made around the medial angle of the eye down to the lateral edge of the nasal bone. The periosteum is separated from this structure: great care being taken to preserve the periorbita, the trochlea and the medial canthal ligament. The eye is mobilised laterally to expose the lamina papyracea and the ethmoid sinuses. These are opened anteriorly and the mucosa over the lateral aspect of the nose is dissected away from the bone and displaced medially. During this part of the procedure the ethmoidal arteries are preserved as far as possible as they lie above the plane of the exposure, below this level the anterior wall of the sphenoid sinus is encountered. This can then be opened in the manner already described and the anterior wall of the pituitary fossa should then be visible.

The limitations of this approach are firstly that it starts from a lateral position and attempts to move medially so that difficulties may occur in orientation. Secondly the floor of the anterior fossa slopes downwards towards the pituitary and forces the plane of surgery inferiorly into the sphenoid sinus thus limiting the exposure of the anterior wall of the pituitary fossa and certainly preventing any attempt to operate on the plane above it. At the conclusion of the operation the cavity is filled with gauze which is led out through the nasal cavity and which is removed over the next few days. Periosteum and skin are sutured and the eyelids are then opened. The immediate post-operative cosmetic effect is not particularly pleasing as there is usually a good deal of swelling, but this settles down over the course of the next few days to leave an acceptable appearence.

The Transantral Transsphenoidal Approach

In this rather roundabout procedure the buccal mucosa is reflected from the anterior wall or the maxillary sinus, which is then removed. This facilitates the resection of the medial bony wall of the sinus to expose the mucosa of the nasal cavity which may be displaced medially to increase the operative field. A lower ethmoidectomy is then performed, as a result of this the anterior wall of the sphenoid sinus is exposed and may be opened to provide a limited exposure to the pituitary fossa and the adjacent clivus (Svien *et al.* 1965, Hamberger *et al.* 1961). It is difficult to manipulate the operating microscope around the cavity. The operation has a sinister reputation for being excessively bloody when compared to the other methods. It is much more time consuming and the considerable cavity that remains requires very large packs that have to be removed piecemeal over a period of several days thus increasing the hospital stay.

Le Fort 1 Maxillotomy

This operation has been a standard part of the maxillofacial repertoire for many years. As with so many other surgical "firsts" the method was described by von Langenbeck (von Langenbeck 1859) as a horizontal osteotomy crossing the maxilla from side to side, at the same level that le Fort subsequently designated as his Type 1 fracture line in 1901 (Drommer 1986). Severe haemorrhage circumscribed its value as a surgical technique during the latter part of the 19th century and the early part of this one, thus limiting visibility and obscuring the surgical detail in the days prior to the operating microscope becoming an everyday tool. It was therefore used only fitfully until the 1930s when it became more widely used in the correction of skeletal deformities of the face; and as one of a series of osteotomies it gained an established role in this context (Drommer 1986). In recent years the author and his colleagues have adapted it for use in another role when they recognised its potential to provide excellent exposure of the central skull base, and in particular the clivus. Not only has it been used for the resection of tumours, but also for treating aneurysms at the junction of the vertebro-basilar arteries, and mid-line basilar trunk aneurysms with considerable success (Uttley *et al.* 1989, Uttley *et al.* 1993).

All the operations are performed under general anaesthesia with orotracheal intubation, care being taken to secure the tube very firmly so that it does not become displaced during the course of the operation. The preliminaries have been described earlier in this chapter. Patients are placed supine on the operating table with a head-up tilt of 15–30° to suit surgical access, operator comfort, and to reduce haemorrhage. The oral cavity is sterilised with an aqueous solution of povidone iodine before an incision is made above the mucogingival reflection, extending from one upper molar area across the midline to the same position on the opposite side of the mouth. A bilateral low level bone cut is then made with an air powered sagittal saw through the malar buttress to the maxillary tuberosity laterally and the nares medially (Fig. 4a,b). This exposes the mucosa of the nasal floor and gives access to the pterigo-maxillary fissure. At this stage the positions of the Luhr compression plates, necessary for accurate reapposition and fixation of the maxilla at the end of the operation, are

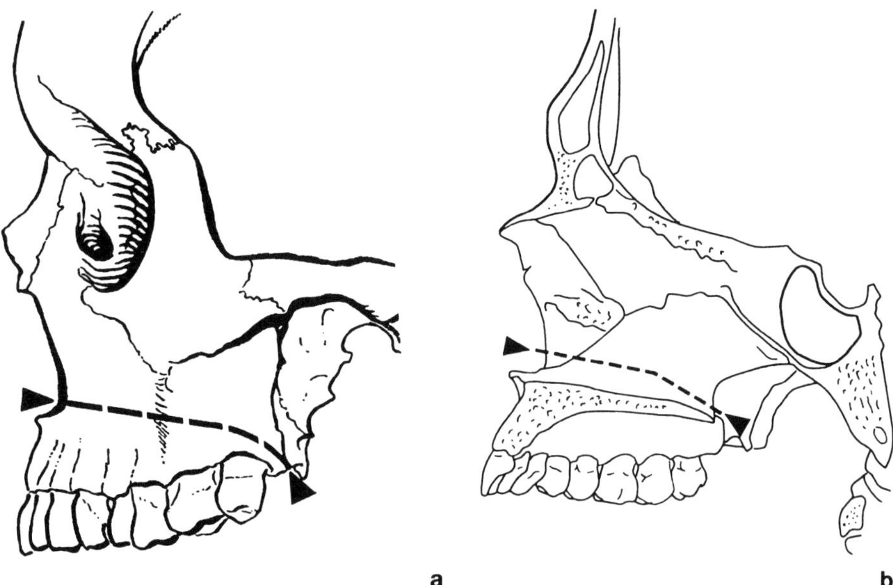

Fig. 4. Osteotomies for le Fort 1 maxillotomy: (a) on lateral aspect of dried skull (dotted line), and (b) through nasal septum on medial aspect of split skull (reproduced by kind permission of the editor of Journal of Neurosurgery)

marked out on either side of the osteotomy. The nasal septum is divided at its inferior midline junction with the maxilla and palate before a curved chisel is used to separate the lateral pterigoid laminae from their maxillary attachment. It now becomes possible to "down fracture" the maxilla maintaining its blood supply, which is generally thought to be dependant on the integrity of the greater palatine arteries. It should be noted that on occasion we have sacrificed one of them, and very rarely both, without postoperative ischaemic consequences, the implication being that sufficient blood supply is maintained through the mucosal blood supply of the faucial pillars. This mobilisation of the maxilla permits the detached portion to be lowered into the oral cavity through a distance equivalent to the normal range of mouth opening from before backwards, which is an important consideration in terms of access, and of even greater value in the edentulous (Fig. 5). The mucosa of the nasal floor is elevated on each side to expose the nasal septum and vomer. The inferior turbinates are excised using heavy scissors and the vomer may be removed to expose the roof of the nasopharynx and the clivus which lies immediately posterior to it. Sometimes the vomer comes away bringing with it the anterior part of the sphenoid sinus, on other occasions it is necessary to remove it piecemeal. It is then possible to insert a modified Dingman gag (Fig. 6) to retract the

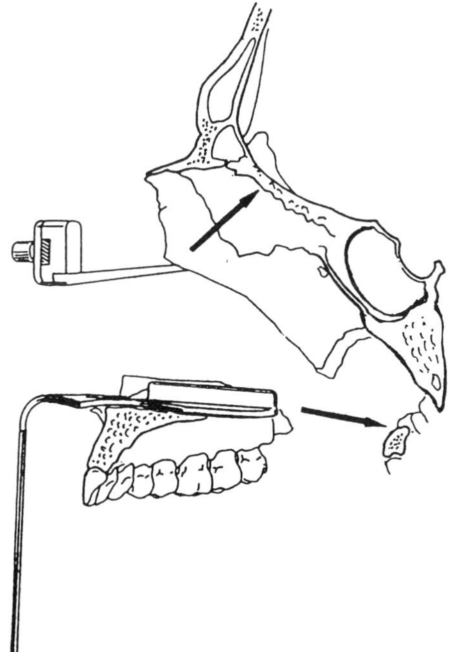

Fig. 5. Detached portion of maxilla lowered into oral cavity. Solid black arrows indicate exposure of skull base (medial aspect of split skull)

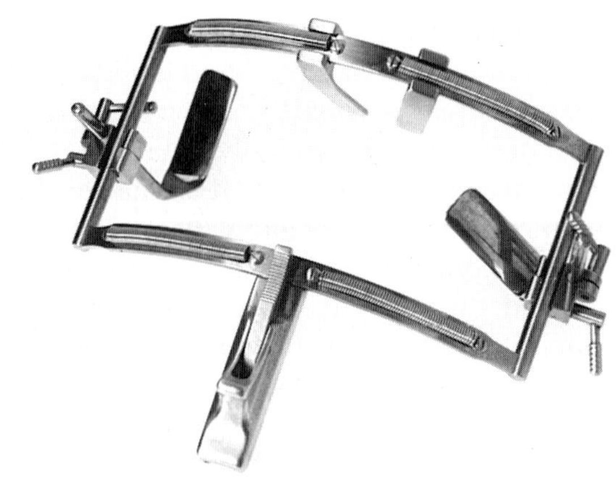

Fig. 6. Modified Dingman gag used in le Fort operation

cheeks laterally and displace the maxilla downwards. With this in position
the mucosa of the posterior pharyngeal wall is exposed, and the midline
structures of the skull base from the middle ethmoids down to the foramen
magnum become accessible. On rare occasions the anterior arch of the
atlas may be reached, usually in the edentulous. The tissues overlying the
clivus are divided by an incision in the midline from above downwards to
its lower border. The posterior pharyngeal wall is very firmly adherent to
the bone in this region. Subperiosteal resection by sharp dissection is usually required before these rather rigid layers can be retracted to each side,
using an instrument of our own design, to expose the whole of the anterior
aspect of the clivus. The compact bone over the pharyngeal surface of
the clivus, together with the underlying spongy bone, may be removed with
a high speed drill and the cutting burr, but when compact bone on the
dural aspect is encountered it is wise to change to a diamond burr, so that
the bone may be removed very gradually and with such delicacy that
the underlying dura is not torn. When the dura is exposed over a small
area it can be separated from the bone to which it is attached quite
readily using a blunt dissector. The bone margins of the exposure may
be enlarged more rapidly now by using a combination of the drill and
Kerrison bone punches. One of the more disagreeable complications arises
as the bone removal edges superiorly, and this takes the form of profuse
venous bleeding from the basal sinuses. To the uninitiated this may be
quite alarming, but control is achieved using either an angled monopolar coagulator to force the dural sinusoid against the bone and then coa-
gulating it, or using a combination of oxidised cellulose mixed with a

sterile absorbable bone sealant to pack the sinusoids (Abseal, Ethicon, Edinburgh). Pathology in the clivus is fairly obvious so that bone removal is continued until normal bone margins are encountered again, or until it is considered that a radical removal has been accomplished and that further dissection is hazardous. Blood is transfused from an early stage to prevent sudden catastrophic losses which could lead to serious hypovolaemic and ischaemic consequences.

Opening the dura may be necessary when tumours extend intracranially e.g. meningiomas, and is always required when dealing with aneurysms. The dural incision may be made in any direction as repair will be achieved using an adhesive "sandwich", not by sutures. The method of dural repair has been dealt with in the introductory section of this chapter, and the reconstitution of the clival defect has also been touched upon there. When these have been accomplished the overlying pharyngeal mucosal edges are approximated and bonded together by means of the fibrin adhesive. The maxilla is replaced and anchored in position with Luhr Vitallium mini-compression plates applied in their pre-determined sites, and after this the buccal mucosa is closed by interrupted black silk sutures.

Post-operative nutrition is maintained with a puncture pharyngostomy through which a pharyngogastric tube is passed and secured to the skin on the side of the neck. The criteria for extubation and discontinuation of the lumbar drain have already been dealt with in the introductory section.

An extension of this procedure has been developed by James and Crockard, and is known as the "open door" or extended maxillotomy (James *et al.* 1991). In this the method is the same as regards the maxillotomy, but in addition the maxilla is divided into two halves from before backwards by a saw cut along the midline suture from above. The bone between the central incisor teeth is divided using a fine osteotome to avoid damage to the adjacent dental roots and the median section is completed by dividing the soft palate in the midline posteriorly. Once more the blood supply to the maxilla proved satisfactory, presumably from the mucoperiosteal vessels, and vascularisation appears to be as generous and forgiving in this situation as it was for the maxillotomy alone. The two separated halves of maxilla not only pass down into the mouth but also swing laterally to afford a better view of the craniocervical junction as well as the clivus. This technique has been of unique value in the management of hitherto untreatable neuraxial compression caused by basilar invagination in cases of osteogenesis imperfecta, and it also has a role to play in the treatment of patients with very long extradural space occupying lesions that extend below the foramen magnum, though much the same exposure may be obtained by combining the standard maxillotomy with a transoral approach and moving the maxilla up and down as required.

Complications (Table 4)

With major surgery of this order it is scarcely surprising that there are a variety of complications, some of them leading to a fatal outcome. Amongst the most mild are cranial nerve lesions, especially involving the sixth cranial nerve in operations at the upper end of the clivus but other cranial nerves may be injured as they pass through their bony foramina, and it is important to bear in mind that the distances from the midline to the foramina measured on a dried skull may have no relevance in situations where there is extensive tumour involvement or bony deformity. Of particular consequence are the lower cranial nerves IX to XII, as damage to these will lead to major difficulties in respect of maintaining an effective airway and a coordinated swallowing mechanism. Patients who suffer this complication live under the perpetual threat of aspiration: rather than being pleasures, eating and drinking become high risk activities, only to be undertaken with the utmost caution and life-long vigilance. The dangers of an aspiration pneumonia cannot be overstated: one of our patients with a clival meningioma succumbed in just this way after what was otherwise a very satisfactory complete excision of the tumour. An over-enthusiastic attack on the tumour may precipitate a premature encounter with the brain stem with deleterious consequences; fortunately this is rare in expert hands.

Major neurological trauma is usually secondary to vascular damage, which may either be delivered directly to the vertebral or basilar arteries during the course of dissection or manipulation, or alternatively to spasm which may occur as a result of mechanical irritation of the vessels, but which is seen more commonly as a consequence of subarachnoid haemorrhage, in the majority of cases where this has its origin in the posterior fossa. If this is seen at angiography, surgery is delayed until such time as

Table 4. *Complications: Transfacial Approaches*

Cranial nerve:	VI	Common
	IX-XII	Serious (Aspiration pneumonia)
Brain stem:	Ischaemic	
CSF fistulae:	Meningitis	
Airway obstruction:	Tracheostomy	
Local:	Facial anaesthesia	
	Dental anaesthesia	
	Palato-nasal fistulae	
	Velo-pharyngeal incompetence	
Mortality:	<4% (Author's series of 62 operations)	

Potential complications of transfacial surgery.

the spasm is judged to have disappeared, because to operate during its developement may lead to potentially catastrophic ischaemic damage. The final way in which vascular damage may occur is when suddenly the vertebo-basilar vessels have to assume a radically new contour following the removal of a major deforming mass. It is a matter of conjecture as to whether this may lead to distortion and mechanical occlusion of the basilar artery itself, or of the small perforating vessels arising from it, but occasionally infarction of the brain stem occurs after otherwise blameless surgery, and this is a plausible mechanism by which it may be mediated.

CSF fistulae have been discussed earlier, and the need for meticulous attention to dural closure has been stressed. The obvious danger of this complication is that meningitis may supervene, and this, even in the era of modern antibiotics, carries a significant morbidity and mortality.

With operations involving the upper respiratory tract there is always the potential danger of airway obstruction developing. Fortunately in our experience tracheostomy is required only rarely, and in these situations it is usually sufficient to begin with a minitracheostomy before contemplating anything more radical.

In terms of purely local damage it is theoretically possible for the viability of whole bone segments to be compromised, causing extensive ischaemic necrosis which would necessitate considerable surgical ingenuity in order to restore aesthetic and functional integrity. In the extended maxillotomy procedure there is the risk of instability developing between the two halves of the palate, which may necessitate further measures to restore essential functional rigidity. It is possible that focal damage to the palate may occur, leading to the formation of a palato-nasal fistula. This is obviously a matter of greater moment when the underlying pathology has been responsible for bone softening. Surgical repair of these fistulae is not usually particularly satisfactory and they are best occluded by a dental plate. Of even greater consequence is the development of velo-pharyngeal incompetence. This is a severe defect not readily treated by any method. It is caused by scarring and shortening of the soft palate which then fails to occlude the nasal passages during the course of swallowing resulting in nasal regurgitation and potential problems in terms of airway management, as well as significant changes in the patient's voice. Some form of palatopharyngoplasty is the best way of dealing with this major complication.

Comparison with Other Methods

In this section the advantages and disadvantages of various other approaches to the clivus are evaluated and compared to the transfacial approaches.

Lateral or posterior fossa approaches are more commonly used for approaching skull base tumours than are the anterior approaches, although the latter are gaining in popularity and being used more extensively. The lateral and posterior approaches are essentially transdural techniques, which means that one has to open the dura overlying the cerebral or cerebellar cortex before having to open the dura yet again for extradural lesions in the clivus. This seems to be an otiose manoeuvre, particularly as there may be difficulties in achieving a CSF proof seal by this type of approach. None of these methods gives consistently troublefree access to the clivus, and none of them afford adequate exposure to the whole of the clivus without a considerable risk of sacrificing major neurovascular structures due to strenuous retraction. It is presumably a long-term familiarity with these methods which leads to their continued employment: they are not exactly ideal for the purpose, and it would appear to be stretching their practical limitations to the utmost to persist in their use unless the circumstances permit of no alternative. It does have the benefit for those who find it difficult to work in a team to continue to work in isolation; but there is nothing to suggest that these methods are so intrinsically superior to the anterior approaches that their benefits may be offset against the increased morbidity that must inevitably accrue to them due to the effect of the greater degree of retraction required for the exposure of the pathology.

The fronto-temporal or pterional approach (Yasargil *et al.* 1978) has been described for rostral clival tumours with extension into the middle fossa, and for tumours located on and around the anterior clinoid processes and extending mainly anteriorly. This route is also suitable for the treatment of most basilar tip aneurysms. Large tumours involving more of the clivus than just the posterior clinoid processes would not be dealt with adequately using this method. Superior access may be obtained using the fronto-zygomatic approach with or without additional local osteotomies, because this reduces the depth of the operating field by 2–3 cm and greatly increases the angle of approach, from being high and acute to low and obtuse on the floor of the middle fossa (Fujitsu *et al.* 1985, Neil-Dwyer *et al.* 1988, Uttley *et al.* 1991). But for the same reasons that limit the pterional approach it is not satisfactory for lesions of the middle and lower clivus. The most useful of the transcranial approaches is the subtemporal transtentorial approach (Malis 1985, Yasargil *et al.* 1980). If necessary the posterior limb of this incision may be extended down over the squamous part of the occipital bone so that a retromastoid lateral suboccipital craniectomy may be performed at the same time, thus giving access to virtually the whole of the ipsilateral aspect of the clivus (Samii *et al.* 1989). The vein of Labbe should be carefully preserved throughout, and Malis (Malis 1985) has suggested a means of leaving this intact whilst still obtaining generous petrosal access, and by the same token it is possible to preserve the sigmoid sinus (Samii *et al.* 1989). The disadvantages of the method are those of any middle fossa approach, namely that brain retraction may lead to epilepsy and aphasia in the dominant hemisphere due to temporal lobe retraction (Yasargil *et al.* 1980). Frequent release of the retractors for short periods is said to minimise this risk, but manoeuvres of this sort tend to interfere adversely with concentration. As one approaches the clivus the risk of causing damage to cranial nerves or to the perforating branches of the vertebro-basilar system appreciably increase. These complications are present to the same extent when one adopts the lateral sub-occipital approach to the clivus (Malis 1985). Indeed the risks to the lower cranial nerves are greater here if one has to operate between and around the multiple tiny roots out of which they are formed. And likewise for vascular damage. If the tumour spreads within the dura to involve the nerve roots and/or vascular structures there is only a remote chance of safely achieving a complete removal, but even in these unfavourable circumstances the lateral sub-occipital approach may act as a means of providing a useful decompression, especially when dealing with indolent meningiomas. In Mayberg's series only 4 (15%) of 26 patients who had a subtotal removal of their meningiomas showed signs of clinical progression, and these cases went on to die (Mayberg *et al.* 1986).

There are a number of extradural lateral approaches which may be used for a limited approach to the clivus. The transcochlear approach introduced by House and Hitselberger (House *et al.* 1976) accomplishes its purpose by extending in an anterior direction the translabyrinthine aperture they had utilised for operations in the cerebellar pontine angle. Clearly this technique must involve mobilisation of the facial nerve which therefore places it in jeopardy. The bone removal extends centrally as far as the ipsilateral internal carotid artery. The method may be used for excising lesions of the petrous apex and tumours directly arising from the adjacent portion of the clivus. It would appear to be satisfactory only for small lesions, and not suitable for the very large lesions that one finds not uncommonly in this region. The operation automatically results in ipsilateral deafness and a significant risk of facial paresis, which is a high price to pay for access, although in mitigation it should be noted that cerebellar and brain stem manipulation is obviously reduced in comparison to the transcranial techniques. The infratemporal fossa approach as described by Fisch (Fisch *et al.* 1979) also involves unilateral deafness, loss of facial sensation due to the division of branches of the Vth cranial nerve, a slight risk of facial paresis, and, in common with all the lateral approaches, it is most suitable for use in tumours at the petro-clival junction rather than those centrally situated in the clivus. Again this method would appear to work best for relatively small lesions rather than for larger ones, due to the limitations imposed on extensive dissection in terms of the depth of the operative field and the restricted angles through which the surgeon has to operate. In over a hundred cases of the infratemporal fossa approach there was a 7% complication rate of CSF fistulae, and approximately half of these cases developed meningitis (Fisch *et al.* 1979). A combined intradural subtemporal and extradural infratemporal preauricular approach has been described which gives access to the ventral portion of the brain-stem between the dorsum sella and the hypoglossal foramen (Sen *et al.* 1990), but it would appear more suitable for lesions of the petrous apex than clival pathology, and suffers from the common restraints on ease of repetition that it shares with the other lateral approaches.

The lateral transtemporal transsphenoidal approach to the skull base avoids some of the morbidity and access problems that may occur with the transcochlear and infratemporal approaches. The tedious dissection associated with these two techniques is replaced by a much more straightforward procedure (Holliday 1986). Although it is essentially an extradural method it could readily be adapted to deal with intradural pathology. It offers the same advantages as the fronto-zygomatic approach in that the zygoma may be mobilised and rotated out of the surgical field, and in addition the temporomandibular joint may be disarticulated and retracted inferiorly to provide access to the infratemporal region. Holliday, who describes the method, records four clival dissections in his series (Holliday 1986).

The use of a high cervical incision offers an alternative lateral approach, but it does involve mobilising the distal portions of the extracranial carotid arteries which may be damaged, and involves the sacrifice of some of the upper cervical nerves. The technique was one of the earliest to be described in the approach to the clivus as it avoided bacterial contamination from the oral cavity (Fox 1967, Stevenson *et al.* 1966, Wissinger *et al.* 1967), and it has been described again in this context more recently (McAfee *et al.* 1987). Even with the additional modification of a labiomandibulotomy the surgical exposure does not permit access to the upper part of the clivus (Biller *et al.* 1981, Krespi *et al.* 1984), though Ammirati *et al.* in a series of cadaveric dissections have extended this approach to encompass a mandibulotomy linked to detachment of the pharynx from the skull base as being the vital elements of a combined oral and cervical attack that gives access to both the midline and the lateral compartments of the skull base, with total exposure of the clivus and cranio-cervical junction, and the added benefit of complete neurovascular control of the internal carotid arteries and lower cranial nerves (Ammirati *et al.* 1993). The original advantage of this lateral extradural method was that CSF leaks occurred into a sterile environment and did not pass into the contaminated nasal and oral cavities, but this has long ceased to be an important consideration with the widespread use of prophylactic antibiotics and effective waterproof seals. With all the lateral approaches, whether they are transcranial or extradural, the major objection to their use in this type of surgery is the considerable difficulty and danger that would be experienced in trying to repeat the operation through dense scar tissue for clinical recurrence, and it is perhaps an index of the hazards involved that none of the authors comment on this crucial aspect of management.

Anterior approaches to the clivus have evolved over the last 20 years as a result of surgeons having to think afresh about pressing clinical problems. These have forced themselves onto the surgical agenda by a revolution in imaging which has changed radically the perception of skull base disorders, together with comparable advances in surgical technology that enable them to be dealt with more effectively. Few of the methods are new. Most of them were described many years ago in other contexts, long before their conscription into the current canon of skull base surgery under the banner of surgical teamwork. This in its turn has been a spur to innovation, and considerable ingenuity has been exercised in determining how to exploit these technical advances most profitably. After the first flush of enthusiasm for each new application there has been a period of retrenchment where more sober counsels have attempted to assess its efficacy against exisiting standards, and this process is reaching a point where reasoned operative protocols are becoming available in certain instances.

The simplest of these methods is of course the transoral approach which was first used for the drainage of retropharyngeal abscesses (Fang *et al.* 1962), but has equally successfully been used in a variety of conditions including resection of the odontoid peg for basilar impression in rheumatoid disease (Crockard *et al.* 1990, Scoville *et al.* 1951), atlantoaxial dislocation (Greenberg *et al.* 1968), congenital anomalies of the craniocervical junction (Gilsbach *et al.* 1983, Menezes *et al.* 1988), excision of extradural (Mullan *et al.* 1966) and intradural (Uttley *et al.* 1989) tumours and clipping of vertebrobasilar aneurysms (Archer *et al.* 1987, Uttley *et al.* 1993). A number of modifications have been made to the method to improve access, namely splitting the palate (Alonso *et al.* 1971, Kennedy *et al.* 1986) or division of the mandible (Arbit *et al.* 1981, Delgado *et al.* 1981, Gilsbach *et al.* 1983, Krespi *et al.* 1988), or both. Even with these improvements access to the clivus is limited by the retracted soft tissue, particularly bilateral retraction of the divided soft palate which interferes with exposure of the upper parts of the clivus so that only the lower 50% of it is readily accessible with these methods. The fear of CSF fistulae and subsequent meningitis has lead some authors to suggest that this should only be used for extradural lesions, but this is a view that cannot be sustained in the light of present practice.

The transbasal approach of Derome (Derome 1988), and the more recently described "extended" transbasal approach using orbital osteotomies (Sekhar *et al.* 1992), give access to the ethmoid sinuses and to the whole of the clivus apart from that portion that lies in the vicinity of the pituitary fossa. Dissections of the lower part of the clivus down to the foramen magnum would appear to be difficult in view of the distances involved and exceptionally long instruments are required for this purpose. The possibility of producing tiny unrecognised dural tears in the anterior fossa and in the clival dura are high, thus great care has to be taken in the repair of both the dura and the floor of the anterior fossa and clivus. In Derome's early work it was suggested that autologous bone grafts should be used for this purpose, but recent work has demonstrated that this is unnecessary and an adequate repair may be achieved using a graft of fat to close the anterior fossa floor, which also reduces the surgical difficulties if the operation has to be repeated (Sekhar *et al.* 1992).

The transsphenoidal approach permits access to the region of the sella and the uppermost part of the clivus, but even if the floor and anterior wall of the sella are removed and attempts to rotate the pituitary forwards are successful, the exposure is confined to the region of the posterior clinoid processes and the adjacent part of the clivus, which is where the basilar venous sinusoids are most prolific. The control of these is notoriously difficult because of the constraints imposed by the restricted access, and thus it would appear sensible to reserve this technique for the purposes of biopsy in this region rather than definitive tumour removal, which may prove costly (Laws 1985). Transethmoidal and transantral approaches to the clivus are even more limited in terms of clival exposure than the transsphenoidal approach and have the disadvantage that they are not true anterior approaches, which may lead to difficulties with orientation during dissection, and although they are well known they are unsatisfactory for the resection of extensive clival lesions.

The transfacial approaches (Curioni *et al.* 1984, Hernandez Altemir 1986) are superior to the transantral approach in that although it is essentially the same pathway that is used, exposure is very much better due to the mobilisation of the cheek and the maxilla being hinged laterally on the zygoma, which enables the microscope to be employed with greater freedom in this situation, although again it is not the most satisfactory means of approaching the clivus.

The more extensive approach of the midfacial degloving operation, offers better access to the central skull base and a wide variety of lesions have been excised using this method (Price *et al.* 1988). The inevitable complications of the method, namely infraorbital and dental sensory loss are relatively minor and usually resolve (Fig. 7).

For reasons outlined earlier the le Fort 1 maxillotomy is the most logical approach for dealing with extensive clival lesions. The method exposes the whole of the clivus including adjacent structures up to the

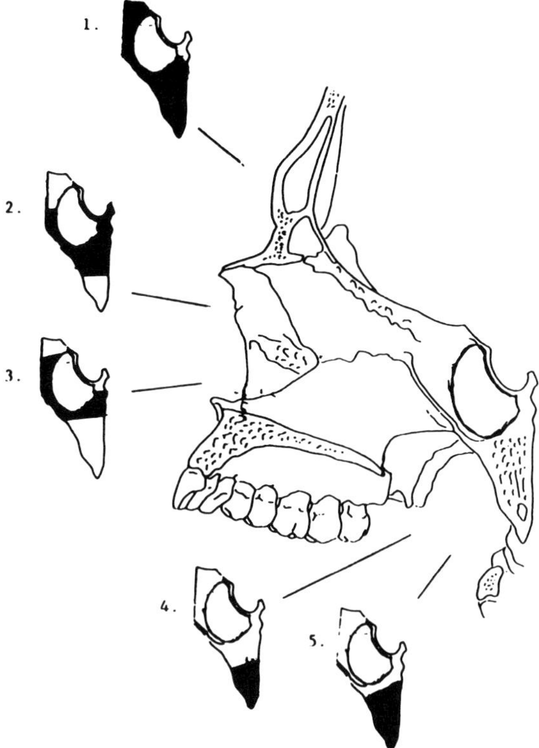

Fig. 7. Clival exposure (shaded black) of anterior approaches: *1* transbasal, *2* transfacial, midfacial degloving, *3* transsphenoidal, transethmoidal, transantral, *4* transoral, and *5* transcervical

middle ethmoid air sinuses (always), and down to the craniocervical junction (infrequently) (Fig. 8). Very often no additional manoeuvres are required, although it is possible to split the palate and/or mandible in dealing with large midline tumours extending above and below the foramen magnum; it may be conveniently combined with the transbasal technique, or even with lateral exposures where circumstances demand it. Recent techiques have helped to render the method extremely safe by enabling CSF fistulae to be obliterated more easily after dealing with intradural lesions, so that the complication rate and mortality are gratifyingly low for the excellent exposure that is obtained (Uttley *et al.* 1989). Finally, and most importantly, bearing in mind the type of pathology that is present in this region, its superiority is demonstrated by the facility with which the method may be repeated over and over again, if it becomes necessary, without increasing the difficulties of surgery or escalating the risks of damage to the neurovascular structures which unfortunately bedevil all the other approaches (Uttley *et al.* 1989).

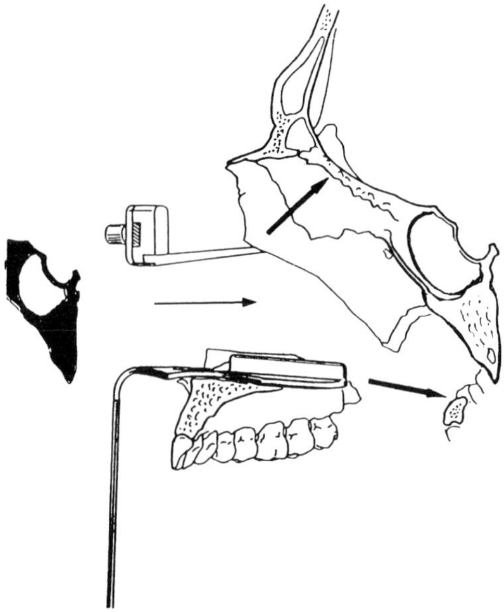

Fig. 8. Clival exposure (shaded black) of le Fort 1 maxillotomy

Conclusions

Recent investigative and surgical developements have kindled a growing interest in skull base surgery and paved the way for a new look at methods for attaining access to lesions in the vicinity of the clivus. A number of operative strategies exist, and their respective merits have been disccussed in this chapter. It would appear that the le Fort I maxillotomy provides optimal exposure of this region, and in its "extended" mode gives access to the adjacent upper cervical spine.

New materials have enabled a waterproof dural closure to be achieved routinely, so that it is possible to operate upon intradural lesions safely.

In view of the pathology encountered in this region operations should be capable of repetition without unduly increasing technical difficulty or escalating the risks of neurovascular damage.

In an ideal world this type of work should be undertaken in designated centres professing a special interest in skull base problems, which are fully equipped to provide up-to-date facilitites for the overall management of patients by a dedicated multidisciplinary team.

Acknowledgements

My grateful thanks to Mrs Rebecca Smith for her help in the preparation of this manuscript.

References

1. Alonso WA, Black P, Connor GH *et al* (1971) Transoral transpalatal approach for resection of clival chordoma. Laryngoscope 81: 1626–1631
2. Ammirati M, Ma J, Cheatham ML, Mei ZT, Bloch J, Becker DP (1993) The mandibular swing-transcervical approach to the skull base: anatomical study. J Neurosurg 78: 673–681
3. Arbit E, Patterson RH Jr (1981) Combined transoral and median labiomandibular glossotomy approach to the upper cervical spine. Neurosurgery 8: 672–674
4. Archer DJ, Young S, Uttley D (1987) Basilar aneurysms: a new transclival approach via maxillotomy. J Neurosurg 67: 54–58
5. Arriaga MA, Janecka IP (1989) Surgical exposure of the nasopharynx: anatomic basis for a transfacial approach. Surg Forum 40: 547–549
6. Biller HF, Shugar JMA, Krespi YP (1981) A new technique for wide field exposure of the base of the skull. Arch Otolaryngol Head Neck Surg 107: 689–702
7. Bohlman HH (1979) Acute fractures and dislocations of the cervical spine—an analysis of three hundred hospitalised patients and review of the literature. J Bone Joint Surg Am 61: 1119–1142
8. Casson PR, Bonnano PC, Converse JM (1974) The midface degloving procedure. Plast Reconstr Surg 53: 102–113
9. Chiari O (1912) Ueber eine Modifikation der Schlofferschen Operation von Tumoren der Hypophyse. Wien Klin Wochenschr 25: 5–6
10. Cook RJ, Uttley D, Wilkins PR, Archer DJ, Bell BA (1994) Prolactinomas in men masquerading as invasive skull base tumours. Br J Neurosurg 8: 53–57
11. Crockard HA, Calder I, Ransford AO (1990) One stage transoral decompression and posterior fixation in rheumatiod atlanto-axial subluxation. J Bone Joint Surg Br 72B: 682–685
12. Crockard HA, Sett P, Geddes JF, Stevens JM, Kendall BE, Pringle JS (1991) Damaged ligaments at the cranio-cervical junction presenting as an extradural tumour: a differential diagnosis in the elderly. J Neurol Neurosurg Psychiatry 54: 817–821
13. Curioni C, Padula E, Toscana P, Maraggia A (1984) The maxillo-cheek flap. Presented at the 7th Congress EAMFS, Paris
14. Delgado TE, Garrido E, Harwick RD (1981) Labiomandibular transoral approach to chordomas of the clivus and upper cervical spine. Neurosurgery 8: 675–679
15. Derome PJ (1988) The transbasal approach to tumours invading the skull base. In: Schmidek HH, Sweet WH (eds) Operative neurosurgical techniques, vol 1. Grune and Stratton, New York, pp 619–633
16. Drommer RB (1986) The history of the "le Fort I osteotomy". J Maxfac Surg 14: 119–122
17. Fang HSY, Ong GB (1962) Direct approach to the upper cervical spine. J Bone Joint Surg Am 4: 1588–1604
18. Fisch U, Pilsbury HC (1979) Infratemporal fossa approach to lesions in the

temporal bone and base of the skull. Arch Otolaryngol Head Neck Surg 105: 99–107

19. Fox JL (1967) Oliteration of midline vertebral artery aneurysm via basilar craniectomy. J Neurosurg 26: 406–412

20. Fujitsu K, Kuwabara T (1985) Zygomatic approach for lesions in the interpeduncular cistern. J Neurosurg 62: 340–343

21. Gilsbach J, Eggert HR (1983) Transoral operations for cranio-spinal malformations. Neurosurg Rev 6: 199–209

22. Greenberg AD (1968) Atlanto-axial dislocations. Brain 91: 655–684

23. Griffith HB, Veerapen R (1987) A direct transnasal approach to the sphenoid sinus. J Neurosurg 66: 140–142

24. Guiot G (1978) In: Fahlbusch R, Werder KV (eds) Treatment of pituitary adenomas. Thieme, Stuttgart

25. Halstead EA (1910) Remarks on the operative treatment of tumors of the hypophysis with the report of two cases operated on by an oro-nasal method. Surg Gynecol Obstet 10: 494–502

26. Hamberger CA, Hammer G, Norlen G, Sjogren B (1961) Transantrosphenoidal hypophysectomy. Arch Otolaryng (Chicago) 74: 2–8

27. Hardy J, Wigser S (1965) Transsphenoidal surgery of pituiary fossa tumors with televised radioflouroscopic control. J Neurosurg 23: 612–619

28. Henderson WR (1939) The pituitary adenomata: a follow-up study of the surgical results in 338 cases (Dr. Harvey Cushing's Series). Br J Surg 26: 811–921

29. Hernandez Altemir F (1986) Transfacial access to the retromaxillary area. J Maxfac Surg 14: 165–170

30. Hirsch O (1910) Endonasal method of removal of hypophyseal tumors. With report of two successful cases. JAMA 55: 772–774

31. Holliday MJ (1986) Lateral transtemporal-sphenoid approach to the skull base. Ear Nose Throat J 65: 153–162

32. House WF, Hitselberger WE (1976) The transcochlear approach to the skull base. Arch Otolaryngol Head Neck Surg 102: 334–342

33. Hout WM, Arafah BM, Salazar R, Selman W (1988) Evaluation of the hypothalamic-pituitary-adrenal axis immediately after pituitary adenectomy: is perioperative steroid therapy necessary? J Clin Endocrinol Metab 66: 1208–1212

34. Huelke DF, O'Day J, Mendelsohn RA (1981) Cervical injuries suffered in automobile crashes. J Neurosurg 54: 316–622

35. Hurwitz LJ, Shepherd WHT (1966) Basilar impression and disordered metabolism of bone. Brain 89: 223–233

36. James JA (1967) Transethmosphenoidal hypophysectomy. Arch Otolaryngol 86: 256–264

37. James D, Crockard HA (1991) Surgical access to the base of skull and upper cervical spine by extended maxillotomy. Neurosurgery 29: 411–416

38. Janecka IP, Sen CN, Sekhar LN, Arriaga MA (1990) Facial translocation: a new approach to the cranial base. Otolaryngol Head Neck Surg 103: 413–419

39. Kanavel AB (1909) Removal of tumors of the pituitary body by an infranasal route. JAMA 53: 1704–1707

40. Kennedy DW, Papel ID, Holliday M (1986) Transpalatal approach to the skull base. Ear Nose Throat J 65: 125–133

41. Krespi YP, Har-el G (1988) Surgery of the clivus and anterior cervical spine. Arch Otolaryngol Head Neck Surg 114: 73–78

42. Krespi YP, Sisson GA (1984) Transmandibular exposure of skull base. Am J Surg 148: 534–538

43. von Langenbeck B (1859) Beitrage zur Osteoplastic—die osteoplastische Resektion des Oberkiefers. In: Reimer, Goshen A (eds) Deutsche Klinik, Berlin

44. Laws ER Jr (1985) Cranial chordomas. In: Wilkins RH, Rengachary SS (eds) Neurosurgery, vol 1. McGraw-Hill, New York, pp 927–929

45. List CF (1941) Neurologic syndromes accompanying developemental anomolies of occipital bone, atlas and axis. J Arch Neurol Psychiatry 45: 577–618

46. Malis LI (1985) Surgical resection of tumours of the skull base. In: Wilkins RH, Rengachary SS (eds) Neurosurgery, vol 1. McGraw-Hill, New York, pp 1011–1020

47. Marks JS, Sharp J (1981) Rheumatoid cervical myelopathy. Q J Med 199: 307–319

48. Mayberg MR, Symon LD (1986) Meningiomas of the clivus and apical petrous bone. Report of 35 cases. J Neurosurg 65: 160–167

49. McAfee PC, Bohlman HH, Riley LH, Robinson RA, Southwick WO, Nachles NE (1987) The anterior retropharyngeal approach to the upper part of the cervical spine. J Bone Joint Surg Am 69: 1371–1383

50. Meijers KA, Cats A, Kramer HP, Lyuendijk W, Onvlee GJ, Thomeer RTW (1984) Cervical myelopathy in rheumatoid arthritis. Clin Exp Rheumatol 2: 239–245

51. Menezes AH, VanGilder JC (1988) Transoral-transpharyngeal approach to the anterior craniocervical junction. J Neurosurg 69: 895–903

52. Mullen S, Naunton R, Hekmat-Panah J, Vialati G (1966) The use of the anterior approach to ventrally placed tumours in the foramen magnum and vertebral column. J Neurosurg 24: 536–543

53. Neil-Dwyer G, Sharr M, Haskell R, Currie D, Hosseini M (1988) Zygomaticotemporal approach to the basis cranii and basilar artery. Neurosurgery 23: 20–22

54. Price JC (1986) The midfacial degloving approach to the central skull base. Ear Nose Throat J 65: 174–180

55. Price JC, Holliday MJ, Kennedy DW, Johns ME, Richtmeier WJ, Mattox DE (1988) The versatile midface degloving approach. Laryngoscope 98: 291–295

56. Redlund-Johnell I (1984) Dislocations of the cervical spine in rheumatoid arthritis. Thesis. Malmo University, pp 69–89

57. Rock JP, Tomecek FJ, Ross L (1993) Transoral surgery: an anatomic study. Skull Base Surg 3: 109–116

58. Rosegay H (1981) Cushings legacy to transsphenoidal surgery. J Neursurg 54: 448–454

59. Samii M, Ammirati MD, Mahran A, Bini W, Sepehrnia A (1989) Surgery of petroclival meningiomas: report of 24 cases. Neurosurgery 24: 12–17
60. Schloffer H (1907) Erfolgreiche Operation eines Hypophysentumors auf nasalem Wege. Wien Klin Wochenschr 20: 621–624
61. Scoville WB, Sherman IJ (1951) Platybasia. Report of ten cases with comments on familial tendencies, a special diagnostic sign, and the end results of operation. Ann Surg 133: 469–502
62. Sekhar LN, Nanda A, Sen C, Snyderman CN, Janecka IP (1992) The extended frontal approach to tumors of the anterior, middle, and posterior skull base. J Neurosurg 76: 198–206
63. Sen CN, Sekhar LN (1990) The subtemporal and preauricular infratemporal approach to intradural structures ventral to the brainstem. J Neurosurg 7: 345–354
64. Spillane JD, Pallis C, Jones AM (1957) Developemental abnormalities in the region of the foramen magnum. Brain 80: 11–53
65. Stapleton SR, Wilkins PR, Archer DJ, Uttley D (1993) Chondrosarcoma of the skull base: a series of eight cases. Neurosurgery 32: 348–356
66. Stevenson GC, Stoney RJ, Perkins RK, Adams JE (1966). A transcervical transclival approach to the vertebral surface of the brain stem for removal of a clivus chordoma. J Neurosurg 24: 544–551
67. Svien HJ, Litzow TJ (1965) Removal of certain hypophyseal tumors by the transantralsphenoid route. J Neurosurg 23: 603–611
68. Uttley D (1993) In: Lynn J, Bloom SR (eds) Surgical endocrinology. Butterworths Heinemann, London pp 171–192
69. Uttley D, Archer DJ, Marsh HT, Bell BA (1991) Improved access to lesions of the central skull base by mobilisation of the zygoma: experience with 54 cases. Neurosurgery 28: 99–104
70. Uttley D, Archer DJ, Taylor WAS, Bell BA (1993) Midline aneurysms of the vertebrobasilar junction: an effective anterior approach. Br J Neurosurg 7: 389–394
71. Uttley D, Moore AJ, Archer DJ (1989) Surgical management of mid-line skull base tumors: a new approach. J Neurosurg 71: 705–710
72. Watkins LD, Uttley D, Archer DJ, Wilkins PR, Plowman N (1992) Giant-cell tumours of the sphenoid bone. Neurosurgery 30: 576–581
73. Wellbourn RB (1986) The evolution of transsphenoidal pituitary microsurgery. Surgery 100: 1185–1190
74. Wilson CB (1984) A decade of pituitary microsurgery. J Neurosurg 61: 814–833
75. Wissinger JP, Danoff D, Wisiol ES, French LA (1967) Repair of an aneurysm of the basilar artery by a transclival approach. Case report. J Neurosurg 26: 417–419
76. Yasargil MG, Mortara RW, Curcic M (1980) Meningiomas of the basal posterior cranial fossa. Adv Tech Stand Neurosurg 7: 3–115
77. Yasargil MG, Smith RD, Gosser JR (1978) Microsurgery of the internal carotid artery and its branches. Prog Neurol Surg 9: 58–121

Presigmoid Approaches to Skull Base Lesions

M. T. Lawton,[1] C. P. Daspit,[2] and R. F. Spetzler[1]

Division of [1]Neurological Surgery and [2]Neuro-Otology, Barrow Neurological
Institute, St. Joseph's Hospital and Medical Center, Phoenix, AZ (U.S.A.)

With 8 Figures

Contents

Introduction

A critical component of many skull base approaches is the safe removal
of the petrous bone (Brackmann *et al.* 1994, Baldwin *et al.* 1994, Spetzler
et al. 1992, Sekhar *et al.* 1994, Al-Mefty *et al.* 1988, Hitselberger and
House 1966, House 1979, Morrison and King 1973). Petrosectomy opens a
corridor of exposure to the center of the skull base. The transpetrosal
approaches include the retrolabyrinthine (Spetzler *et al.* 1994), translabyrinthine (Brackmann *et al.* 1992, House 1979, Morrison and King 1973),
transcochlear (House and Hitselberger 1976), and middle fossa approaches
(House and Shelton 1992, Brackmann *et al.* 1994). Still, exposure gained
from these approaches can be limited medially at the region of interest or
inadequate for larger lesions. Therefore, transpetrosal approaches have
been used in combination with other approaches to gain even more exposure. For example, the combined supra- and infratentorial approach joins
the subtemporal and transpetrosal exposures (Daspit *et al.* 1991, Spetzler

et al. 1992, Spetzler *et al.* 1991, Hitselberger and House 1966) and the far-lateral combined supra- and infratentorial approach adds to them the far lateral exposure (Baldwin *et al.* 1994, Heros 1986, Sen and Sekhar 1990, Sen and Sekhar 1991, Spetzler and Grahm 1990b, Baldwin *et al.* 1995). We have continued to experiment with combination approaches, and one that has proven useful is the orbitozygomatic-combined supra- and infratentorial approach. This chapter reviews the surgical anatomy and techniques involved with the transpetrosal approaches, discusses the various combination approaches that use petrosectomy as their foundation, and identifies the current indications for these techniques.

The Transpetrosal Approaches

We categorize the temporal bone dissection into three variations: retrolabyrinthine, translabyrinthine, and transcochlear (Table 1). The retrolabyrinthine approach removes temporal bone between the semicircular canals anteriorly and the posterior fossa dura on the posterior aspect of the temporal bone. The semicircular canals are skeletonized, but not violated, to maximize this working space. The translabyrinthine approach removes the semicircular canals, which causes loss of hearing (Brackmann *et al.* 1992, House 1979). Their removal increases the exposure anteriorly to the internal auditory canal (IAC). The transcochlear approach requires the facial nerve to be dissected from its bony canal and transposed to gain access to the cochlea for its removal (House and Hitselberger 1976). This approach enables almost complete removal of the petrous bone, with maximum exposure of the brain stem and clivus. The three types of temporal bone dissections represent a graduated increase in the amount of petrous bone resected with a corresponding increase in anterior exposure. The price of this increased exposure is progressively greater sacrifice of function of the seventh and eighth cranial nerves.

Extended Retrolabyrinthine Approach

The patient is positioned supine with the head turned away from the lesion, bringing the midline parallel to the floor and inclined slightly downward.

Table 1. *Preservation of Cranial Nerve Function*

Approach	Hearing	Facial nerve
Retrolabyrinthine	Preserved	Preserved
Translabyrinthine	Sacrificed	Preserved
Transcochlear	Sacrificed	Transient paralysis or paresis

The mastoid bone becomes uppermost in the operative field. A shoulder roll under the ipsilateral shoulder minimizes neck rotation. The skin is incised at the zygoma 1 cm anterior to the tragus and curves gently around the ear to the mastoid tip. The scalp flap is retracted inferiorly with fish-hooks and a Leyla bar (Spetzler 1988).

Basic mastoidectomy is performed first. We prefer the MedNext (Med-Next Co., Riviera Beach, FL) high-speed drill over the Osteon (Zimmer Assoc., Santa Barbara, CA) drill used previously because it is more powerful, weighs less, and has less torque. The operating microscope and suction-irrigation are essential. An initial cut is made along the temporal line, the ridge that continues from the superior border of the zygomatic arch posteriorly to the mastoid cortex, marking both the inferior limit of temporalis muscle insertion and the floor of the middle fossa (tegmen of the temporal bone). A second cut is made perpendicularly, running inferiorly to the mastoid tip immediately behind the posterior canal wall. Mastoid cortex is then removed widely and rapidly with a large burr. It is important that the neurotologist remove superficial bone extensively, because residual bone along the posterior canal wall or mastoid tip constricts operating space, limits viewing angles, and obscures anatomical landmarks. Bone in the sinodural angle and covering the sigmoid sinus is removed completely to allow retraction of the sinus posteriorly.

The sigmoid sinus, middle fossa dura, and sinodural angle between them are the first important landmarks. The superior petrosal sinus lies deep to the sinodural angle and represents the posterior-superior margin of the temporal bone. Dissection into the mastoid antrum reveals the horizontal semicircular canal, which leads the surgeon to other anatomy, including the external genu of the facial nerve medially and inferiorly, the posterior semicircular canal posteriorly, and the epitympanum and superior semicircular canal anteriorly. The posterior and superior semicircular canals are skeletonized, drilling as far anteriorly as possible (Fig. 1). Resection of temporal bone above and below the otic capsule exposes medial middle fossa dura, the superior petrosal sinus, and the jugular bulb. A large dural surface is thereby exposed which, when opened, accesses the cerebellopontine angle. The retrolabyrinthine approach provides excellent exposure of the angle but does not provide exposure of the anterior brain stem.

Translabyrinthine Approach

The translabyrinthine approach is used when greater exposure is needed. The initial part of this approach is the same as the retrolabyrinthine approach. The neurotologist proceeds by removing all three semicircular canals and skeletonizing the posterior half to two-thirds of the IAC

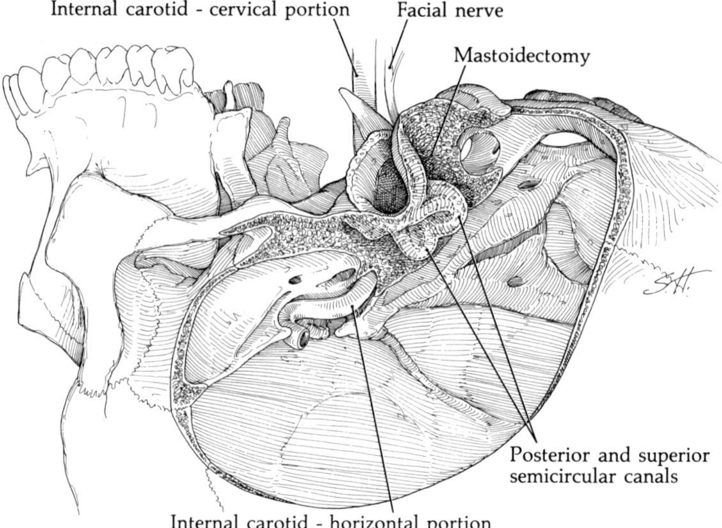

Fig. 1. The extended retrolabyrinthine approach consists of mastoidectomy and skeletonization of the semicircular canals. [With permission of Barrow Neurological Institute®]

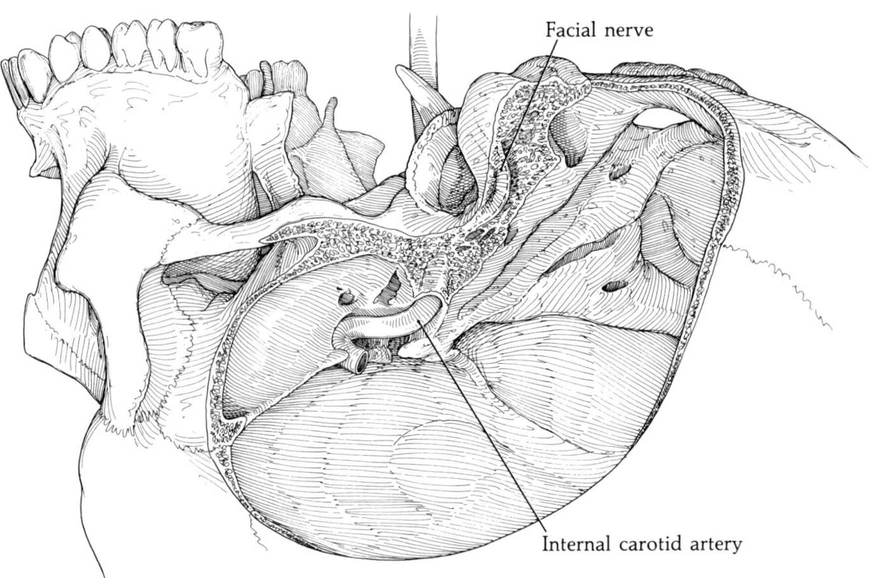

Fig. 2. The translabyrinthine approach removes the semicircular canals and skeletonizes the descending segment of the facial nerve and internal auditory canal. [With permission of Barrow Neurological Institute®]

(Fig. 2). The medial walls of the vestibule and superior semicircular canal ampulla represent the lateral wall of the IAC fundus, so minimal bone removal at this location exposes IAC. The superior vestibular nerve lies posterosuperiorly in the canal and is encountered first. This nerve is separated from the facial nerve anterosuperiorly by a shelf of bone, Bill's bar. Therefore, the superior vestibular nerve is an important landmark in identifying the facial nerve as it exits the IAC and courses anteriorly to the geniculate ganglion. The facial nerve is guarded carefully throughout the drilling with the aid of facial nerve monitoring. It is skeletonized with a diamond bit along its horizontal (tympanic) segment, external or second genu, and descending (mastoid) segment. The nerve is left in its thinned bony canal to minimize risk of injury. Additional exposure is gained by removing bone anteriorly and medially above the IAC in Kawase's triangle. Typically, the sigmoid sinus is unroofed to the jugular bulb to maximize inferior exposure beneath the IAC.

After this extensive bone removal, the exposure is more anterior than that of the retrolabyrinthine approach. The cerebellopontine angle, anterolateral brain stem, and inferior clivus are visualized. However, the exposure is obtained at the expense of ipsilateral hearing and has an increased risk of cerebrospinal fluid (CSF) leakage.

Transcochlear Approach

The trancochlear approach is a forward extension of the translabyrinthine approach that mobilizes the facial nerve, removes the cochlea, and opens into the cerebellopontine angle to expose anterolateral brain stem and clivus (House and Hitselberger 1976). This approach gives the maximum exposure that can be achieved by a transpetrosal approach by essentially resecting the entire petrous bone (Fig. 3).

The initial procedure is the same as for the translabyrinthine approach, except the external auditory canal is transected and oversewn in two layers. The facial nerve is skeletonized along its course from its entrance into the internal auditory canal to its exit from the stylomastoid foramen. An extended facial recess opening is performed. The facial recess is a tract of air cells bounded medially by the descending segment of the facial nerve, laterally by the chorda tympani, and superiorly by the fossa incudis. Opening the facial recess exposes the middle ear space, the stapes and incus, the promontory of the cochlea, Jacobson's nerve, and the horizontal segment of the facial nerve. The facial recess is opened into the epitympanum and the ossicles are removed. The chorda tympani is sectioned inferiorly at its origin from the descending portion of the facial nerve, allowing the facial recess to be extended inferiorly to the hypotympanum and retrofacial area. The greater superficial petrosal nerve is sectioned anteriorly at its origin

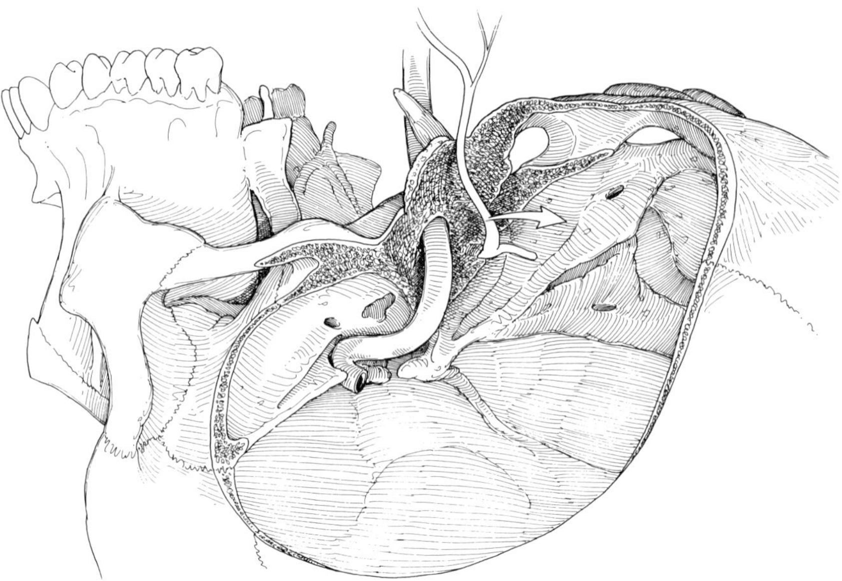

Fig. 3. The transcochlear approach requires transposition of the facial nerve posteriorly and removal of the cochlea. [With permission of Barrow Neurological Institute®]

from the geniculate ganglion. These maneuvers free the facial nerve, which is transposed posteriorly after dissection from its bony canal.

The cochlea is then drilled out completely, beginning with the promontory that houses the basal turn. Bone removal is carried forward to the septum between the basal turn and the internal carotid artery. The internal carotid artery and internal jugular vein leave the carotid sheath and enter the skull base in proximity to each other. The jugulocarotid septum, a ridge of bone that separates the carotid artery as it turns anteriorly from the jugular vein as it turns posteriorly, is removed to expose the jugular bulb completely. The close relationship of the ninth, tenth, and eleventh cranial nerves must be remembered to avoid injuring them. During the extensive drilling of the temporal bone, the dura of the internal auditory canal is kept intact to protect this part of the facial nerve.

When the drilling is completed, the entire tympanic portion of the temporal bone is removed. Superiorly, the superior petrosal sinus is exposed from the sinodural angle laterally to Meckel's cave medially. Inferiorly, the inferior petrosal sinus and jugular bulb are exposed. Bone removal extends medially to the clivus and anteriorly to the internal carotid artery and periosteum of the temporomandibular joint. The bone surrounding the carotid artery can be removed superiorly to the middle fossa floor and medially to the siphon, thereby creating the exposure needed for a saphenous vein bypass graft from the petrous segment to supraclinoid segment of the carotid artery, if necessary (Spetzler *et al.* 1990a).

The transcochlear approach gives the greatest exposure of the trans-petrosal approaches. A wide triangular corridor is opened leading directly to the clivus. The approach sacrifices hearing and increases the risk of CSF leakage. Mobilization of the facial nerve increases the risk of facial paresis or paralysis (Spetzler *et al.* 1994, Spetzler *et al.* 1992).

The Combination Approaches

Combined Supra- and Infratentorial Approach

There are three essential components of the combined approach (Daspit *et al.* 1991, Spetzler *et al.* 1994, Spetzler *et al.* 1992, Spetzler *et al.* 1991, Hitselberger and House, 1966). First, one of the temporal bone dissections described above is performed. Second, a supra- and infratentorial cra-niotomy is made that crosses the transverse sinus. Third, the tentorium is divided to connect the supra- and infratentorial compartments. Extensive exposure of the medial petrous and clival regions and associated neuro-vascular structures is obtained with minimal brain retraction.

When the neuro-otologist has completed the temporal bone drilling, an edge of middle fossa dura is exposed above the petrosectomy defect and an edge of posterior fossa dura is exposed behind the sigmoid sinus (Fig. 4). These epidural locations serve as burrholes for a subtemporal-suboccipital craniotomy that crosses the transverse sinus. A large dural surface is ex-posed with visualization of the transverse, sigmoid, and superior petrosal sinuses. Before the dura is opened, the brain is relaxed with hyperventila-tion, mannitol, and removal of CSF through a lumbar drain. The dura is incised anteriorly over the temporal lobe and curves posteriorly and infe-riorly to the superior petrosal sinus below where it enters the sigmoid sinus. A second dural incision is made inferiorly in front of the sigmoid sinus, curving up to the superior petrosal sinus. The superior petrosal sinus is cauterized or clipped and divided. The surgeon should be aware of a low-lying vein of Labbé that could be injured during the dural opening.

The sigmoid sinus may be sacrificed if the contralateral transverse and sigmoid sinuses are patent angiographically and communicate with the ipsilateral transverse and sagittal sinuses through a patent torcular hero-phili. As an added assurance, sigmoid sinus pressures are measured before and after test occlusion of the sigmoid sinus. We have observed no eleva-tions of more than 7 mm Hg when angiographic patency of the sinuses has been confirmed (Spetzler *et al.* 1992). If the pressure were to rise by more than 10 mm Hg with test occlusion, the sinus should be kept intact. These measurements are made after the superior petrosal sinus has been divided.

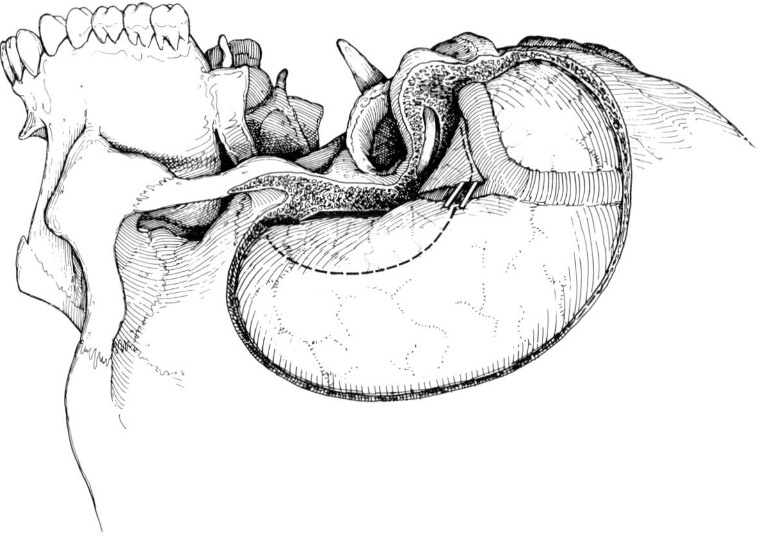

Fig. 4. The dural incision for the combined supra- and infratentorial approach crosses the superior petrosal sinus below where it enters the sigmoid sinus, thereby preserving the sigmoid sinus. [With permission of Barrow Neurological Institute®]

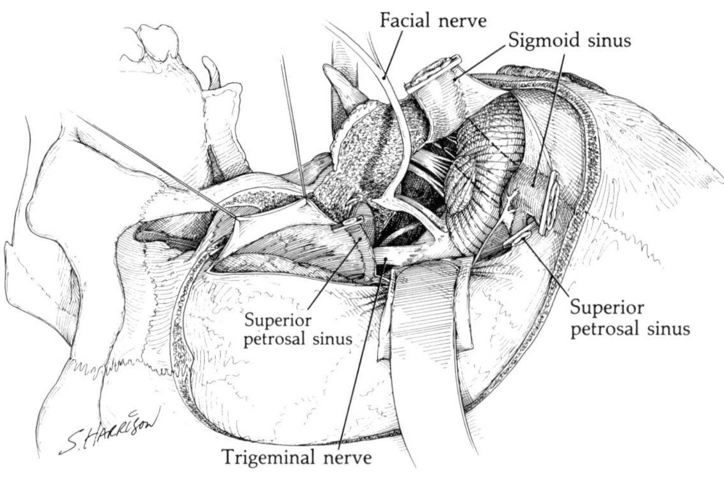

Fig. 5. Incising the tentorium medially to the tentorial incisura exposes the cranial nerves, brain stem, vasculature, and clivus. Note that the sigmoid sinus has been divided. [With permission of Barrow Neurological Institute®]

The sigmoid sinus can be sacrificed safely when these angiographic and hemodynamic criteria are met. It is divided below its confluence with the superior petrosal sinus. The vein of Labbé consistently and reliably enters the transverse sinus above this junction and will therefore drain contralaterally. Notwithstanding these safety concerns, division of the sigmoid sinus is only necessary when additional exposure is needed and we have not sacrificed the sigmoid sinus in more than 3 years.

When the dural incisions are completed and the superior petrosal sinus has been divided, the tentorium is incised medially to the tentorial hiatus, posterior to the fourth cranial nerve (Fig. 5). This crucial maneuver connects the supra- and infratentorial compartments and relaxes neural structures. The posterior temporal lobe is elevated, while the surgeon is careful to preserve the vein of Labbé which is tethered to the transverse sinus. The petrous region, clivus, brain stem, cranial nerves, and vessels of the posterior circulation are well visualized. The lesion is accessed by working between adjacent cranial nerve bundles. The approach gives wide exposure along the skull base from the foramen magnum to above the dorsum sella with minimal brain retraction.

Far Lateral-Combined Supra- and Infratentorial (Combined-Combined) Approach

Occasionally petroclival lesions span the entire length of the posterior fossa from above the petrous apex to below the foramen magnum. For these lesions, a combination approach joining the transpetrosal, subtemporal, and far-lateral approaches overcomes the limitations of just a transpetrosal approach (Baldwin *et al.* 1994, Baldwin *et al.* 1995). This approach is the most extensive of the combination approaches and is referred to as the "combined-combined" approach. The far-lateral approach has been well-described elsewhere/Spetzler *et al.* 1994, Heros 1986, Sen and Sekhar 1990, Sen and Sekhar 1991, Spetzler and Grahm 1990b) but is simply a lateral extension of a unilateral suboccipital approach that removes additional lateral occipital bone, the inferior foramen magnum, the posterior half of the condyle, and the arch of the first cervical vertebra. Bone removal gives a more anterior angle to the inferior clivus and upper cervical region, enabling access to the anterolateral brain stem, lower cranial nerves, and the vertebrobasilar junction. When used with the combined supra- and infratentorial approach, the entire petroclival region is exposed.

An important modification to the far-lateral approach is the patient's position (Spetzler *et al.* 1994, Spetzler and Grahm 1990b). We use a modified park-bench position with the patient on his or her side, lesion side upward. The operating table is extended by placing a 3/4-inch plastic board under the mattress and pulling both the mattress and board 20 cm beyond the edge of the table. The patient is positioned so that the dependent arm hangs over the extended end of the table, cradled in a padded sling in the gap between the Mayfield head holder and its attachment to the table. This position improves venous return, minimizes brachial plexus compression, and enables better positioning of the head.

Unlike other transpetrosal approaches, the head is not placed in the straight lateral position. Three maneuvers position the head optimally: (1) flexion in the anteroposterior plane until the chin is one finger's breadth from the sternum, (2) rotation 45° away from the side of the lesion (*down*), and (3) lateral flexion 30° down toward the opposite shoulder. The clivus is then perpendicular to the floor, allowing the surgeon to look down the axis of the basilar artery and work between horizontally arrayed cranial nerves. The ipsilateral mastoid process becomes the highest point in the operative field, and the posterior cervical-suboccipital angle is opened maximally to increase the surgeon's operating space.

The hockey-stick incision used for the far-lateral approach is enlarged, beginning anteriorly at the zygoma, coursing superiorly around the pinna and toward the inion, and ending inferiorly in the midline at C4. A myocutaneous flap is elevated to expose the lateral temporal bone, mastoid, posterior cranium, and laminae of C1 and C2. A cuff of nuchal fascia is left to reattach the cervical muscles at the end of the procedure.

Bone removal consists of four parts: petrosectomy, C1 laminotomy, craniotomy, and condylar expansion. The neuro-otologist first drills the temporal bone. Rotation of the head can be adjusted during the petrosectomy to bring the head parallel to the floor to facilitate drilling. The arch and lateral mass of C1 are exposed, and the vertebral artery is dissected along its course from the transverse foramen to its dural entry point. The arch of C1 is removed with the Midas Rex (Midas Rex™, Inc. Fort Worth, TX) drill. The lateral cut is made at the sulcus arteriosus, and additional atlantal bone is removed until the transverse foramen is reached. If necessary, the foramen can be opened dorsally and the artery mobilized. The craniotomy cut then connects the foramen magnum with the anterior margin of the petrosectomy overlying the inferior temporal lobe, crossing the transverse sinus. A second cut connects the lateral foramen magnum with the posteroinferior margin of the petrosectomy, immediately behind the sigmoid sinus. The underlying dural sinuses are dissected carefully from the bone flap, which is then removed. Finally, the lateral aspect of the foramen magnum, jugular tubercle, and posteromedial two-thirds of the occipital condyle are removed. The extreme lateral removal of bone minimizes retraction and maximizes exposure of the anterior brain stem along this route.

The dura can be opened either in two flaps in front of and behind the sigmoid sinus to preserve this structure or in a single flap that sacrifices the sigmoid sinus. The two dural flaps are simply the standard openings for the combined approach plus the standard opening for the far-lateral approach. The latter opens the dura in the midline at the C1 level and extends laterally in an L shape below the dural entry point of the vertebral artery and extends superiorly to the sinodural angle. The lateral cuts enable the dura and vertebral artery to be pulled laterally against the margin of the craniotomy. When the presigmoid dural opening of the combined approach is completed, two windows of exposure are opened on either side of the preserved sigmoid sinus. In contrast, sacrificing the sigmoid sinus and crossing it below the sinodural angle join these two incisions to create a single flap extending from the anterior margin of the craniotomy over the temporal lobe, across the sigmoid sinus, and down to the C1 level (Fig. 6). When the tentorium is incised to the hiatus, a large unobstructed opening is created that exposes the anterolateral brain stem from the midbrain to the upper cervical spinal cord (Fig. 7). Arachnoid dissection reveals the second through twelfth cranial nerves, both vertebral arteries, posteroinferior cerebellar arteries, anterior spinal artery, vertebrobasilar junction,

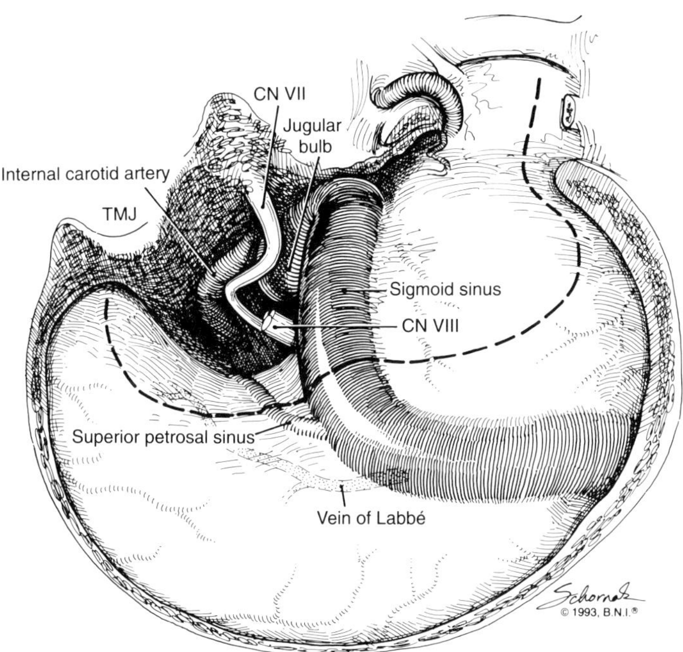

Fig. 6. The dural opening for the far-lateral-combined supra- and infratentorial ("combined-combined") approach. Alternatively, the dura can be opened in two flaps in front of and behind the sigmoid sinus to preserve this structure. (From Baldwin HZ, Miller CG, van Loveren HR *et al.* (1994) J Neurosurg 81: 60–68.)
[With permission of Journal of Neurosurgery]

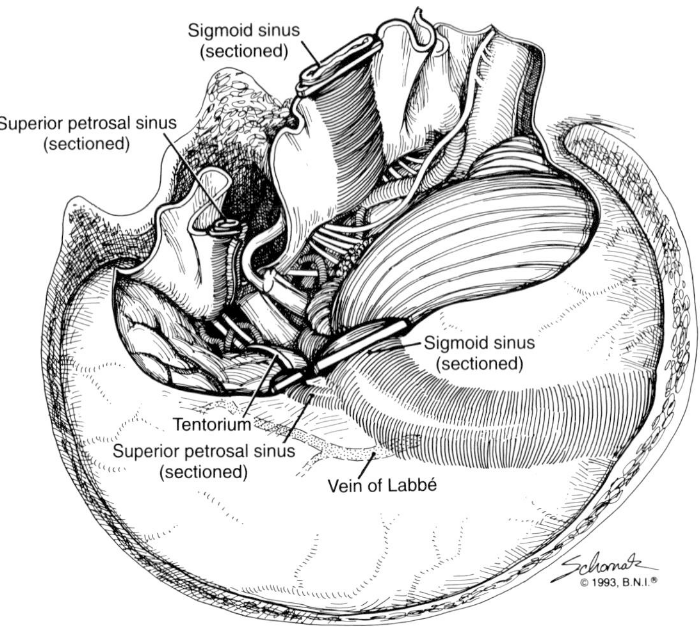

Fig. 7. An overview of the exposure provided by the far-lateral-combined supra- and infratentorial ("combined-combined") approach. (From Baldwin HZ, Miller CG, van Loveren HR *et al.* (1994) J Neurosurg 81: 60–68.) [With permission of Journal of Neurosurgery]

basilar artery, and the entire length of the clivus (Fig. 8) (De Oliveira *et al.* 1985). Division of the dentate ligaments facilitates surgical manipulation of neural structures.

The Orbitozygomatic-Combined Supra- and Infratentorial Approach

We have continued to experiment with new combination approaches to provide the exposure needed for complex skull base lesions. An approach that we have used extensively in recent years is the orbitozygomatic approach (Hakuba *et al.* 1986, Hakuba *et al.* 1989, McDermott *et al.* 1990, Ikeda *et al.* 1991, Lee *et al.* 1993). The technique removes the superior orbital rim and roof, lateral orbital rim and wall, and zygomatic arch in a single piece to allow downward retraction of the globe and an upward viewing angle to the anterior brain stem. It is ideal for gaining added exposure of the basilar artery terminus for high-riding aneurysms. We began using this approach mainly for such lesions and have had good results. The orbitozygomatic approach also provides a route to cavernous malformations that surface on the anterior midbrain. In addition, remov-

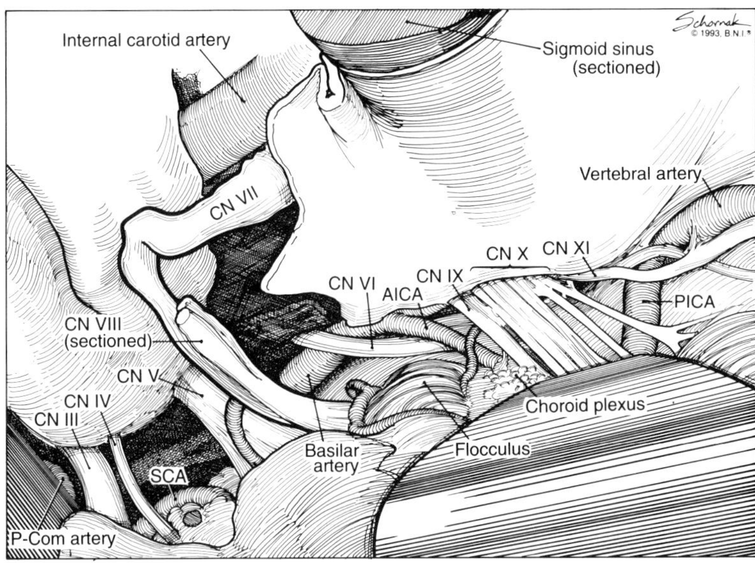

Fig. 8. A close-up view of the exposure provided by the far-lateral-combined supra- and infratentorial ("combined-combined") approach. (From Baldwin HZ, Miller CG, van Loveren HR *et al.* (1994) J Neurosurg 81: 60–68.) [With permission of Journal of Neurosurgery]

ing the zygoma gives the surgeon wide exposure of the middle fossa and an upward angle to medial lesions. When the orbitozygomatic craniotomy is combined with the combined supra- and infratentorial approach, the anterior, middle, and posterior fossae are widely exposed. A lesion at the center of the skull base encasing important arteries and cranial nerves can be accessed from various angles to optimize the dissection of these structures.

Current Indications for Transpetrosal Approaches

We have developed a plan for selecting the best approach or combination of approaches for dealing with petroclival lesions (Table 2). The critical factors are lesion location, size, pathology, and the patient's preoperative neurological function. Classically, the clivus is divided into thirds, and lesions located in the upper third are treated with a pterional or subtemporal approach. This orbitozygomatic approach has largely supplanted the pterional/subtemporal approach at this institution, but we routinely drill down lateral temporal bone as part of the orbitozygomatic craniotomy to provide subtemporal exposure if needed. Lesions confined to the middle third of the clivus are accessed through one of the transpetrosal approaches, and lesions of the lower third of the clivus are exposed through a far-lateral craniotomy.

Table 2. *Selection of Appropriate Approach*

Approach	Lesion location
Orbitozygomatic	upper 1/3 of the clivus
Transpetrosal	middle 1/3 of the clivus
Retrolabyrinthine	CP angle
Translabyrinthine	CP angle and anterolateral brain stem
Transcochlear	CP angle and anterior brain stem
Far lateral	lower 1/3 of the clivus
Combined	upper 2/3 of the clivus and middle cranial fossa
Combined-combined	entire clivus and middle cranial fossa
Orbitozygomatic-combined	upper 2/3 of clivus, entire middle cranial fossa, and anterior cranial fossa

CP cerebellopontine.

Usually, small lesions can be exposed adequately with one of these approaches. However, larger lesions are more likely to need one of the combination approaches. If the lesion involves the entire clivus and foramen magnum, the combined-combined approach may be required.

Once a decision has been made to drill the temporal bone, the surgeon must estimate the amount of temporal bone resection needed to obtain adequate exposure. This evaluation is balanced with an assessment of preoperative neurological function, specifically the function of the seventh and eighth cranial nerves. When the patient has good preoperative hearing and the surgeon wants to preserve it, temporal bone removal is limited to a retrolabyrinthine drilling. This approach exposes only the cerebellopontine angle and not the anterolateral brain stem, but it preserves both hearing and facial nerve function. Patients with poor preoperative hearing are well suited to translabyrinthine drilling, which gives anterolateral exposure of the brain stem at the expense of hearing and an increased risk of CSF leakage. When large lesions compressing the brain stem produce preoperative hearing loss and facial nerve deficits, a transcochlear approach is ideal. The increased exposure of the anterior brain stem is often critical, and preoperative deficits lessen the impact of the greater risk of facial paresis or paralysis.

Pathology is an important factor in selecting the approach. Vascular lesions typically require a more focused area of exposure. The pial surface of a cavernous malformation and the neck of an aneurysm must be visualized adequately (Sekhar *et al.* 1994). Such visualization can often be accomplished through more limited exposures that spare the patient extensive temporal bone drilling. In contrast, tumors typically require wide exposure and extensive temporal bone resection is unavoidable, as is the case with meningiomas, chordomas, chondrosarcomas, glomus tumors, and skull base carcinomas. However, some tumors are soft and more easily removed, and less exposure is needed for their removal. Schwannomas, epidermoids, and dermoid tumors may be dealt with through a more conservative craniotomy (Yasui *et al.* 1989).

References

1. Al-Mefty O, Fox JL, Smith RR (1988) Petrosal approach for petroclival meningiomas. Neurosurgery 22: 510–517
2. Baldwin HZ, Miller CG, van Loveren HR, Keller JT, Daspit CP, Spetzler RF (1994) The far lateral/combined supra- and infratentorial approach. A human cadaveric prosection model for routes of access to the petroclival region and ventral brain stem. J Neurosurg 81: 60–68
3. Baldwin HZ, Spetzler RF, Wascher TM, Daspit CP (1995) The far lateral-combined supra- and infratentorial approach: Clinical experience. Acta Neurochir (Wien) 134: 155–158
4. Brackmann DE, Green JD (1992) Translabyrinthine approach for acoustic tumor removal. Otolaryngol Clin North Am 25: 311–329
5. Brackmann DE, House JR, III, Hitselberger WE (1994) Technical modifications to the middle fossa craniotomy approach in removal of acoustic neuromas. Am J Otol 15: 614–619
6. Daspit CP, Spetzler RF, Pappas CTE (1991) Combined approach for lesions involving the cerebellopontine angle and skull base: Experience with 20 cases—preliminary report. Otolaryngol Head Neck Surg 105: 788–796
7. De Oliveira E, Rhoton AL, Jr, Peace D (1985) Microsurgical anatomy of the region of the foramen magnum. Surg Neurol 24: 293–352
8. Hakuba A, Liu S, Nishimura S (1986) The orbitozygomatic infratemporal approach: A new surgical technique. Surg Neurol 26: 271–276
9. Hakuba A, Tanaka K, Suzuki T, Nishimura S (1989) A combined orbitozygomatic infratemporal epidural and subdural approach for lesions involving the entire cavernous sinus. J Neurosurg 71: 699–704
10. Heros RC (1986) Lateral suboccipital approach for vertebral and vertebrobasilar artery lesions. J Neurosurg 64: 559–562
11. Hitselberger WE, House WF (1966) A combined approach to the cerebellopontine angle. A suboccipital-petrosal approach. Arch Otolaryngol 84: 267–285
12. House WF, Hitselberger WE (1976) The transcochlear approach to the skull base. Arch Otolaryngol 102: 334–342
13. House WF (1979) Translabyrinthine approach. In: House WF, Luetje CM (eds) Acoustic tumors, Vol 2: Management. University Park, Baltimore
14. House WF, Shelton C (1992) Middle fossa approach for acoustic tumor removal. Otolaryngol Clin North Am 25: 347–359
15. Ikeda K, Yamashita J, Hashimoto M, Futami K (1991) Orbitozygomatic temporopolar approach for a high basilar tip aneurysm associated with a short intracranial internal carotid artery: A new surgical approach. Neurosurgery 28: 105–110

16. Lee JP, Tsai MS, Chen YR (1993) Orbitozygomatic infratemporal approach to lateral skull base tumors. Acta Neurol Scand 87: 403–409
17. McDermott MW, Durity FA, Rootman J, Woodhurst WB (1990) Combined frontotemporal-orbitozygomatic approach for tumors of the sphenoid wing and orbit. Neurosurgery 26: 107–116
18. Morrison AW, King TT (1973) Experiences with a translabyrinthine-transtentorial approach to the cerebello-pontine angle. J Neurosurg 38: 382–390
19. Sekhar LN, Kalia KK, Yonas H, Wright DC, Ching H (1994) Cranial base approaches to intracranial aneurysms in the subarachnoid space. Neurosurgery 35: 472–483
20. Sen CN, Sekhar LN (1990) An extreme lateral approach to the intradural lesions of the cervical spine and foramen magnum. Neurosurgery 27: 197–204
21. Sen CN, Sekhar LN (1991) Surgical management of anteriorly placed lesions at the craniocervical junction—an alternative approach. Acta Neurochir (Wien) 108: 70–77
22. Spetzler RF (1988) Two technical notes for microsurgery. BNI Quarterly 4: 38–39
23. Spetzler RF, Fukushima T, Martin N, Zabramski JM (1990a) Petrous carotid-to-intradural carotid saphenous vein graft for intracavernous giant aneurysm, tumor, and occlusive cerebrovascular disease. J Neurosurg 73: 496–501
24. Spetzler RF, Grahm T (1990b) The far-lateral approach to the inferior clivus and the upper cervical region: Technical note. BNI Quarterly 6: 35–38
25. Spetzler RF, Daspit CP, Pappas CTE (1991) Combined approach for lesions involving the cerebellopontine angle and skull base: Experience with 30 cases. Skull Base Surg 1: 226–234
26. Spetzler RF, Daspit CP, Pappas CTE (1992) The combined supra- and infra-tentorial approach for lesions of the petrous and clival regions: Experience with 46 cases. J Neurosurg 76: 588–599
27. Spetzler RF, Hamilton MG, Daspit CP (1994) Petroclival lesions. Clin Neurosurg 41: 62–82
28. Yasui T, Hakuba A, Kim SH, Nishimura S (1989) Trigeminal neurinomas: Operative approach in eight cases. J Neurosurg 71: 506–511

Anterior Approaches to Non-Traumatic Lesions of the Thoracic Spine

A. Monteiro Trindade and J. Lobo Antunes

Hospital Santa Maria, Lisbon (Portugal)

With 32 Figures

Contents

Introduction

The decision on which approach to choose when dealing with pathology involving the thoracic spine depends on a number of factors such as the topography of the lesion, its extension, its relationship with the neural structures, its probable nature, its texture and vascular supply, the degree of resection one wishes to accomplish, and the need to stabilize the spine. Furthermore, the age and clinical status of the patient, and the prognosis of the disease, as well as the experience of the surgeon, should also be taken in consideration. It is clear that the simpler and the less traumatic the procedure, the better it is tolerated by the patient, who, particularly in cases of infectious or neoplastic processes, is often quite sick.

The posterior approaches, through a standard laminectomy, are not suitable for lesions involving the vertebral bodies, or located anteriorly to the cord, be they intra or extradural. The exposure achieved by a laminectomy gives limited access, not allowing a radical removal, or an adequate decompression of the cord, and may cause significant morbidity [16].

The anterior approaches to the thoracic spine, particularly through a thoracotomy, were initially developed to treat Pott's disease, in which it was found to be ideal to achieve all the objectives: cleaning of the septic foci, wide decompression, and secondary stabilization [11, 30]. This approach was later adopted to deal with infections of other aetiologies, tumours, complex fractures, congenital anomalies, vascular disorders, and various degenerative conditions such as the sinister thoracic herniated disc [1, 10, 30, 34, 48, 50, 76]. In this review, we will not deal with the traumatic pathology, and will use the herniated disc as the paradigm of the lesion to be approached anteriorly, although other surgical alternatives will be briefly discussed.

The anatomic peculiarities of the various segments—superior, mid and lower—, and the nature of the pathology, may require distinct avenues of approach. We emphasize the absolute requirement of a wide exposure, good visibility, and the use of microsurgical techniques and instrumentation.

For the upper thoracic spine from T1 to T3 the anterolateral, transpleural exposure through a thoracotomy is usually inadequate. A useful alternative is the median transsternal approach.

For the mid thoracic spine we prefer a transpleural route. The side of the thoracotomy depends on where is the bulk of the pathology located, and its nature. One should enter one or two intercostal spaces above the level, so a perpendicular view to the area involved is gained. One may also choose the space related to the lesion, so the rib directly connected to the pathology may be resected.

For the lower thoracic segments and the thoracolumbar transition we prefer a thoracoabdominal route, with a transpleural access through the 10th intercostal space, releasing the diaphragm at its costal attachment and exposing the upper lumbar vertebras retroperitoneally after section of the pillars of the diaphragm. This approach is easier on the left side, because of the difficulty of retracting the liver on the right side.

In this review we shall describe briefly the surgical anatomy relevant to the various surgical procedures, the general operative steps, the modifications dictated by the kind of pathology one has to deal with, and the complications the surgeon may have to face, based on our experience of more than sixty procedures for various kinds of disease process.

Surgical Anatomy

To approach the thoracic spine through an anterior route a detailed knowledge of the regional anatomy is indispensable [45]. During our description of the various operative procedures, we will point out the anatomical details we feel should be taken in consideration. Here we will emphasize the main general morphological features we deem particularly revelant (Figs. 1, 2).

1. The vertebral body has roughly a triangular shape. The posterior wall is markedly concave, the midline being 2–4 mm deeper than the lateral contours.

2. The width of the pedicle at its insertion, represents about half of the width of the body.

3. The head of the rib is connected to the articular facets present in the lateral surface of the vertebral body. These are two independent joint surfaces, which are separated by the posterolateral portion of the intervertebral disc. The inferior articular surface—which is numbered the same

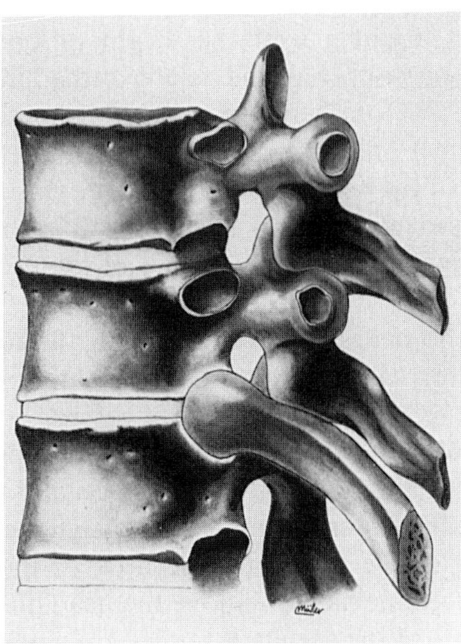

Fig. 1. Diagram of the lateral thoracic spine at the T7 to T9 segments. Note the relationships between the rib and the articular facets on the body and transverse process. The foramen and posterior aspect of the disc are hidden by the rib

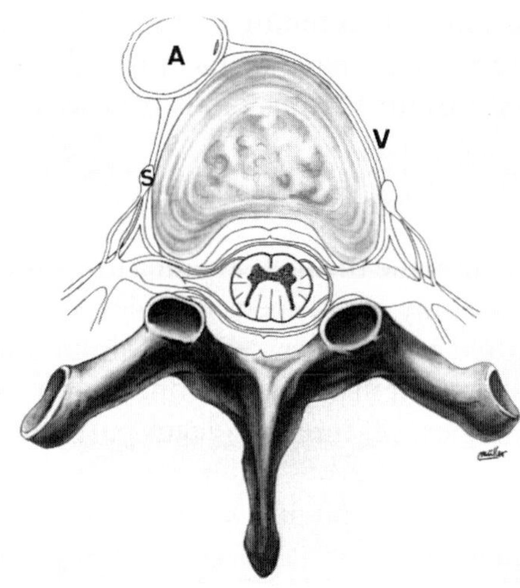

Fig. 2. Diagram depicting the relationships between the vascular and neural structures and the vertebra. Note: 1. The concavity of the posterior surface of the body. 2. The cord is anchored by short dural sleeves, and is central or slightly anterior, making it vulnerable to anterior compression. *A* aorta, *S* sympathetic trunk, *V* segmental vessels

way as the rib—has a height which is slightly larger than the pedicle, and its posterior limit corresponds to the point of insertion of the pedicle. Its height represents about a $\frac{1}{3}$ of the height of body. In contrast the superior facet represents only half the height of the inferior facet.

4. The intervertebral foramen is circumscribed anteriorly mostly by the vertebral bodies. In fact only $\frac{1}{3}$ corresponds to the intervertebral disc.

5. The insertion of the head of the rib is made through the radiate ligaments which are fused with lateral ligaments that connect the vertebral bodies. The area of insertion occupies $\frac{1}{2}$ or $\frac{1}{3}$ of the height of the vertebral body.

6. At the lower thoracic spine the 12th, 11th and occasionally the 10th rib are articulated only with the respective vertebral body and marginally with the disc.

7. The rib is also connected with the transverse process of the corresponding vertebra. The anterior limit of this union and the costal tuberosity where the corresponding inferior costotransverse ligament inserts, outline the posterior border of the foramen. The neck of the rib thus hides the pedicle, so to expose it, one has to remove the head and neck of the rib.

8. Lateral surfaces of the vertebral bodies are markedly concave.

9. The anterior longitudinal ligament is strongly adherent to the anterior contour of the disc, and more loosely attached to the bone surface. It thins out laterally, where it fuses with the expansions of the costovertebral

ligaments. Its thickness, elasticity, and resistance, makes it an excellent point of reference as the bone is progressively removed in cases of neoplastic or infectious pathology.

10. The posterior longitudinal ligament is also thicker in the midline. Its fibers are axially oriented, and this explains the possible occurrence of longitudinal lacerations following, for instance, hyperflexion of the spine.

11. The intervertebral disc has a height that corresponds to $\frac{1}{3}$ or $\frac{1}{4}$ to the height of the adjacent vertebras.

12. The thoracic spinal canal is almost cylindrical. The normal thoracic kyphotic curvature results from the wedge configuration of the bodies and discs. The pedicles are strictly oriented in a straight anteroposterior plane.

13. Between T4 and T7 the aorta has a close relationship with the left lateral surface of the vertebral bodies. It then moves medially to occupy a more anterior position, and at the level of the diaphragm is strictly prevertebral.

14. The superior hemiazygos vein occupies, on the left side, a position lateral to the aorta receiving collateral branches down to the 6th or 7th interspace. The azygos vein is lateral to the oesophagus on the right side, running inferiorly to join the superior vein cava at the 4th interspace. At the point where it turns medially it may receive some branches, which may be divided if necessary.

15. The segmental arteries run horizontally following the concavity of the vertebral body. At the level of the foramen they bifurcate into a radiculomedullary and an intercostal branch. There may be an anastomosis between adjacent vessels at this level.

16. The principal medullary artery, the artery of Adamkiewicz, is located on the left side in about 60% of the cases, and originates mostly between T9 and T11. This should be kept in mind when approaching the lower thoracic segment.

17. The sympathetic chain runs vertically, and lies on top of the heads of the ribs, at the anterior edge of the foramina. From the intercostal nerves the chain receives rami communicantes. Section of a few of these will be of no functional consequence as long as the major chain is preserved. From the inferior thoracic ganglia larger trunks are derived; these constitute the splanchnic nerves, and should be spared.

We deliberately omit the anatomical details of the posterosuperior mediastinum or of the thoracolumbar transition and the reader should consult the literature on the subject. Some of these procedures should be performed as a team approach with thoracic or general surgeons, if one is not familiar with the anatomical details and safe surgical routes in these areas.

Anterior Surgical Approaches [1, 10, 16, 30, 34, 42, 48, 49, 62, 75, 76]

Thoracotomy

For the left transthoracic approach the patient is placed in right lateral decubitus with a 30° posterior rotation. Adequate padding is placed under the right axilla, the right leg is flexed and the left is held semiflexed. The left upper limb is elevated and the patient is held securely with wide adhesive tape and a variety of supporting devices.

The left hemithorax, and the iliac crest are scrubbed. The cutaneous incision extends from the lateral border of the paraspinal muscles, to slightly beyond the anterior axillary line close to the chondrocostal joint (Fig. 3). The subcutaneous tissue and fat are incised with cautery down to the underlying muscles. The latissimus dorsi is dissected bluntly and cut, following the cutaneous incision. Underneath it, the serratus is released from the rib cage and sectioned; the lateral border of the trapezius may also have to be divided. The 6th or the 7th ribs are then identified, and the periosteum is separated with care not to harm the neurovascular bundle laying in the inferior groove.

The rib is then sectioned at the level of chondrocostal joint and at the posterior angle and the pleural cavity entered. A Gausset retractor is then placed and the lung gently collapsed manually and displaced anteriorly, thus exposing the posterolateral gutter and the aorta. The appropriate area is then identified with the help of an image intensifier. The following

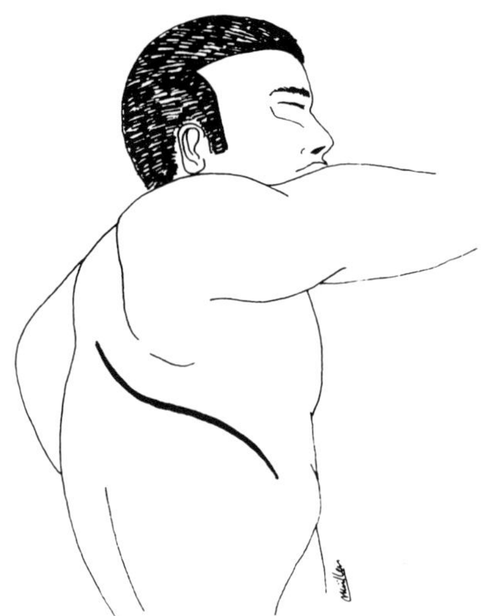

Fig. 3. Classic thoracotomy incision (6th or 7th interspaces) for a right side approach

surgical steps vary depending on the nature of the lesion and will be discussed in the ensuing sections.

After the lesion is dealt with, the pleura is closed, and the thoracic cavity drained in the usual fashion with two independent tubes. The periosteum and the intercostal muscles are closed with running sutures and the wall muscles closed in separate planes with reabsorbable material. The drains are kept with low pressure suction for 3 to 4 days.

Toraco-Abdominal Approach [27, 75, 76, 79]

To expose the T11 T12 and upper lumbar vertebrae, we open the 10th intercostal space, with or without rib resection. Once the pleura is opened and the lung collapsed, the diaphragm is sectioned from within about 1.5 cm of its posterior costal insertion to the lateral pillar. With digital blunt dissection a retroperitoneal plane is developed and the viscera displaced anteriorly and secured with a Doyen retractor.

The section of the arcuate ligament exposes completely the thoraco-lumbar transition. Care should be taken to preserve the sympathetic chain.

Transsternal Approach [1, 6, 34, 39, 48, 51, 62, 65, 72, 73]

This approach to the anterior upper thoracic spine may be undertaken through a skin incision that follows the anterior border of the sterno-cleido-mastoid muscle and is prolonged downwards to the level of the xyphoid process, or through a T incision in which the horizontal limb follows the lower cervical crease [39].

The strap muscles may have to be divided at their clavicular insertion, and the clavicle may be detached from the sternum on one side. After the pretracheal and precervical fascia are divided a sternotomy is done. After exposure and gentle retraction of the thymus, the left innominate vein is ligated and divided. The dissection then proceeds through the space between the left common carotid on one side, and the innominate artery, trachea, oesophagus and thyroid on the other. The anterior surface of the thoracic spine down to T5 is thus exposed.

Another alternative, the so-called "trap door" exposure, may be adopted. In this procedure the sternum is split down to the fourth inter-space, and the incision carried out laterally through the fourth interspace [51]. This is entered after ligation of the internal mammary vessels, splitting of the pectoralis major muscle, and incision of the intercostal muscles. The dissection in the neck follows the anterior border of the sterno-cleido-mastoid, transecting the omohyoid muscle, until the carotid sheath is visualized. All major vessels are dissected and isolated, the vagus, recurrent laryngeal nerve and phrenic nerves are identified. The trachea, larynx, thyroid, and oesophagus are gently displaced and the vertebral bodies exposed. This approach will give good anterior visualization, as well as a nice anterolateral approach on the side of the exposure.

Quite recently, a lateral approach combining a cervicotomy and a standard thoracotomy, with a costal flap situated at the level of the scapula, was also proposed [19]. The reader is referred to the original paper for the technical details of this complex procedure.

In any of these procedures a multidisciplinary approach is strongly recommended. It should be kept in mind that the surgeon is working between very delicate structures, with substantial risk of injuring the left recurrent laryngeal nerve, and is approaching the anterior column, with the dural tube completely hidden, so that the dissection has to proceed very cautiously.

Other Surgical Approaches

Although the main subject of this chapter is the transthoracic approaches to the spine, brief mention should be made of two alternative routes.

Transpedicular Approach

This was first proposed by Patterson and Arbit [52] for herniated discs; it may be used for laterally placed lesions [37], but gives limited access to midline hard discs or osteophytes.

This exposure is made through a midline incision, and subperiosteal dissection of the paraspinal muscles. After correct identification, the joint is partially removed with small Kerrison rongeurs and drills and the uppermost half of the pedicle of the inferior vertebral body, which is adjacent to the disc, is removed with fine drills. The disc is then identified. Care should be taken not to injure the root. The disc may then be entered with a #11 blade and part of its content removed. The space may be further enlarged with drills, and by carving the vertebral plates, particularly of the inferior body. With a small reverse curette and variety of other tools, the posterior longitudinal ligament may be brought into the cavity, and the disc fragments retrieved. This may be possible with soft, easily dissectable pieces, but the visualization is limited. If there are intradural fragments it may be necessary to open the dura, and this may require a laminectomy, but again, utmost care is required.

Posterolateral Thoracotomy [25, 28, 31, 35, 38, 44, 61, 66, 67, 81]

This approach is a modification of the classic costotransversectomy first performed by Menard in 1900. This type of thoracotomy is undertaken with the patient in a $\frac{3}{4}$ prone position. A paramedian, longitudinal or arciform incision is done, and the muscles are cut parallel to the midline, exposing at least two ribs, the lower one being the reference to the involved disc. The ribs are then isolated subperiosteally to the posterior tubercle, exposing 7 or 8 cm of the rib, which is then cut. The transverse processes are also removed. The parietal pleura is separated by blunt dissection, and the space should again be identified by appropriate image techniques. The superior $\frac{2}{3}$ of the adjacent pedicle is then removed and the juxta-foraminal segment of the disc visualized. As in the transpleural routes this intersomatic opening may be enlarged, and the disc material is removed as previously described. If the pleura is injured inadvertently, it should be promptly sutured, and no drainage is required.

We believe that the angle of vision is less favorable than with the transthoracic approach and the exposure of the anterior dural surface more constrained. This approach may also be indicated in infectious processes, when there is not a major intracanal component, or a major reconstructive procedure is not required [30, 57].

Herniated Thoracic Disc

Although the true incidence of herniated thoracic discs is difficult to ascertain, they represent less than 1% of all operated herniated discs. Of these, 50% are at the T8 T9 and T9 T10 interspaces, this pathology being exceedingly rare above the T4 level [38, 53, 59, 60, 61, 81].

They usually occur between the ages of 30 to 60, with a peak between 45 and 55 years. Interestingly, most of these patients will not demonstrate striking degenerative changes at either the cervical or lumbar segments but, quite often, there will be calcifications of the nucleus pulposus of the involved disc, and sometimes of the adjacent ones, without decrease in its height. Asymptomatic calcified intervertebral thoracic discs are frequently found in middle aged people but the risk of herniation is certainly extremely low.

From both the clinical and pathological points, it is useful to distinguish three different entities. The acute herniated disc is usually median, large, and heterogeneous in appearance (Figs. 4–6). Quite often there is a history of trauma, a few weeks prior to the sudden onset of the symptoms. This suggests a two step mechanism with an initial disruption of the annulus and laceration of the posterior longitudinal ligament, which is usually linear, axial, and close to the midline. Following additional motion, probably with an axial or flexion vector, there is extrusion of the degenerated disc material. Since the dural sac is anchored anteriorly by the short nerve roots, the dural sac is distended over the disc material, which is contained at this level, and this also facilitates its penetration into the

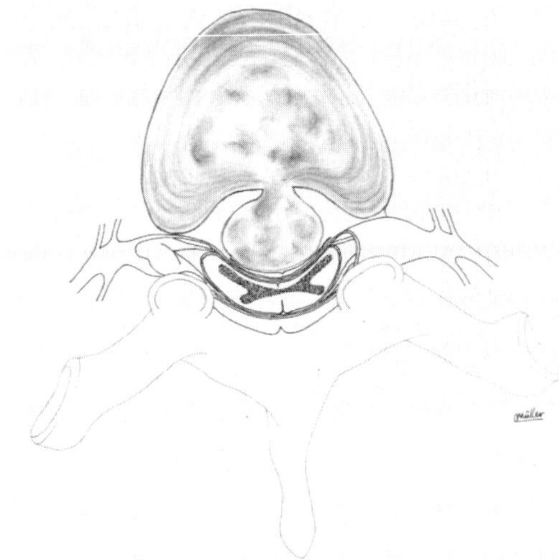

Fig. 4. Soft, central, extruded disc occupying half of the area of the spinal canal. Note that the fragment is "embraced" by the dura, tented by the emerging nerve roots

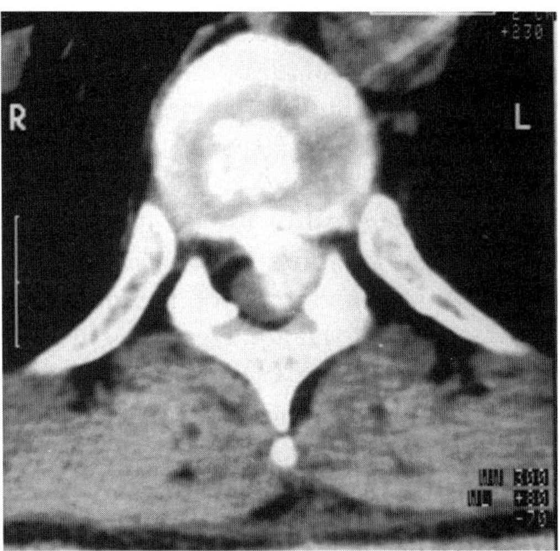

Fig. 5. CT. Horizontal cut at T9–T10 interspace demonstrating a calcified disc with a large herniated fragment, extruded through the posterior longitudinal ligament

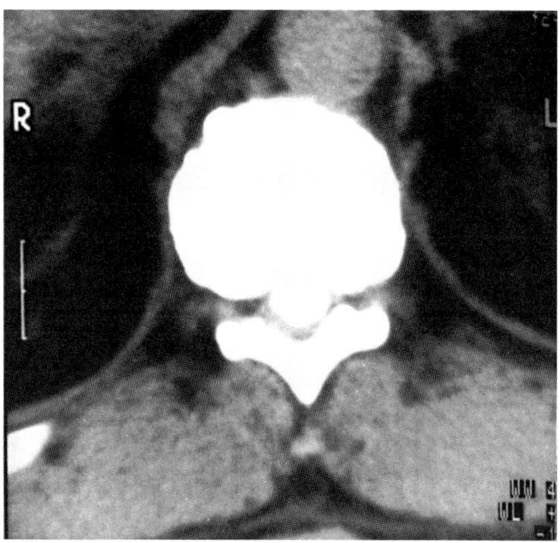

Fig. 6. CT. Horizontal cut—midline hard herniated disc at T10–T11

subdural space. In our experience, in only one instance was there a descending migration of the extruded fragment (Figs. 7, 8). The herniated material consists of creamy or liquid whitish material, and fragments with the typical appearance of degenerated fibrous cartilage.

The clinical history is often biphasic, with an initial history of violent direct trauma or fall. Except for acute, localized, midline pain, which subsides spontaneously or with strong analgesics, there are no other neurologic symptoms or signs. After a period of two to eight weeks, following a movement of flexion or rotation of the spine, a sudden severe neurological deficit, affecting both the motor and sensory pathways, develops, often without pain. Quite commonly the deficit is not symmetrical, and the patient presents a Brown-Séquard syndrome, even when imaging demonstrates a midline lesion. The sensory level corresponds to the level of the pathology. Compression of the corresponding spinous processes may induce acute pain or a Lhermitte's sign. Sphincter control is also lost. We have observed a symmetrical motor deficit only in the cases where diagnosis was delayed, or following an ill advised thoracic laminectomy. In less severe cases the motor pattern is segmental, involving the flexors of the thigh or the extensors of the leg and foot. Two cases presented an asymmetric posterior column syndrome, interpreted as a demyelinating disease. The prognosis is obviously much better in such patients. Acute pain, with an intercostal nerve radiation, with or without pyramidal signs, is rarer, even when the fragment is laterally located.

In some cases the evolution is subacute, and the neurological picture is progressive, slowly or in a stepwise fashion, although a sudden deteriora-

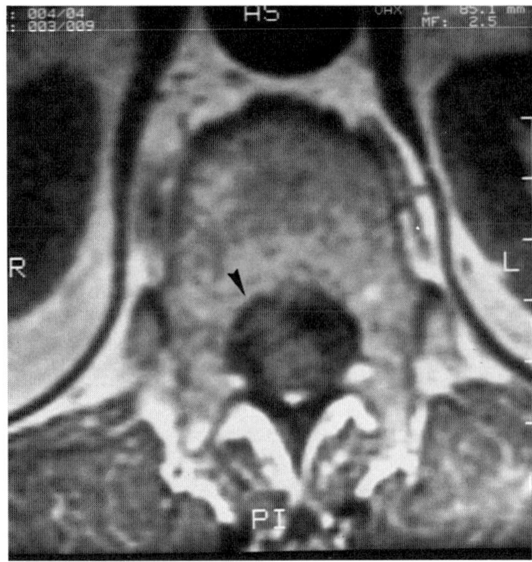

Fig. 7. MR. Horizontal cut at T10 level. Note the inferiorly migrated fragment (arrow)

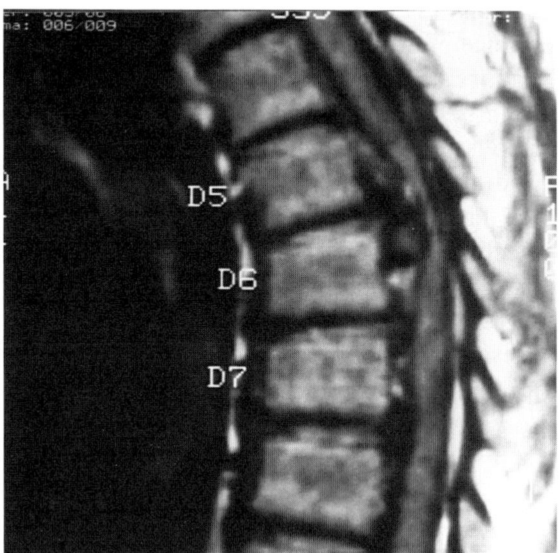

Fig. 8. MR. Sagittal cut at the T6 level. In this case there were multiple herniated disc fragments, one of which migrated inferiorly

tion may follow a fall or a sudden effort. As a rule, the motor deficit is not as pronounced, the sensory level not as clearly defined, and unilateral radicular pain quite striking. In such cases the herniated disc is usually asymmetrical, posterolateral or foraminal. The extruded component is not as pronounced but there are osteophytic spurs, which elevate the posterior longitudinal ligament. In our experience these changes are present at the lower thoracic segments, in congenitally narrowed canals, and may be aggravated by calcified ligamenta flava. A vascular component due to compression of a radicular artery cannot be excluded.

Chronic herniated discs, calcified osteophytic lesions, cause a progressive, slowly evolving picture suggestive of compressive myelopathy. There may be previous episode of spine trauma, and recurrent episodes of pain, ascribed to "rheumatism" or mechanical factors. The lesions responsible are true osteophytic spurs, that grow inside the canal from the vertebral plates, displacing the posterior longitudinal ligament, which may be partially calcified (Fig. 9). In addition, one may find small calcified nodules originating in the ligament itself, or in previously extruded disc material.

In more than half of cases of acute herniated discs calcification of the nucleus pulposus of one or more intervertebral discs is found. This is clearly seen in sagittal radiographs, as areas of hyperdensity, fluffy in appearance, with irregular contours, reaching the posterior border of the disc [31]. When there is a single disc involved this is usually the symptomatic one. When there is more than one calcified, only one of them is the cause of the neurological symptoms. On plain radiographs is quite difficult

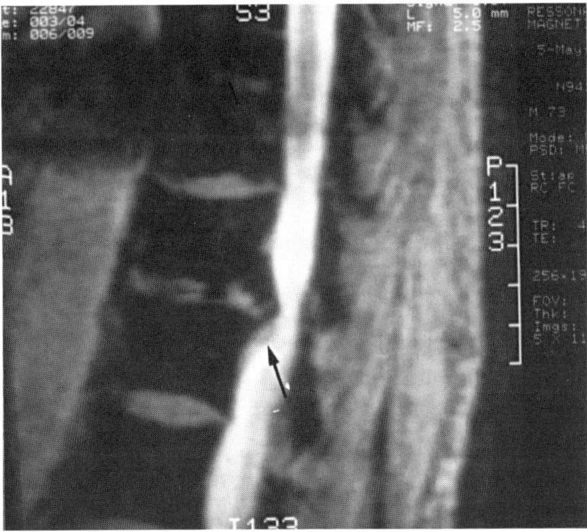

Fig. 9. MR. Sagittal cut. Hard herniated disc at T11–T12 level, in a 73 year old man with a small soft component (arrow)

to evaluate how extensively the canal is compromised by osteophytic spurs, although conventional linear tomography may be of help.

Computerized tomography is most helpful [4], and demonstrates the calcification of the disc material and how it impinges upon the neural structures. In acute cases the intracanalar lesion is spherical, with high density, displacing the cord. Unless sagittal reconstructions are made, extrusions below the disc level are hard to diagnose. In some cases the disc material is isodense with the neural structures, and may be difficult to identify, particularly when the lesion is small and occupies a lateral, paraforaminal position. In such cases the intrathecal injection of contrast may help to demonstrate the lesion.

Magnetic resonance is, of course, the technique of choice, identifying the lesion, its exact location, its characteristics, its relationship with the neural structures, and the presence of migrated fragments.

Surgical Treatment

The initial steps for the transthoracic approach were described previously. Once the thoracic cavity is entered we have to identify correctly the disc space involved. We use the image intensifier and an antero-posterior projection. To avoid possible errors it is preferable to begin counting from the last lumbar segment upwards, and identify the last rib and the T12 vertebra. The disc space is then entered with a needle (G14) which is visualized with fluoroscopy. One can also palpate the ribs below the level of the pathology, and, occasionally, osteophytic spurs are so clearly visible that we have no doubt about the interspace we are aiming at.

Following the correct identification, the collapsed lung and if necessary the diaphragm are gently held with the help of malleable retractors, which are secured with a Gausset retractor. The operating microscope is then brought into the field.

The pleura is then incised, and it is important to call the attention to the fact that the approach is somewhat different for the T6 T7 to the T9 T10 levels, than for the lower thoracic levels. In fact, in the upper segments, the head of the rib articulates with both vertebral bodies, so that the most posterolateral part of the disc cannot be visualized. In this case, the pleural incision should start approximately 4 cm lateral to the foramen, and should run medially to the anterior third of the lateral surface of the vertebral body. It is then enlarged as a T following the longitudinal axis, thus exposing the vertebral bodies. Care is to be taken to save the circumferential vessels, as well as the sympathetic chain, and the splanchnic nerves. To this effect, the incised pleura is carefully lifted and separated from the underlying tissues with blunt dissection. At the T10–T11 and T11–T12 levels the heads of the ribs articulate with the lateral face of the respective vertebral body, 1 to 3 mm below the vertebral plate. Here we prefer to make a double T, the horizontal incisions following the ribs adjacent to the involved space and then completed with a longitudinal cut that goes slightly beyond the exposed vertebral bodies. The pleural flaps are then suspended with 2-0 silk sutures (Fig. 10).

Once the areolar tissue that lies underneath the pleura is exposed, the head of the rib, the neck, and the superior tuberosity are identified with a blunt dissector. The vascular bundle that runs horizontally on top of the vertebral body is followed to the foramen, and the sympathetic chain isolated. Quite often the branch that exits through the foramen, joining the chain slightly below, has to be divided, so that the sympathetic chain is released, and slightly pulled forwards with a vessel loop, thus uncovering the foramen and the head of the rib. Using bipolar coagulation and gentle dissection, the bone structures and the costovertebral and costransverse ligaments are exposed. These are sectioned with a #11 blade, and with a small curette the joint space is identified, and the rib slightly separated from the vertebra. The head of rib and its neck are then removed with rongeurs, thus exposing the joint surfaces of the vertebral bodies and the

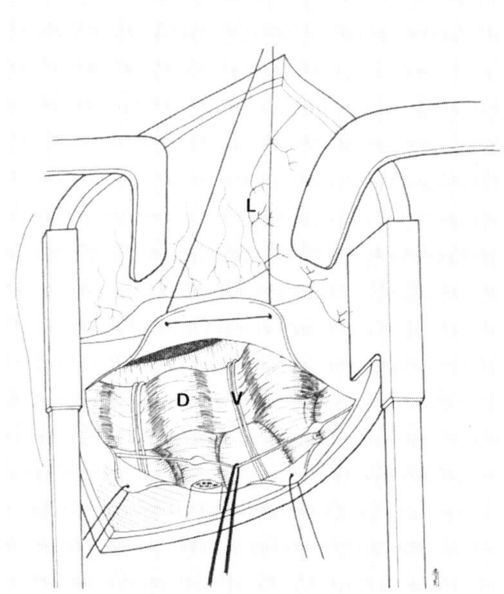

Fig. 10. Transthoracic approach—operative diagram. The lung (*L*) is collapsed, and the pleura widely opened and held by stiches. The sympathetic chain is gently displaced. Note the aorta and segmental vessels (*V*), running along the lateral surface of the vertebral bodies. The prominence of the disc (*D*) is clearly seen

disc. For the lower levels (T10, T11, T12) there is usually no need to resect the rib.

The disc space is easily identified by its lateral bulge and the annulus is incised with a #11 blade. The disc space is entered and the degenerated material removed with small pituitary rongeurs. We usually avoid at this point the most posterior part of the space which is limited by the annulus and the posterior longitudinal ligament, structures which are usually fused. The cartilage plates are curetted. Using high speed drills of various diameters we proceed to enlarge the intervertebral space. We usually begin at the point were the ribs articulate, enlarging it to a square of about 1 cm in size, extending to a depth of 1.5 cm (Fig. 11a, b). Hemostasis is easily achieved with bone wax. With careful drilling, under constant irrigation, we are left with a very thin lamina of bone underneath the posterior longitudinal ligament which can be removed with small curettes (Fig. 12). One should keep in mind the concavity of the posterior surface of the vertebral body. After this maneuvre is completed, the residual annulus and ligament, as well as the posterolateral lip, are removed with the drill or fine Kerrison rongeurs.

Most the acute herniated thoracic discs are extruded and enter the epidural space through a small defect in the ligament. Occasionally, liquefied, whitish material enters back into the space created in the vertebral bodies. With a blunt hook the orifice of the extrusion is identified and carefully enlarged with a fine straight Kerrison rongeur or, alternatively, the ligament is incised starting at the foramen, gently pushing the ligament anteriorly (Fig. 13). The disc material can then be removed with a variety of different instruments (Figs. 14, 15). This step should proceed very cautiously, as the dura might have been transgressed and a fragment of disc is lying in the anterior subarachnoid space.

Some of the larger acute herniations have the configuration of small spheres, which have carved a niche in the anterior surface of the dural sac. Any attempt to pull the dural sleeve should be avoided. One should start by removing the visible component without any manipulation of the dura. As the dura expands slowly, we are then able to inspect it for the presence of any defect through which a small arachnoidocele may prorude. Very rarely there is a small intradural fragment which should be removed. We have not observed a massive intradural extrusion, nor have we found a piece within the subarachnoid space. In such cases, the dural sac may be opened longitudinally, but of course a wider exposure is necessary. Any small dural defect may be sutured or closed with a small piece of muscle secured in place with fibrin glue.

The chronic thoracic discs may result from either a calcification of a previously herniated "soft" disc, or from osteophytic spurs associated with a calcified posterior ligament. As a rule, they are more frequent at the

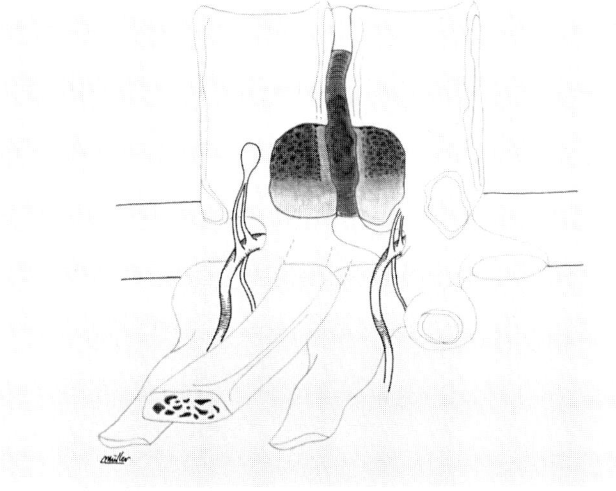

a

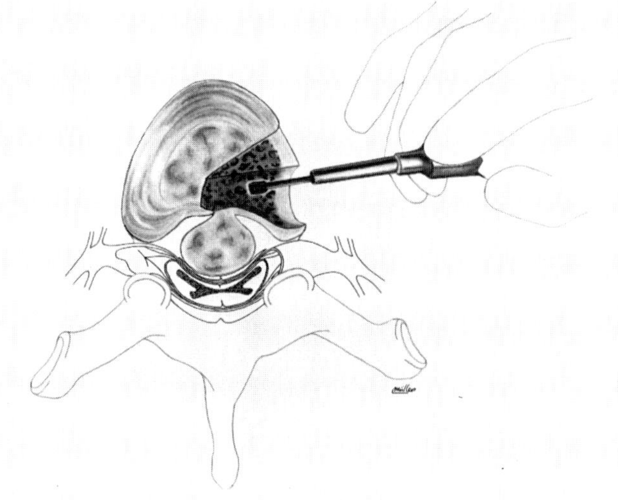

b

Fig. 11. (a, b) After the intersomatic disc is removed the adjacent bodies are drilled down to the posterior cortical bone. The intercostal nerves and rami communicantes are also depicted

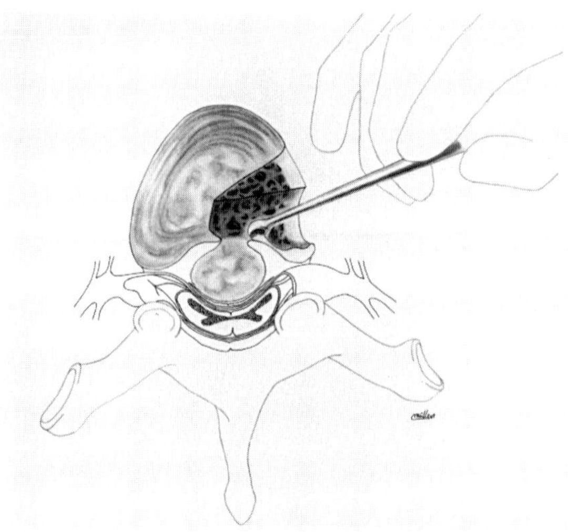

Fig. 12. The posterior cortical bone is being removed with a small curette

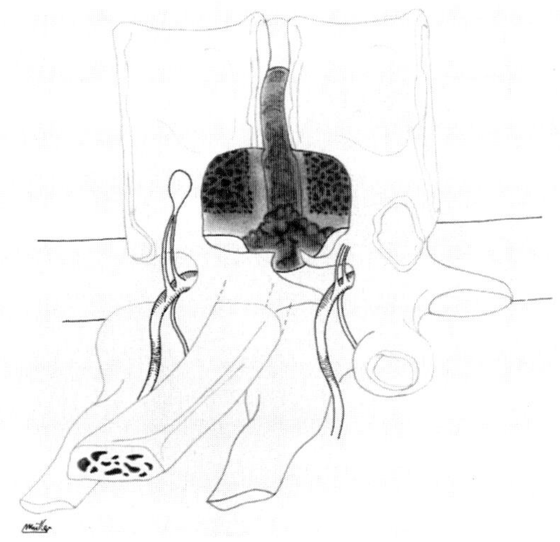

Fig. 13. The extruded fragment comes into view after opening the posterior longitudinal ligament

lower segments, occupy the whole width of the disc space, and occur in
congenitally narrow spines (Fig. 9). Exceptionally, they are eccentric and,
together with calcified, hypertrophic ligamenta flava, may lead to an asymmetrical compression of the neural structures (Fig. 16). We do feel that
the transthoracic route affords a much safer approach to these most
treacherous lesions, and strongly advise against posterior or posterolateral
techniques.

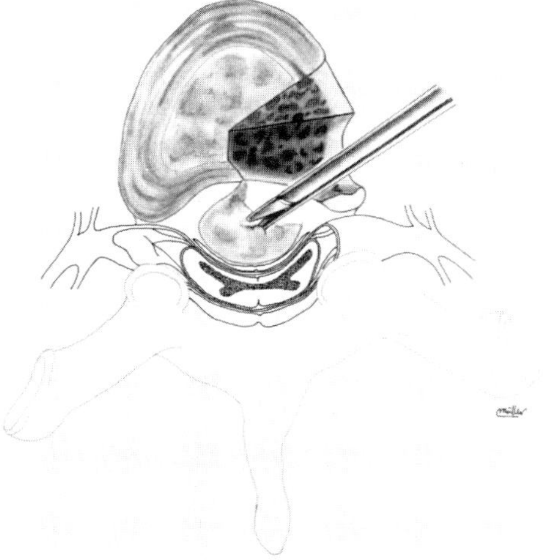

Fig. 14. The extruded piece is removed under direct vision with pituitary rongeur, allowing clear visualization of the anterior dura

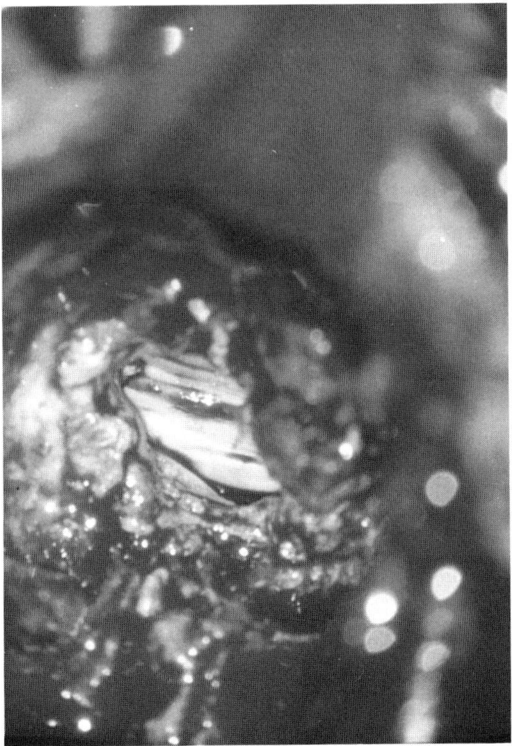

Fig. 15. Transthoracic approach to the T9–T10 disc—operative photograph. The disc has been removed, and the ventral dura is exposed

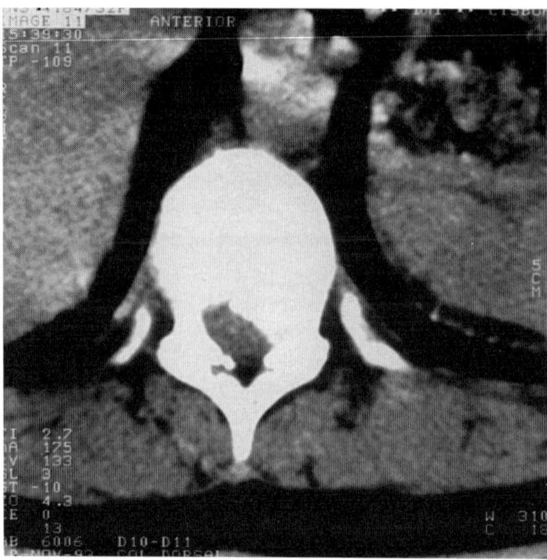

Fig. 16. CT. Horizontal cut at the T10–T11 interspace, showing a hard lateral
herniated disc in a 38 year old woman

Hemostasis of epidural venous plexus is sometimes quite tedious, but
may be achieved with bipolar coagulation and small pieces of surgicel or
microfibrillar collagen.

In two of our cases the herniated fragment migrated caudally, and this
had been clearly visualized by the pre-operative image studies. In such
cases, we had to enlarge our bone window, and remove a larger segment of
the posterior ligament. In most cases, there is no need to perform an
arthrodesis either with autologous bone or instrumentation, and we simply
fill the space in the vertebral bodies with Gelfoam. The edges of the parietal
pleura are then approximated with separate 2/0 Vycril sutures, and the
wound closed as described previously.

Tumours

In the last decade, neoplasms of the spine have become an area of increasing interest. This is due, in part, to the development of image techniques and particularly magnetic resonance, which allow an earlier diagnosis and a detailed evaluation of the topography of the pathological process,
and the introduction of more reliable stabilization techniques, allowing
more radical resections. About 50 to 60% of all tumour pathology of the
spine is localized to the thoracic segment and primary tumours represent
about 5–10%. The diversity of histological types is explained by the multiple cell lines that can be the source of neoplastic proliferation. The

remaining 85–90% of the tumours in this location are secondary or metastatic deposits. The great majority of these originate in the vertebral body, and invade the anterior epidural space, causing neural compression. The incidence of these lesions thus justifies the interest in alternative anterior surgical approaches to the thoracic spine [54, 60, 63, 68, 71 ,76].

Clinical awareness of this pathology has also increased in recent years, and the diagnosis is now made, quite often, in the early stages of the natural history. Pain is the hallmark of these lesions and may start insidiously or, more rarely, quite suddenly. It may be persistent or intermittent, with typical nocturnal exacerbation, or aggravated by motion or certain postures. It may be localized or follow an intercostal irradiation. There may be a local muscle spasm, associated with a scoliotic tilt, or, less often, a conspicuous local deformity. More dramatic presentations, with spontaneous fractures and sudden catastrophic neurological deficits, are less frequent [3, 64].

The neurological signs may initially be absent but, as the disease evolves, a Brown-Séquard syndrome, or a more symmetrical neurological deficit leading to paraplegia, will ultimately develop.

Appropriate image studies are indispensable [5, 18]. In most cases there is a variable degree of bone destruction, and the more malignant the tumour, the larger the erosion [21]. Less aggressive neoplasms will have a geographical pattern with a well defined outer margin. In many instances, there are areas of calcification, which in tumours of cartilaginous origin are flocculent or fleck like, or will have a onion pell pattern in cases of Ewing's sarcoma or osteogenic sarcoma. CT scan and MRI are indispensable to assessment of the degree of bone destruction and compression of the neural structures and the extension of the soft tissue component. Spinal angiography should be performed when a vascular lesion—aneurysmal bone cyst, hemangioma, or certain metastases—is suspected, or if one wants to define better the vascular anatomy of the cord. Pre-operative embolization is extremely helpful in cases of vascular tumours [80].

Benign tumours of the spine include, among others, osteoid osteomas, osteoblastomas, osteochondromas, chondromas, fibromyxochondromas, hemangiomas, eosinophilic granulomas, aneurysmal bone cysts, and giant cell tumours [3, 13, 15, 22, 32, 43, 54, 60, 64]. The majority of these lesions affect mainly the posterior neural arch. The most notable exception is the vertebral hemangioma, also the most common tumour, albeit asymptomatic in the great majority of the cases. Indeed vertebral hemangiomas are present at autopsy in about 10% of cases, and only rarely cause neurological manifestations. This may occur when the lesion expands inside the canal, leads to collapse of the body and subsequent angulation, or bleeds. As a rule, this lesion remains confined to the body, but may extend to the neural arch, or may erode the cortical bone, thus extending to the adjacent paraspinal space or the vertebral canal. Treatment is required in cases of persistent intolerable pain, neurological deficit, or threatening vertebral instability. Low dose radiotherapy, embolization with supraselective angiographic techniques, vertebroplasty either through a transpedicular or a transsomatic approach with various substances, and radical surgery may all be considered [20, 80].

Giant cell tumours or osteoclastomas may cause substantial bone destruction, leading to instability and tend to recur if not excised radically, so that an aggressive surgical strategy is advisable.

As we mentioned before, the remaining benign tumours usually start in the posterior neural arch and are dealt through dorsal or posterolateral approaches. In Fig. 17 we show an exception to this general rule, a giant aneurysmal bone cyst which required a thoracotomy, resection of two ribs, and partial removal of the vertebral body without secondary arthrodesis.

Metastatic tumours are much more frequent than primary malignant neoplasms [6, 7, 12, 17, 24, 47, 54, 69, 77, 82] (Fig. 18). It should be emphasized that one in every five patients with a malignant neoplasm will develop secondary deposits in the spine, and this incidence is even higher in autopsy studies. These bony metastases are the third most frequent location, after lung and liver, and the most common sources are lung, breast, prostate, kidney and thyroid. The lumbar segment is more frequently affected followed by the mid and low thoracic spine. Not infrequently we are dealing with a solitary lesion, confined to the vertebral body, thus

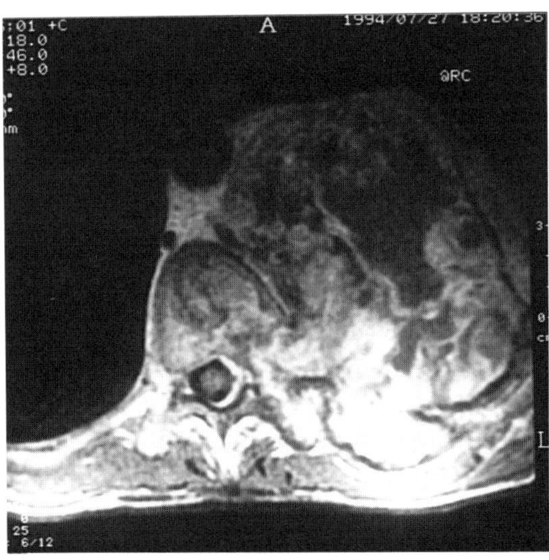

Fig. 17. MR. Horizontal cut. Giant aneurysmal bone cyst destroying the rib, pedicle and part of the body

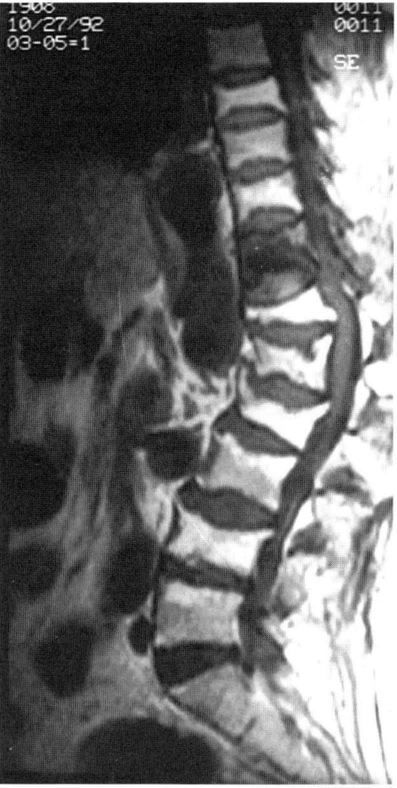

Fig. 18. MR. Sagittal cut. Metastatic collapse of T11 in a patient with severe osteoporosis

justifying aggressive radical excisions [7, 70]. Metastases in the vertebral bodies may remain silent and be detected only by imaging [24]. Collapse of the vertebral body, epidural extension of the lesion and vascular compromise of the cord are responsible for the neurological compromise in these cases [12, 17, 21].

The group of primary malignant tumours includes the plasmocytoma, Ewing's sarcoma, osteogenic sarcoma, chordoma, chondrosarcoma, fibrosarcoma, lymphoma (Hodgkin and non-Hodgkin), and angiosarcoma [71, 77, 78]. Plasmocytomas are probably the most common among the primary malignant tumours [56] (Fig. 19). The spine is involved in approximately 50% of all skeletal lesions. The process usually starts in the vertebral body, extending to the pedicles, and more rarely to the neural arch. As the tumour expands, the cortical bone is eroded, and disappears, and the displaced bony fragments, often seen in metastatic deposits, are not present. The ligaments are displaced by the expanding lesion, which appears as a homogeneous, moderately contrast-enhancing mass in both CT and

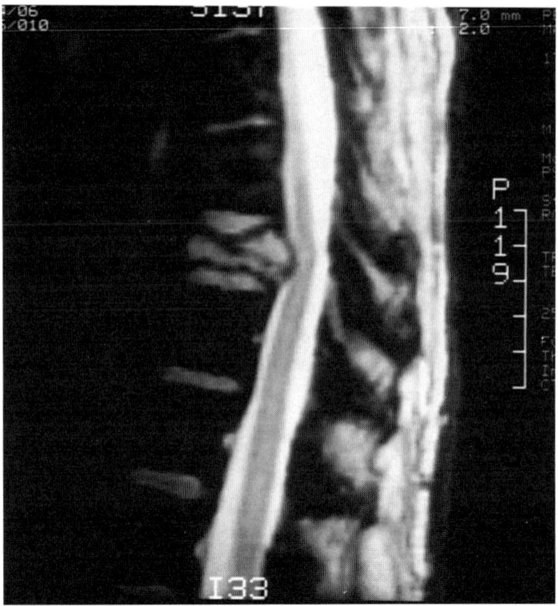

Fig. 19. MR. Sagittal cut. Plasmocytoma of the T9 vertebra. Note the collapse of the body with excellent perservation of the disc

MRI scan. The clinical course may be quite rapid, due to the collapse of the vertebral body, angulation of the spine, or the development of an epidural mass, and may be associated with signs and symptoms of the systemic illness typical of multiple myeloma [23, 33, 41, 56, 74].

Osteosarcomas may occur spontaneously or develop in a patient with Paget's disease, with a previously benign irradiated bone tumour, or other predisposing lesions [15, 46] (Fig. 20). It represents about 6.4% of all primitive tumours of the spine. These are destructive lesions, which may contain areas of calcification. Radical surgical resection is advisable.

Chondrosarcomas seem to show predilection for the thoracic spine. Radiographically, they may present as a pure osteolytic lesion, or with areas of increased density, with a reticular or punctiform appearance. About half of them are confined to the body, while in the other half the joint processes, the pedicles and the neural arch are involved. Radical excision followed by adjunctive therapy is the treatment of choice.

Other less common lesions of mesodermal origin are the fibrosarcomas and the malignant fibrous histiocytomas. They cause variable degrees of local erosion and expansion into the paravertebral space. Ewing's sarcoma occurs in young patients and affects the spinal column in about 5% of the cases. Chemotherapy followed by radical surgery is currently the proposed treatment. Chordomas are exceedingly rare in the thoracic spine and re-

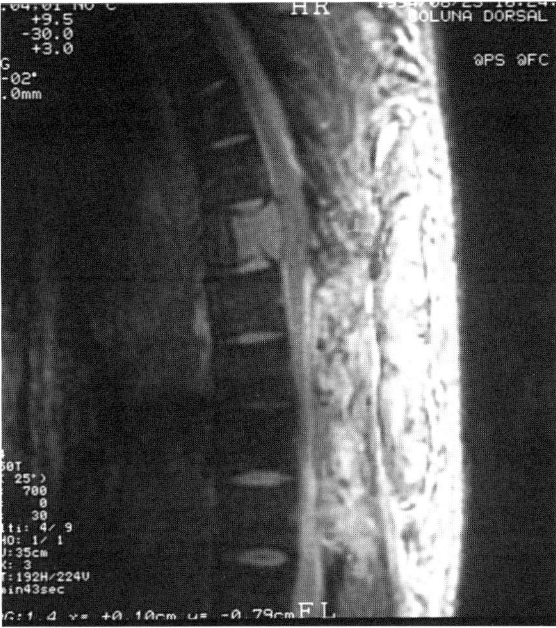

Fig. 20. MR. Sagittal cut. Osteosarcoma in a 44 year old man

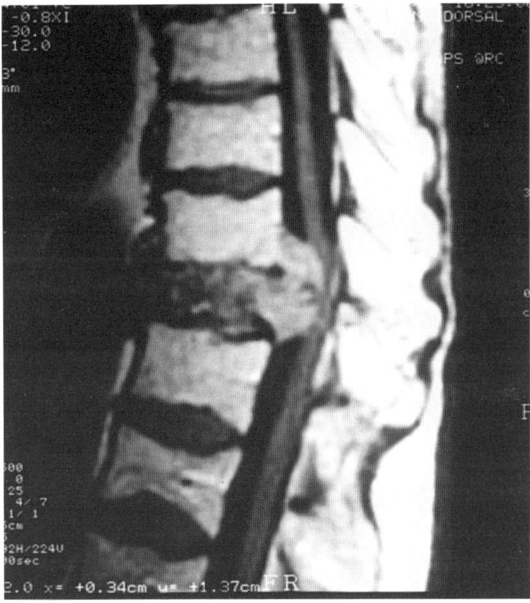

Fig. 21. MR. Sagittal cut. Chordoma of the T7 vertebra. The tumour has caused destruction of the adjacent discs. There is major invasion of the canal following complete destruction of the posterior longitudinal ligament

quire wide surgical resection (Fig. 21). Lymphomas may cause rapid and extensive destruction of one or two adjacent vertebral bodies, with collapse and spinal cord compression. They may also present with an exophytic mass invading the adjacent structures, or grow into the canal. Chemotherapy and/or radiotherapy are mandatory, but surgery may be indicated, particularly when there is instability of the spine.

Surgical Treatment

The surgical approach to the neoplastic lesions of the thoracic spine has to be planned according to the topography of the tumour, and usually has to give wider access than when dealing with degenerative or infectious processes. Thus, it is imperative that the relationship of the tumour with both the prevertebral and intraspinal structures be clearly defined pre-operatively, and that the exposure allows the radical removal of the lesion and, when required, the stabilization of the spinal column [28, 34, 48, 50, 55, 72, 73].

As mentioned before, high thoracic lesions at the T1 and T2 levels, and eventually at C7 and T3, should be approached anteriorly through a cervicosternal approach [39, 51, 75] since transaxillar [39] or suprasternoclavicular techniques do not afford the wide exposure necessary in these cases. The transthoracic transpleural routes are quite adequate for lesions between T3 and T9. The choice between a left or a right approach should be made according to the degree of paravertebral expansion and the topography of the bone pathology (foraminal encroachment, destruction of the adjacent rib, pedicle, or articular facets, or invasion of the retropleural or retrovertebral space). At the T10 to T12 level, and at the thoracolumbar transition (T12 to L2) we prefer a combined thoraco-abdominal approach, opening the pleural cavity [27].

Once the involved segment of the spine is exposed it is usually easy to identify the tumour by the bulge of the parietal pleura. The pleura is coagulated along the posterior segment of the adjacent ribs, for about 3 cm and is incised to the vertebral bodies, and separated from the underlying neoplasm, thus exposing the adjacent foramen and the exit of the neurovascular bundles. Dissection is carried out bluntly over the vertebral bodies and the pleura is suspended with 2.0 silk sutures.

Once the limits of the vertebral lesion are defined, the intact discs above and below are identified and removed with curettes. The vascular bundle is coagulated or ligated with clips and sectioned at the transition between the anterior and lateral aspects of the vertebral body, and pulled gently off the lateral ligaments displaced by the tumour.

When there is a significant exophytic component or major invasion of the paravertebral spaces it is often necessary to start by removing the tumour, before the vertebral body is clearly identified. In such cases, and particularly with large masses, care should be taken to spare the intercostal vessels to prevent ischemia of the neural structures. One can however, divide vessels over the anterolateral surface of the vertebral bodies without problems, if the foraminal branches of the intercostal arteries are spared. We have often resorted to the use of preoperative angiography to obtain the necessary information on the vascular anatomy. Intraoperative monitoring of sensory evoked potentials is also done routinely.

Once the lateral surface of the tumour is exposed, it is coagulated extensively with bipolar cautery. We then open a square window of about 1 cm^2 in size, and try to remove with suction and a variety of rongeurs as much tumour as possible. This is a crucial step, particularly in very vascular or soft tumours. Pre-operative embolization is, of course, most useful. Care should be taken not to put pressure on the posterior surface. We can then achieve a temporary hemostasis, and proceed to delineate the contour of the neoplasm, starting at the level of the intact disc spaces, identifying the foraminal structures, the posterior face of the body and the posterior longitudinal ligament. It may help to remove, partially or totally, the pedicle of the affected vertebra, regardless of whether it is invaded or not, using a small oblique Kerrison rongeur or a microdrill.

Removal continues gradually from the periphery of the tumour to the area initially decompressed. A total excision can thus be achieved. Occasionally, such as in cases of plasmocytoma, it may be possible to leave parts of the vertebral body that appear to be intact.

Greatest care is required to remove any tumour that protrudes into the canal. Manipulations should always be away from the dural sac, and the epidural vessels carefully coagulated, although this may be quite tedious.

The choice of technique to reconstruct the vertebral body depends on the nature, prognosis, and local extension of the tumour, and will be discussed separately.

Infections

We will consider here only the pyogenic spondylitis and spondylodiscitis, including Pott's disease. The indication for an anterior transthoracic approach arises when there is anterior spinal cord compression, a large anterior collection of pus, or the need to proceed with correction of a deformity and stabilization of the spine [2, 29, 30, 40, 57, 58].

It is well established that both tuberculous and non-tuberculous pyogenic infections of the spine are being diagnosed with increasing frequency, due to a number of biologic, immunological and socio-economic factors. Tuberculous spondylitis (Pott's disease) is reappearing even in countries where tuberculosis was thought to have been irradicated. In more ad-

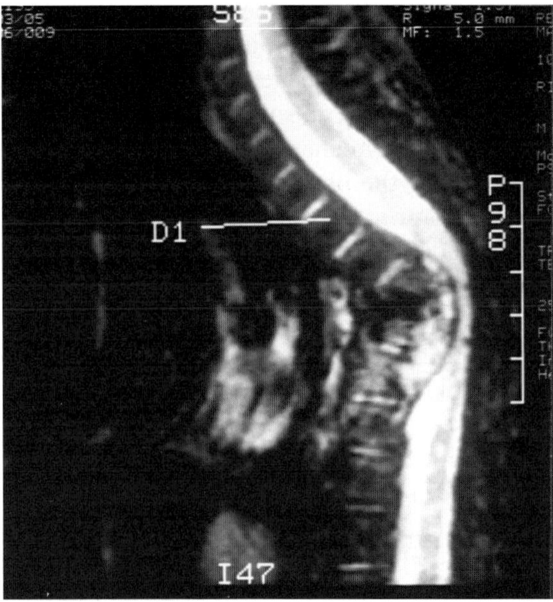

Fig. 22. MR. Sagittal cut. Pott's disease in a two year old boy involving T3 to T5 vertebral bodies. This patient had already undergone a laminectomy at another institution, which contributed to the kyphotic deformity (see Fig. 28 for the post-operative result). The boy had only a mild paraparesis

vanced countries, it affects mainly the elderly, debilitated or immuno-supressed, and we have noted a predominance in the fifth decade, although we have treated a number of young children (Fig. 22). The thoracic segments below D9 are the ones more often involved, but the segment between D4 and D6 is another site of election. The infection usually starts at the anterior part of the vertebral body, and spreads to the adjacent vertebrae often destroying the disc space. The destructive process may affect 3 or 4 vertebrae. Atypical forms include involvement of a single vertebral body—simulating a metastatic deposit—or the posterior arch, and the epidural abscess. The disease may be the result of an acute infec-tion or the reactivation of an old focus in the vertebral body. The disc space is infected quite early, the infection spreading to the bodies above and below, with the development of an abscess with multiple, sequestered fragments, initially contained by the longitudinal ligaments (Fig. 23). As the erosion of the cortical bone advances, the body collapses, and simulta-neously a paravertebral abscess may form (Fig. 24). It is at this stage that the neurological symptoms appear, as the result of several factors: the intraspinal expansion of the abscess, the angulation of the spine with a kyphotic deformity, and, probably, vascular compromise with obstruction

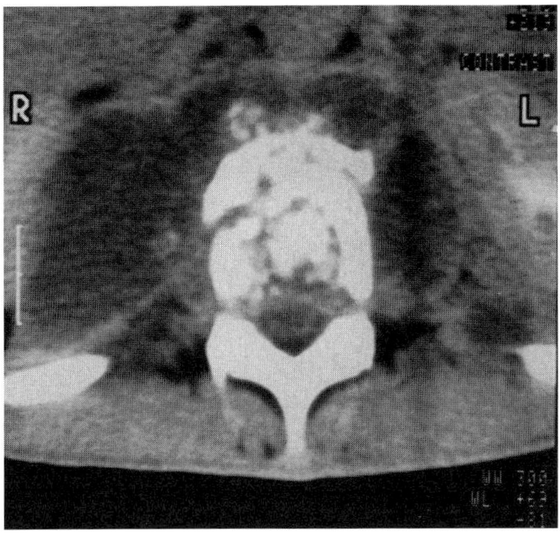

Fig. 23. CT. Horizontal cut. Pott's disease. Extensive destruction of the disc and body with multiple sequestra and a voluminous paravertebral abscess. There is also an anterior epidural purulent collection

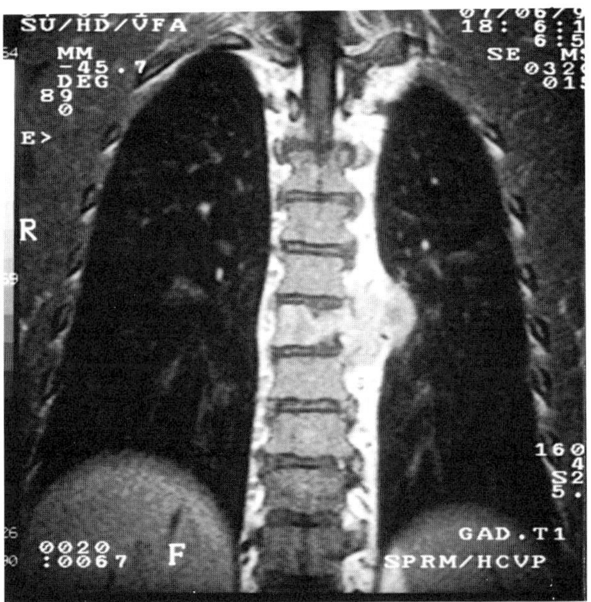

Fig. 24. MR. Coronal cut. Pott's disease. There is a paraspinal abscess at the T7 level with relative sparing of the bone structures. The discs are intact

of the venous drainage. The typical "cold abscess" may displace the parietal pleura, and extend down several segments, reaching the diaphragm, or even below it. More rarely, rupture may occur into the pleural cavity or through the paravertebral muscles, to the subcutaneous space. Clinically, tuberculosis of the spine will present as a subacute or chronic disorder, with non-specific back pain with a mechanical component; only late in the evolution do neurological symptoms appear, quite often associated with systemic signs of infection.

Pyogenic spondylitis or spondylodiscitis of the thoracic spine will rarely cause a severe destructive process that will justify a major surgical intervention to drain the infectious focus and the spine. In contrast, we have observed this in the lumbar spine, where the degree of destruction is similar to Pott's disease. Of interest is that in four patients we have detected a mixed flora where the mycobacterium was found in association with Staphylococcus, Pseudomonas, Serratia and Streptococcus (Fig. 25) Although we have a large experience with Brucella spondylitis we have not yet found the need to approach these infections transthoracically. Staphylococcus aureus (Fig. 26) is the most common offending agent, but Proteus, Escherichia coli and other Enterobacteria may also be isolated. A previous history of sepsis, phlebitis, furunculosis or urinary infection may be present.

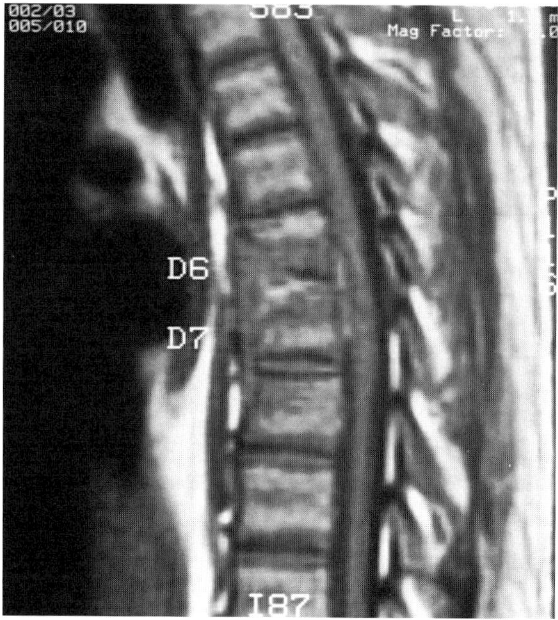

Fig. 25. MR. Sagittal cut. This 25 year old man had a mixed infection—Mycobacterium and Serratia—spondylitis

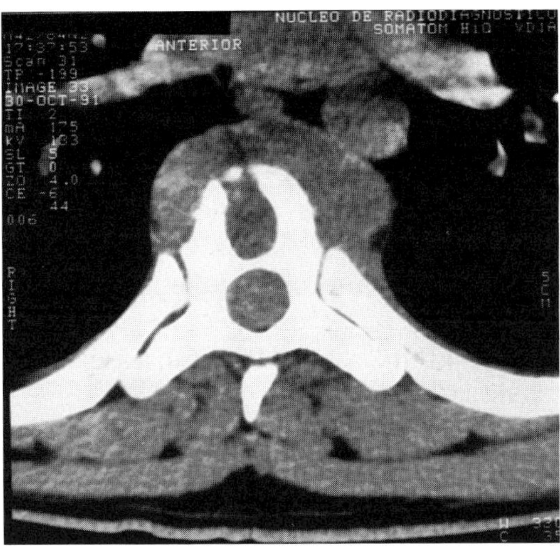

Fig. 26. CT. Horizontal cut. Staphylococcus spondylitis. In this case there was erosion of the body but no sequestra, associated with a circumvertebral abscess

The early diagnosis of a vertebral infection is virtually impossible. At later stages, three to four weeks after the onset, diminution of the disc space, disappearance of the cortical bone of the vertebral plates, and irregularity of the bodies with areas of hypodensity associated with foci of calcification are quite characteristic. Later, reduction in height of the vertebral body and secondary angulation may develop.

CT scan changes in Pott's disease are quite typical. The structure of the vertebral body virtually disappears, with multiple sequestra within heterogeneous areas of hyper and hypodensity, partially contained by the ligaments, and associated with pockets of isodense or slightly hyperdense material. The disc is not identifiable and the spinal canal may appear occupied by bone fragments and purulent material. In most cases the pedicles remain intact. The presence of paraspinal abscesses is pathognomonic. In contrast, in non-tuberculous infections the bone sequestra are smaller, do not project beyond the limit of the cortical bone, even when this has disappeared, and the collection of purulent material in the. paravertebral spaces is not as large. The dural and neural structures are usually better preserved. In these cases, the intravenous injection of contrast may outline a capsule, and the epidural component is more clearly visualized.

All these changes are also clearly documented by MRI, with gadolineum enhancement, which is now the image technique of choice. The volume, extension and compressive effect is well demonstrated, which is of crucial interest in planning the surgical approach.

Surgical Technique

As mentioned before, the major goals of any surgical procedure for an infectious process of the spine are the cleaning of the contaminated area, decompression of the neural structures, and stabilization and correction of the spinal deformity. In some cases, needle biopsy guided by CT is quite useful to confirm the diagnosis.

The levels most commonly affected are the mid and lower thoracic, and the approach has to be planned accordingly. In general, only two adjacent vertebrae are involved, but in cases of Pott's disease, more than two vertebrae may be affected.

The side of approach is dictated by the extension of the purulent collection into the paravertebral spaces, and once the area is exposed the focus of infection is easily identified. We begin by aspirating the purulent material for the appropriate microbiological studies. Some degree of decompression is immediately obtained. The pleura is then coagulated and incised in a T fashion, the horizontal branch following the axis of the spine so that the adjacent vertebral bodies are exposed completely. In tuberculous processes the pleura is often quite thick and adherent to the underlying structures requiring patient blunt and sharp dissection.

The identification of the various anatomical structures is not easy at times, so it may help to start at the disc space following the axis of the neck and head of the rib, which may be resected following division of the ligaments. The residual disc material is removed gradually, and the adjacent, partially destroyed vertebral bodies, are similarly cleaned using small angled and straight curettes and rongeurs. The identification of the pedicle and the limits of the foramen is an important step for the delineation of the posterior surface of the body, but this may not be possible until a large decompression of the vertebral bodies and disc is achieved. The anterior and posterior longitudinal ligaments are useful landmarks, and may be preserved due to their unusual thickness. After a thorough cleaning of the infected area, a thin shell may persist posteriorly. We are always concerned about the possibility of secondary compression, so we like to remove it.

The procedure is usually easier than for neoplastic processes, as the evacuation of pockets of pus, and the removal of bone sequestra or cartilage pieces, may be performed safely. In chronic lesions, however, the existence of areas of sclerotic reaction may require the use of high-speed drills. The curettage of the bone should proceed until a normal looking structure, judged by its aspect, consistency and bleeding characteristics is found. Hemostasis usually does not pose any difficulty.

The cavity thus formed is often quite irregular in contour, so it has to be shaped to accept a bone graft, usually from rib or iliac bone. In tuberculosis and brucellosis we always irrigate the exposed area with warm saline containing rifampicin and we place gelfoam impregnated with antibiotic on the surgical bed.

Once the bone graft is secured the pleura is approximated with reabsorbable sutures and a drain is left in the pleural cavity.

Stabilization Techniques

Whenever more than a half of the volume of a vertebral body is removed, structural reinforcement of the weakened segment is recommended [8]. The transthoracic approach spares the posterior elements, so a "replacement" procedure usually suffices. The material used to fill the gap created by the procedure varies according to the pathology.

When there is a previous deformity and simultaneous compromise of the posterior pillar, as it is often the case in Pott's disease, simultaneous or sequential anterior and posterior stabilization procedures may be required. We will not dwell on the various devices that have been introduced in recent years, as every surgeon seems to have his favourite [14, 20, 26, 28, 42, 50, 55, 70, 79].

In most cases of degenerative disc pathology, the amount of the bone removed is usually limited, and there is no need to place a graft. If we are concerned by the presence of severe osteoporosis we usually place an autologous bone graft, using rib struts (Figs. 27, 28). One or two segments are

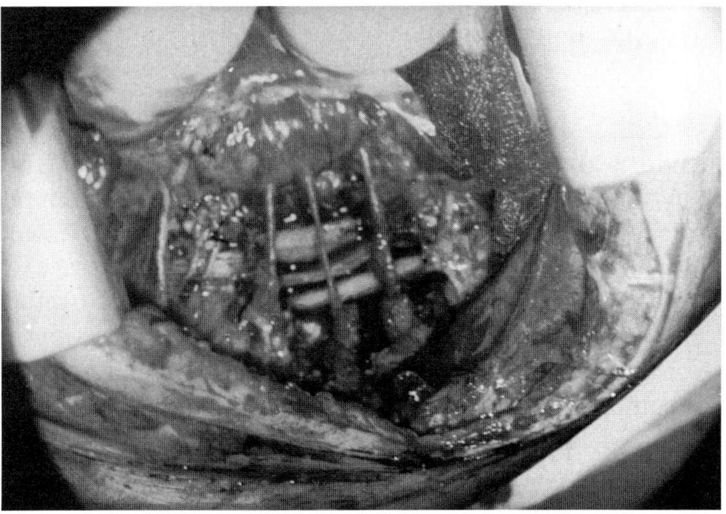

Fig. 27. Intra-operative view of patient depicted in Fig. 22 after removal of the diseased vertebral bodies and correction of the deformity. Rib struts are inserted in the gap. Note the perserved segmental vessels

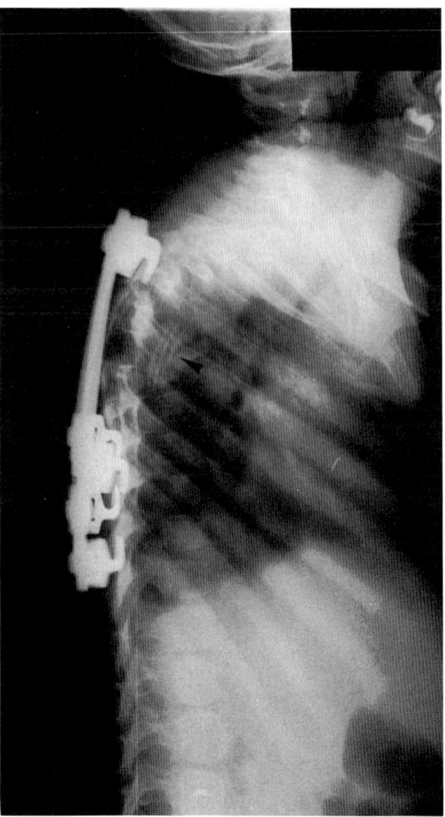

Fig. 28. Post-operative radiograph of patient depicted in Fig. 22. Stabilization was performed anteriorly with rib struts (arrow), and posteriorly with TSRH instrumentation

cut to fit into a groove carved in the lateral wall of the vertebrae. The parietal pleura, sutured on top of the area, will hold the graft in place.

The wide resection required in cases of infection, which often entails the removal of one or two bodies and three discs, makes it necessary to place a graft between the intact bodies. A bundle of rib struts, held together with a titanium or steel wire, may be carefully impacted in the spongy bone of the superior and inferior bodies. We have also used quadrangular blocks fashioned from the iliac crest. This may be held in place with a titanium plate.

When dealing with neoplastic processes in patients with limited prognosis we have used acrylic (methyl-methacrylate) stabilized by Steinmann pins introduced vertically in the adjacent vertebral bodies (Figs. 29, 30).

In benign tumours we again use a block of autologous bone, which is secured with multiperforated lateral plates, which in addition will have a

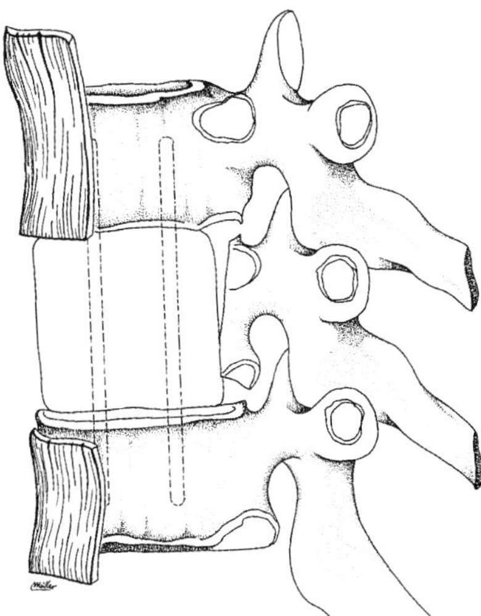

Fig. 29. Stabilization with methyl-metracrylate and Steinmann pins. The posterior longitudinal ligament may be perserved or removed

compressive effect, such as the titanium Z Plates-ATL (Figs. 31, 32). These have the advantage of MR compatibility. We have also used these in association with acrylic in some malignant lesions which run a more protracted course.

Operative Complications

Among the intra-operative complications, probably the most disturbing is the excessive bleeding that may occur, which may increase neurological deficit, not only because of ischemia of the cord, but also because it makes the surgical removal of the offending lesion much more hazardous. Hemorrhage may be due to injury to a major vessel, or come from the lesion itself. We believe that pre-operative angiography is extremely useful, and should be followed by embolization in the case of very vascular tumours. The use of a "cell-saver" device may be of great assistance.

The removal of lesions with an extension into the spinal canal is often difficult, because the normal anatomical landmarks may be obscured by residual pathology or bleeding, and the axis of vision is often not optimal. Neurological deterioration may thus be the result of the rough handling of the neural structures, or of inadequate technique such as the placement of excessive amounts of hemostatic material. Good visualization, meticulous technique and the use of the operative microscope and appropriate instrumentation should minimize these risks. The principle that only after an adequate internal decompression is achieved, should one deal with the edge of the lesion, should be kept in mind.

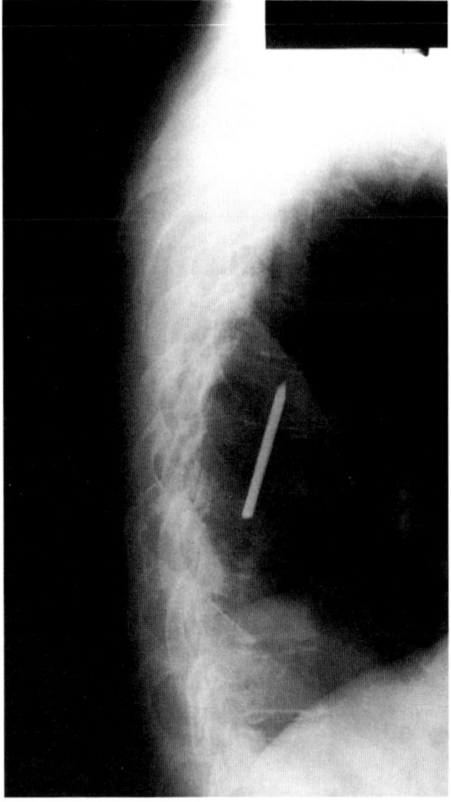

Fig. 30. Stabilization with methyl-metracrylate and Steinmann pins in a patient with metastatic disease

The penetration of the dura either by the pathological process or by the surgeon, may be the source of a CSF leak, and this should be immediately recognized and repaired with sutures or, when not possible, sealed with fragments of muscle and fibrin glue.

Collapse of the lung, if done atraumatically should cause no untoward problems. Pleural laceration should be meticulously repaired. We have had no excessive bleeding into the pleural cavity, as we carefully check the hemostasis in all cases.

Complications from the stabilization procedures should not occur if the graft or prosthetic material is correctly inserted. We favour the use of a corset in the ensuing three to six months, in every case in whom one or more vertebral bodies are removed. The application of the various prosthetic materials may however be hazardous. Adequate protection of the dura and copious irrigation are mandatory when acrylic is used. In addition, placement of pins or plates should be carefully planned. We have not

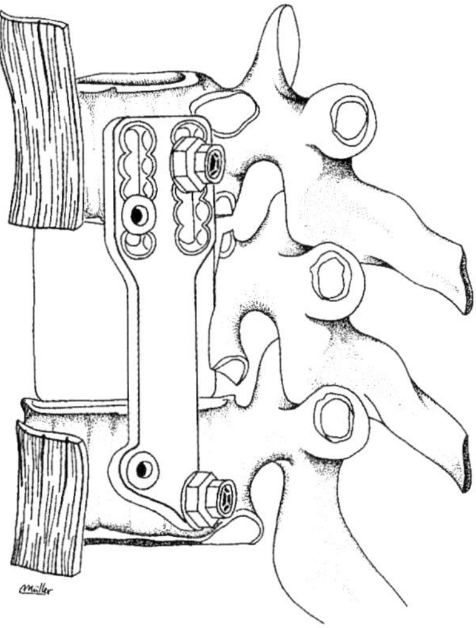

Fig. 31. Stabilization with a lateral plate. Usually four screws are inserted, affording excellent compressive stabilization

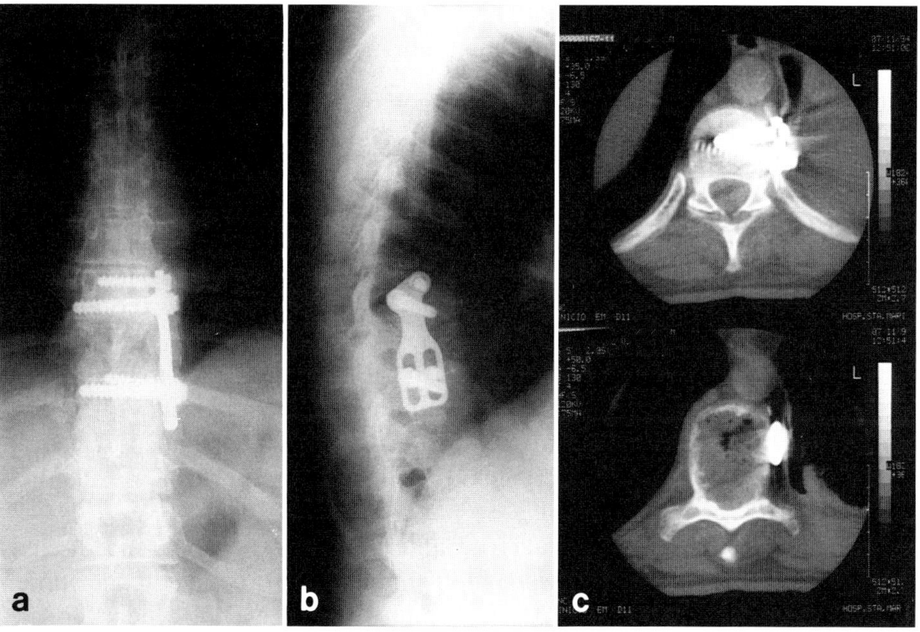

Fig. 32. Stabilization with methyl-metacrylate and a Z plate—ATL. Same patient as Fig. 19. (a) AP radiograph. (b) Lateral radiograph. (c) CT. Horizontal cut. Note that the plate is placed laterally and secured by screws inserted in the intact adjacent vertebral bodies

yet reoperated a patient due to displacement of the prosthesis. In cases of Pott's disease we have observed lateral displacement of the rib segment used in the intersomatic arthrodesis, but no instability or overgrowth of the bone callus was encountered.

During the post-operative period medical complications may supervene, particularly in patients with neoplastic or infectious disorders since they are often quite ill. Poor healing in areas of previous irradiation, metabolic disturbances, respiratory infections, renal insufficiency, and phlebitis should all be promptly recognized and treated [36, 50, 73, 79].

Aggressive antibiotic coverage is particularly important in cases of Pott's disease. Two of our patients died following surgery from disseminated infection. Adequate pre-operative pulmonary care is crucial to prevent subsequent respiratory difficulties.

Despite the fact that a great number of our patients had significant risk factors in about 60 transthoracic approaches, we had only three fatalities— one from pulmonary embolism and two from dissemination of a tuberculous infection.

Conclusions

In conclusion, in our view, the choice of a transthoracic approach for nontraumatic lesions of the spine is based on three main grounds:

1. The need to have a sufficiently wide exposure, with good visualization of the operative area, which allows the removal "in toto" of any pathology which impinges upon the dural sac. This is particularly important in cases in which there is a marked deformity and potential compromise of the neural elements by a lesion emerging from the vertebral body or the disc space.

2. The need to remove simultaneously the intrathoracic expansion of a lesion primarily located in the spinal column, such as happens in infectious processes or voluminous tumours that destroy one or more vertebral bodies, some of which are in close proximity to important mediastinal structures.

3. The need the reconstruct the anterior column, when the disease itself, or the decompressive procedure, threaten the stability of the spine. Anterior stabilization will suffice in many instances but whenever the middle and posterior columns are compromised, posterior stabilization may be necessary, and this can be done simultaneously or in successive interventions.

Following these general principles, we feel that the transthoracic route is particularly suitable for degenerative pathology be it a soft disc, an osteophyte or a calcified ligament, which by their size, texture and localization, make a posterior or posterolateral route hazardous. We will not deny the fact that extrapleural posterolateral approaches in the hands of experienced surgeons, may be equally effective, but we do believe that, when there are no clear medical contraindications, the transpleural approach is a more reliable procedure with very little morbidity.

The increase in incidence of infectious spondylitis, and particularly Pott's disease, makes it mandatory for the neurosurgeon to be familiar with these techniques. Here again, these procedures allow a wide exposure and the achievement of excellent stabilization in a single procedure.

The same statements could be made, "mutatis mutandis", for the neoplastic disorders of the spine, which often develop in the anterior bone elements. We certainly feel much more comfortable in dealing with a vascular neoplasm in a wide field, than when we are confined in our approach.

Some disadvantages should be pointed out, and perhaps the most significant is the need to violate the pleural space, with its attending complications. Good preparation and aggressive postoperative care will minimise the risks. It is also true that whenever there is a component of posterior compression, and when there is a need to stabilize posteriorly, this route cannot be used.

We will emphasize again the necessity of carefully planning the surgery. Whenever possible the exact nature of the pathology should be determined beforehand, and needle biopsy guided by CT may be very valuable. Furthermore, detailed imaging studies, including of course MRI, are indispensable in all cases, and spinal angiography should be used in cases of suspected vascular lesions or when information on the vascular supply of the cord is of interest.

All this anatomic information is of crucial importance, particularly in cases in which the surgeon has to deal with the pathology before reliable anatomic landmarks come into view. Quite often, the surgeon has to move expediously, but without ever losing reference points that are crucial for the safe pursuit of his goals.

It is often assumed that these are difficult procedures, because some of the initial steps are not intrinsically "neurosurgical" in nature, requiring manoeuvres and the use of tools we are not familiar with, and work in the vicinity of structures such as the lung or the aorta which we consider "tiger country". But these are additional reasons why a multidisciplinary approach, particularly when gaining experience with these procedures, is of great importance. The cooperation of a skilled anesthesia team is also required.

It is our opinion that when good clinical sense, careful planning, detailed anatomical knowledge, precise operative technique, and a multidisciplinary team are combined, transthoracic approaches to the spine are safe and quite effective. We strongly believe that we, neurosurgeons, have to be familiar with them, because no other specialty is so well prepared to improve or preserve the neurological function so dramatically threatened in these patients.

Acknowledgements

We want to thank Carlos Cabral, MD and Jorge Mineiro, MD for their skilled surgical collaboration, and Mr. Daniel Müller for his beautiful illustrations.

References

1. Anderson TM, Mansour KA, Miller JI (1993) Thoracic approaches to anterior spinal operations: anterior thoracic approaches. Ann Thorac Surg 55: 1447–1452
2. Antunes JL (1992) Infections of the spine. Acta Neurochir (Wien) 116: 179–186
3. Antunes JL (1991) Tumours of the vertebral column. Neurocirugia 2: 198–201
4. Arce CA, Dohrmann GJ (1985) Thoracic disc herniation. Improved diagnosis with computed tomography scanning and a review of the literature. Surg Neurol 23: 356–361
5. Beltran J, Noto AM, Chakeres DW, *et al* (1987) Tumours of the osseous spine: staging with MR versus CT. Radiology 162: 565–569
6. Birch R, Bonney G, Marshall RW (1990) A surgical approach to the cervicothoracic spine. J Bone Joint Surg (Br) 72: 904–907
7. Black P (1979) Spinal metastasis: current status and recommended guidelines for management. Neurosurgery 5: 726–746
8. Benzel EC (1993) The anatomic basis of spinal instability. Clin Neurosurg 41: 224–241
9. Breslau RC (1983) Transaxillary approach to the upper dorsal spine. In: Watkins RG (ed) Surgical approaches to the spine. Springer, Berlin Heidelberg New York Tokyo, pp 58–63
10. Capener N (1954) The evolution of lateral rachotomy. J Bone Joint Surg (Br) 28: 173–179
11. Cauchoix J, Binet J (1957) Anterior surgical approaches to the spine. Ann R Coll Surg Engl 21: 237–243
12. Chade HO (1976) Metastatic tumours of the spine and spinal cord. In: Vinken PJ, Bruyn GW (eds) Handbook of clinical neurology, vol 20. North Holland, Amsterdam, pp 415–434
13. Clough JR, Priece CHG (1968) Aneurysmal bone cyst. J Bone Joint Surg 50B: 116–127
14. Crockard HA, Ransford AO (1990) Stabilization of the spine. Adv Techn Stand Neurosurg 17: 154–188
15. Dahlin DC, Unni KK (1983) Bone tumours, 4th ed. Thomas, Chicago
16. Dohn DF (1980) Thoracic spinal cord decompression: alternative surgical approaches and basis of choice. Clin Neurosurg 27: 611–623

17. Dunn RC, Kelly WA, Whons RNW, *et al* (1980) Spinal epidural neoplasia. A 15 year review of the results of surgical therapy. J Neurosurg 52: 47–51
18. El-Khoury GY, Moore TE, Kathol MH (1990) Radiology of the thoracic spine. Clin Neurosurg 38: 261–295
19. Fessler RG, Dietze DD, MacMillan M, *et al* (1991) Lateral parascapular extrapleural approach to the upper thoracic spine. J Neurosurg 75: 349–355
20. Feuerman T, Dwan PS, Young RF (1986) Vertebrectomy for treatment of vertebral hemangioma without pre-operative embolization. J Neurosurg 65: 404–406
21. Findlay GFG (1987) The role of vertebral body collapse in the management of malignant spinal cord compression. J Neurol Neurosurg Psychiatry 50: 151–154
22. Friedlaender GE, Southwick WO (1982) Tumours of the spine. In: Rothman RH, Simeone FA (eds) The spine. Saunders, Philadelphia, pp 1037–1039
23. Friedman M, Kim TH, Panahon AM (1976) Spinal cord compression in malignant lymphoma: treatment and results. Cancer 37: 1485–1491
24. Galasko CSB (1982) Mechanisms of lytic and blastic metastatic disease of bone. Clin Orthop 169: 20–27
25. Garrido E (1980) Modified costotransversectomy: a surgical approach to ventrally placed lesions in the thoracic spinal canal. Surg Neurol 13: 109–113
26. Hall DJ, Webb JK (1991) Anterior plate fixation in spine tumour surgery: indications, technique and results. Spine 16 [Suppl 3]: 580–583
27. Heitmiller RF (1988) The left thoracoabdominal incision. Ann Thorac Surg 46: 250–253
28. Hernigou P, Dupar F (1994) Lateral exposure of the cervicothoracic spine for anterior decompression and osteosynthesis. Neurosurgery 35: 1121–1125
29. Hitchon PW, Osenbach RK, Yuh WT, *et al* (1990) Spinal infections. Clin Neurosurg 38: 373–387
30. Hodgson AR, Stock FE, Fang HSY, *et al* (1960) Anterior spinal fusion: the operative approach and pathologic findings in 412 patients with Pott's disease of the spine. Br J Surg 48: 172–178
31. Hulme A (1960) The surgical approach to thoracic intravertebral disc protusions. J Neurol Neurosurg Psychiatry 23: 133–137
32. Janin Y, Epstein JA, Carras R, *et al* (1981) Osteoid osteomas and osteoblastomas of the spine. Neurosurgery 8: 31–38
33. Kempin S, Sundaresan N (1990) Disorders of the spine related to plasma cell dyscrasias. In: Sundaresan N, Schmidek HH, Schiller Al, *et al* (eds) Tumours of the spine. Saunders, Philadelphia, pp 214–225
34. Kittle CF (1988) Which way in? The thoracic incision. Ann Thorac Surg 45: 234
35. Larson SJ, Holst RA, Hemmy DC, *et al* (1976) Lateral extracavitary approach to traumatic lesions of the thoracic and lumbar spine. J Neurosurg 45: 628–637
36. Lazio BE, Staab M, Stamhough JL, *et al* (1993) Latissimus dorsi rupture: an unusual complication of anterior spine surgery. J Spinal Disord 6: 83–86

37. Lesoin F, Jomin M (1985) Posterolateral approach to thoracic disk herniations through transversoarthropediculectomy. Surg Neurol 23: 375–379
38. Lesoin F, Rousseaux M, Autricque A, *et al* (1986) Thoracic disc herniations: evolution on the approach and indications. Acta Neurochir (Wien) 80: 30–34
39. Lesoin F, Thomas CE, Autricque A, *et al* (1986) A transsternal biclavicular approach to the upper thoracic spine. Surg Neurol 26: 253–256
40. Lifeso RM, Harder E, McCorkell SJ (1985) Spinal brucellosis. J Bone Joint Surg 67B: 345–351
41. Loftus CM, Michelsen CB, Rapaport F, *et al* (1983) Management of the plasmocytomas of the spine. Neurosurgery 13: 30–36
42. Lobosky JM, Hitchon P, McDonnell DE (1984) Transthoracic anterolateral decompression for the thoracic spinal lesions. Neurosurgery 14: 26–30
43. MacCarty C, Dahlin D, Doyle J, *et al* (1981) Aneurysmal bone cysts of the neural axis. J Neurosurg 18: 671–677
44. Maiman D, Larson S, Luck E, *et al* (1984) Lateral extracavitary approach to the spine for thoracic disc herniation: report of 23 cases. Neurosurgery 14: 178–182
45. Maiman DJ, Pintar FA (1990) Anatomy and clinical biomechanics of the thoracic spine. Clin Neurosurg 38: 296–324
46. McKenna RJ, Schwinn CP, Soong KY, *et al* (1966) Sarcomata of the osteogenic series; an analysis of 552 cases. J Bone Joint Surg 48A: 1–26
47. Manabe S, Tateishi A, Mitsutoshi A (1989) Surgical treatment of metastatic tumours of the spine. Spine 14: 41–47
48. McElvein RB, Nasca RJ, Durham WL, *et al* (1988) Transthoracic exposure for anterior spinal surgery. Ann Thorac Surg 45: 278–283
49. Mitchell RL (1990) The lateral limited thoracotomy. J Cardiovasc Surg 99: 590–596
50. Moore AJ, Uttley D (1989) Anterior decompression and stabilization of the spine in malignant disease. Neurosurgery 24: 713–717
51. Nazzaro JM, Arbit E, Burt M (1994) "Trap door" exposure of the cervicothoracic junction. Technical notes. J Neurosurg 80: 338–341
52. Patterson RH, Arbit E (1978) A surgical approach through the pedicle to protruded thoracic discs. J Neurosurg 48: 768–772
53. Perot PL, Munro DD (1969) Transthoracic removal of midline thoracic disc protusions causing spinal cord compression. J Neurosurg 31: 452–458
54. Perrin RG, McBroom RJ (1990) Thoracic spine tumours. Clin Neurosurg 38: 353–372
55. Perrin RG, McBroom RJ (1988) Spinal fixation after anterior decompression for symptomatic spinal metastasis. Neurosurgery 22: 324–327
56. Raven RW, Willis RA (1949) Solitary plasmocytoma of the spine. J Bone Joint Surg 31B: 369–375
57. Rezai AR, Lee M, Cooper PR, *et al* (1995) Modern management of spinal tuberculosis. Neurosurgery 36: 87–98
58. Richardson JD, Campbell DL, Grover FL, *et al* (1976) Transthoracic approach for Pott's disease. Ann Thorac Surg 21: 552–556

59. Ridenour TR, Haddad SF, Hitchon PW, *et al* (1993) Herniated thoracic disc: treatment and outcome. J Spinal Disord 6: 218–224
60. Schmorl G, Junghanns H (1975) The human spine in health and disease. Grune and Stratton, New York
61. Sekhar L, Jannetta P (1983) Thoracic disc herniations: operative approaches and results. Neurosurgery 12: 303–305
62. Sicard A (1970) Chirurgie du rachis—voies d'abord des corps vertebraux. In: Sicard A, Mansay L (eds) Nouveau traité de technique chirurgicale, Tome II. Masson et Cie, Paris, pp 44–64
63. Siegal T, Siegal T (1985) Surgical decompression of anterior and posterior malignant epidural tumours compressing the spinal cord: a prospective study. Neurosurgery 17: 424–432
64. Simeone F (1990) Spinal tumours in adults. In: Youmans J (ed) Neurological surgery, 3rd ed. Saunders, Philadelphia, pp 3531–3547
65. Smith TK, Stallone RJ, Yee JM (1979) The thoracic surgeon and anterior spinal surgery. J Thorac Cardiovasc Surg 6: 925–928
66. Steck JC, Dietze DD, Fessler RG (1994) Posterolateral approach to intradural extramedullary thoracic tumours. J Neurosurg 81: 202–205
67. Stillerman CB, Weiss MH (1990) Management of thoracic disc disease. Clin Neurosurg 38: 325–352
68. Sundaresan N, DiGiacinto GV, Hughes JE, *et al* (1991) Treatment of neoplastic spinal cord compression: result of a prospective study. Neurosurgery 29: 645–650
69. Sundaresan N, Krol G, DiGiacinto G, *et al* (1990) Metastatic tumours of the spine. In: Sundaresan N, Schmidek HH, Schiller AL, *et al* (eds) Tumours of the spine: diagnosis and clinical management. Saunders, Philadelphia, pp 279–304
70. Sundaresan N, Galicich JH, Lane JM, *et al* (1985) Treatment of neoplastic epidural cord compresion by vertebral body resection and stabilization. J Neurosurg 63: 676–684
71. Sundaresan N, Krol G, Hughes JEO (1990) Primary malignant tumour of the spine. In: Youmans J (ed) Neurological surgery, 3rd ed. Saunders, Philadelphia, pp 3548–3573
72. Sundaresan N, Shah J, Foley KM, *et al* (1984) An anterior surgical approach to the upper thoracic vertebrae. J Neurosurg 61: 686–690
73. Sundaresan N, Schmidek HH, Schiller AL, *et al* (1990) Tumours of the spine. Diagnosis and clinical management. Saunders, New York
74. Valderama JAF, Bollough PG (1968) Solitary myeloma of the spine. J Bone Joint Surg 50B: 82–90
75. Watkins RG (1983) Surgical approaches to the spine. Springer, Berlin Heidelberg New York Tokyo
76. Weinstein J (1989) Surgical approaches to spine tumours. Orthopaedics 12: 897–905
77. Weinstein J, Malain R (1982) Tumours of the spine. In: Rothman RH, Simeone FA (eds) The spine. Saunders, Philadelphia, pp 1279–1318
78. Weinstein JN, Mclain RF (1987) Primary tumours of the spine. Spine 12: 843–851

79. Westfall SH, Akbarnia BA, Merenda JT, *et al* (1987) Exposure of the anterior
    spine. Technique, complications and results on 85 patients. Am J Surg 154:
    700–704
80. Whiteman MH, Braun IF, Kochan JP (1994) Interventional neuroradiology
    for spine column tumours. In: Rea G (ed) Spine tumours. AANS, Chicago,
    pp 37–58
81. Young S, Karr G, O'Laoire S (1989) Spinal cord compression due to thoracic
    disk herniation: results of microsurgical posterolateral costotransversectomy.
    Br J Neurosurg 3: 31–38
82. Zerick W, Fessler RG, Cahill Dw (1994) Metastatic spine tumours: an
    overview. In: Rea G (ed) Spine tumours. AANS, Chicago, pp 7–22

The Far Lateral Approach to Lumbar Disc Herniations

F. Porchet, H. Fankhauser, and N. de Tribolet

Department of Neurosurgery, University of Lausanne (Switzerland)

With 16 Figures

Contents

Introduction

The diagnosis of extreme lateral lumbar disc herniation (ELLDH) as a cause of lumbar radiculopathy was first described by Abdullah in 1974 [1]. This discal pathology has been recognized for many years as an occasional cause of negative disc exploration and immediate failure of classical disc surgery in sciatica [1, 18, 24, 25, 29, 31, 30, 31, 33, 35, 41]. Only since the introduction of computed tomography (CT) for the diagnosis of lumbar disc disease have the characteristics of ELLDH become fully appreciated [3, 6, 13, 17, 23, 30, 32, 47]. Myelography alone was an insufficient diagnostic tool to detect this specific pathology. With the rapid development of neuroradiologic diagnostic imaging, including magnetic resonance imaging (MRI) [13, 32], recognition of this particular type of lumbar disc disease has increased its incidence, ranging from 0.7% to 11.7% of the total operated herniated discs [1, 22, 24, 45]. In a recent review of our series of patients with lumbar disc disease we found an overall incidence of ELLDH of 5.8% over a period of 8 years [38]. 78% of all ELLDH occured at the L4-L5 and L5-S1 levels, with an almost equal frequency, but the overall incidence of ELLDH per level varied relative to the level of the pathological disc.

Parallel with the improvement in neuroradiological imaging, the surgical techniques were modified with a particular interest in microsurgery [10, 28, 42, 46, 50]. The advantage of microdissection is brilliant coaxial illumination, together with the high magnification it affords, allowing meticulous preparation in the depth with minimal retraction.

Using the microscope, the approach to ELLDH was restudied [11, 12, 14, 16, 21, 27, 43]. In the past, ELLDH were usually reached in the course of an extended interlaminar approach, including total removal of the facet joint [1, 2, 22, 24, 29, 35, 39, 41]. There is justified concern about the removal of a potentially important structure, although single facetectomy does not necessarily lead to gross radiological instability. The enlarged interlaminar approach with medial removal and undermining of the facet joint remains a satisfactory technique to handle some of the far lateral lumbar disc herniations. ELLDH however protrude or extrude in a lateral and cranial direction and come to lie underneath the dorsal root ganglion or even between the upper pedicle and the nerve root. This region is difficult to reach by undermining the facet joint without compromising the strength of the facet.

Before 1985 we performed total facetectomy, but we now favour the lateral transmuscular or paramuscular route as the least invasive possible. This approach has long been known to orthopaedic and neurological surgeons for the aim of intertransverse fusions, excision of occasional disc herniations [44, 49] or ganglionectomies [34].

Clinical Presentation

The clinical presentation of ELLDH has been discussed in several articles [3, 18, 29, 39, 45, 40] but in the earlier literature there is some disagreement concerning the frequency and presentation of ELLDH at different levels. We analysed the clinical signs and symptoms and physical parameters in a retrospective review of the clinical records of 178 cases operated for ELLDH in our department between January 1982 and December 1989

[38]. The overall incidence of ELLDH compared to the number of para-median lumbar disc herniations during the same period of time was calculated as 5.8%. Of a total of 226 disc herniations in the upper lumbar spine (L2-L3 and L3-L4) there were 39 ELLDH with an incidence of 17.2%. In the lower lumbar spine (L4-L5 and L5-S1) we noted 139 ELLDH among a total of 2821 disc herniations which corresponds to an incidence of 4.9%. Assuming that all classical paramedian disc herniations cause a lower root syndrome and all ELLDH cause an upper root syndrome we calculated the probability of an ELLDH for each nerve root syndrome: there was a 4.4% probability of an ELLDH in L5 radiculopathies, a 32.2% probability in L4 radiculopathies and even a 43.6% probability in L3 radiculopathies. The age and sex distribution did not differ from classical disc herniations, with a peak incidence in the sixth decade. The first and dominant clinical sign of radiculopathy was leg pain, either of the sciatic, the femoral or the diffuse type. We did not find a typical pain radiation in the expected dermatomal segment in every case of ELLDH, which is in contrast with the findings of Epstein *et al.* [12], who noted an unequivocal pain distribution in patients with diagnosis of ELLDH. We must emphasize, however, that leg pain in all ELLDH was strictly unilateral.

Observations concerning low back signs and symptoms in patients with ELLDH differ widely from author to author. Abdullah [1] and Osborne [33] described absence of low back pain in their first series. Several other authors [12–14, 18, 22, 24, 45] confirmed the presence of low back signs in the majority of their cases with eventually reproduction of pain by lateral bending towards the side of the lesion. 158 patients out of 178 (88.8%) in our series complained of low back pain of various degrees. It is worth emphasizing however that ELLDH at upper lumbar levels (L2-L3, L3-L4) usually produce no or minor low back signs.

The mechanism of amplified compression of the nerve root caused by nerve traction test remains unchanged in extreme lateral lumbar disc diseases. The femoral nerve traction test should therefore be positive in all ELLDH at or above the level L4-L5 because of upper nerve root compression. Knowledge concerning the relative increased incidence of ELLDH at upper lumbar levels, combined with a positive femoral traction test on physical examination, should raise the degree of suspicion of ELLDH. More than 30% of femoral pain syndromes but less than 5% of sciatica pain syndromes are due to ELLDH.

Motor and sensory deficits do not differ in ELLDH as compared to classical paramedian disc herniation.

There are no specific clinical characteristics of ELLDH but, rather, a clinical constellation including advanced age, pain pattern of the femoral type with positive femoral nerve traction test, minor low back pain and a monoradicular motor deficit of an upper lumbar nerve root.

Anatomical Review

The relationship between bone structures, ligaments, vascular structures, intervertebral discs and nerve roots in the lumbar spine, and especially in the lateral interpedicular compartment (LIPC), is rather complex, but is well described in different texts [4, 5, 7–9, 19, 20, 26, 36, 37, 40, 44]. There exists some confusion about different nomenclatures of this lateral zone: Macnab [25] introduced the term "hidden zone" describing in a general way the concerned region. Terms like intervertebral canal, intervertebral foramen, foraminal zone, subarticular zone, far-out zone or extracanalicular zone are not always well defined. We adopted the term lateral interpedicular compartment (LIPC) since the "intervertebral canal" is a 3 dimensional area demarcated primarily by the pedicles. The entrance and exit of this compartment are "foramina".

Paravertebral Muscles and Fasciae

The paravertebral muscles are covered dorsally by the cross-hatched posterior layer of the thoracolumbar fascia and the longitudinally orientated fibres of the erector spinae aponeurosis (ESA). Between these two layers some adipose tissue can be found (Fig. 1). Immediately ventral to the ESA are the lumbar erector spinae muscles, laterally, and multifidus muscle medially. The lumbar erector spinae are composed of the lumbar fibres of the longissimus thoracis, medially, and the iliocostalis lumborum, laterally. The lumbar fibres of the longissimus and iliocostalis are attached to the transverse processes and their accessory process. The multifidus muscle is attached to the mamillary process and the articular capsule and covers the facet joint (Fig. 2). The ideal surgical approach therefore is transmuscular between the multifidus and the longissimus (Fig. 1). Underneath these major muscles, the smaller intertransversarii mediales and laterales muscles extend between adjacent segments (Fig. 1). The intertransversarius medialis muscle runs from the accessory process and the mamillo-accessory ligament to the next lower mamillary process and covers the isthmic area dorsally (Fig. 2). The intertransversarius lateralis muscle courses between two adjacent transverse processes lateral to the operative exposure. The intertransverse ligament (ITL) is a fascial sheet between the transverse processes just anterior to the intertransverse muscles and has a distinct horizontal and vertical leaf (Figs. 1–3). This ligamental (ITL) tissue ranges from a thin membranous to a thick ligamentous structure sometimes difficult to separate from the intertransversarius lateralis muscle. Immediately ventral to the horizontal and lateral to the vertical leaf lies the psoas muscle (Fig. 1). We distinguish therefore 3 compartments formed by the ITL: antero-laterally the compartment with the psoas and the nerve plexii,

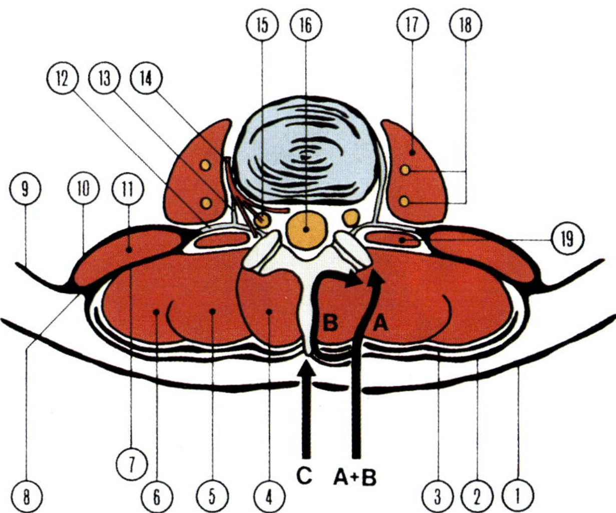

Fig. 1. Axial schematic of the lumbar spine. *1* skin, *2* thoracolumbar fascia, *3* erector spinae aponeurosis, *4* multifidus muscle, *5* longissimus muscle, *6* iliocostalis muscle, *7* middle layer of thoracolumbar fascia, *8* lateral raphe, *9* aponeurosis of m. transversus abdominis, *10* anterior layer of thoracolumbar fascia, *11* quadratus lumborum muscle, *12* horizontal leaf of intertransverse ligament (ITL), *13* vertical leaf of ITL, *14* lumbar artery medial to vertical leaf, *15* emerging nerve, *16* thecal sac, *17* psoas muscle, *18* nerve plexi, *19* intertransverse muscle. The ITL is continous with the anterior and middle layer of the thoracolumbar fascia. *A* transmuscular approach, *B* paramuscular approach, *C* midline approach

antero-medially the lateral interpedicular compartment (LIPC) and adjacent structures, and posteriorly the intertransversarii and posterior paraspinal muscles.

The Lumbar Arteries and Veins

The lumbar arteries arise from the back of the aorta in front of each of the upper four lumbar vertebrae, and pass backwards around the related vertebral body, covered by the tendinous arch of the psoas muscle. Upon reaching the level of the LIPC, the artery divides into several branches to supply the paravertebral muscles, the zygoapophysial joints and eventually the abdominal wall. Opposite the intervertebral foramen, the lumbar artery (LA) courses between the emerging nerve, medially, and the vertical leaf of the ITL, laterally (Fig. 1), and gives off 3 medially directed branches. These are the anterior spinal canal branch, the posterior spinal canal branch and the radicular artery. After giving off these branches, the LA penetrates the horizontal leaf of the ITL along with the accompanying veins. This penetration site is an important landmark for the lateral limit of the surgical

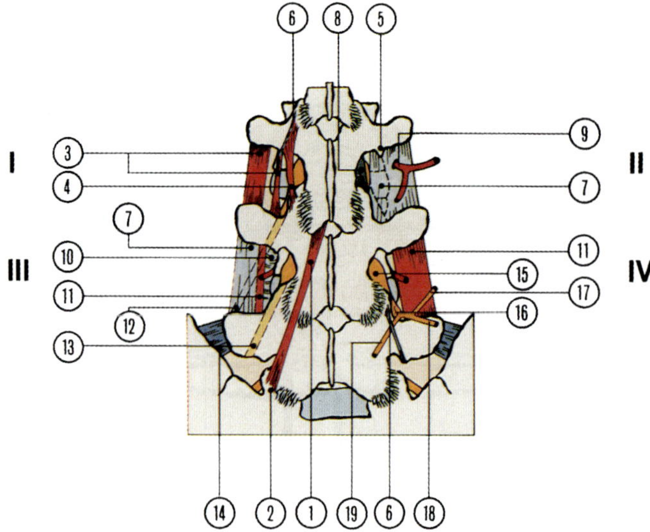

Fig. 2. Posterior view of lumbar spine. *1* multifidus muscle, *2* mamillary process.
I The medial intertransverse m. *4* arises from the accessory process *5*, the mamillo-
accessory "ligament" *6* and the mamillary process, and attaches to the mamillary
process of the vertebra below. The lateral intertransversi *3* course between the
transverse processes (TPs) lateral to the operative exposure. *II 9* Lumbar artery
LA, *7* horizontal leaf of the ITL, *8* lateral border of yellow ligament. *III* After
removal of part of horizontal leaf. LA medial to vertical leaf *10*, exiting dorsal *13*
and ventral *12* rami within the psoas muscle *11*, iliolumbar ligament *14*. *IV* ITL removed. Dorsal root ganglion *15*, dorsal ramus *16* and its lateral *17* intermediate *18*
and medial *19* branches. The medial branch passes beneath the mamillo-accessory
ligament. These branches innervate the paraspinal muscles, posterior vertebral
elements and skin

exposure. Veins accompanying the arteries and rich anastomoses of venous
plexii are found in the intertransverse space.

Lumbar Spinal Nerves and Their Relationship to the LIPC

Each spinal nerve is connected centrally to the spinal cord by a dorsal and
ventral root, separated by a septum but enclosed in a common dural
sheath. Peripherally, at the exit of the LIPC, each spinal nerve divides into
a large ventral ramus and a smaller dorsal ramus. The ventral ramus
courses lateral to the caudal pedicle, where it crosses the vertical leaf of the
ITL to enter the psoas muscle (Figs. 3, 4). The spinal nerve itself is consequently quite short and no longer than the width of the lateral interpedicular compartment in which it lies. The dorsal root ganglion (DRG) is
located within the LIPC immediately inferior to the cranial pedicle, and the
subarachnoid space terminates just proximal to the DRG.

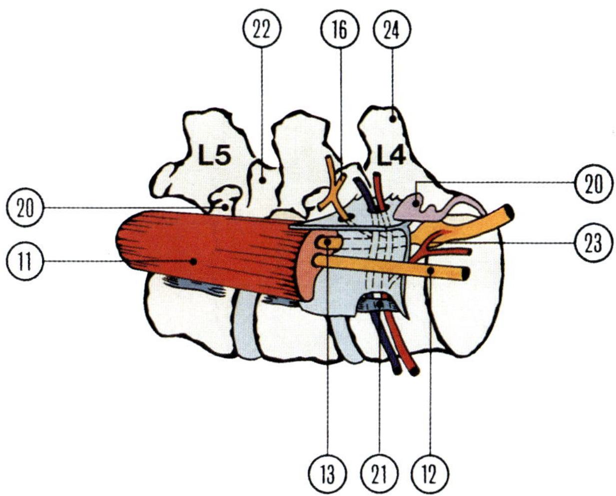

Fig. 3. Right oblique view of lumbar spine. The psoas muscle arises from the anterior aspect of the TPS *20*, lateral aspect of intervertebral disc, and the fibrotendinous arch *21* over the lateral concave side of the body. It courses anterior to the TPs and sacral ala into the pelvis. The exiting ventral ramus is medial to the vertical leaf of the ITL until it pierces it to enter the psoas muscle. The dorsal ramus pierces the horizontal leaf and trifurcates near the junction of the caudal superior articular process *22* and TP. The LA and the lumbar veins pierce the vertical leaf by passing deep to the arch. Radicular artery *23*, spinous process *24*

The relationship between bone structures and lumbar nerves changes in the cranio-caudal direction (Figs. 5, 6A and B). This leads to important alterations in the course of the lumbar nerves. The origins of the pedicles from the vertebral bodies are shifted more antero-laterally from L1 to L5 (Fig. 6B) and simultaneously the TPs originate more anteriorly from the pedicles. The horizontal width of the pedicles increases in the caudal direction due to an increase in their diameter and the change in the orientation of their long axis from vertical at L1 to oblique at L5 (Fig. 6A). The width of the LIPC consequently increases in the caudal direction and in parallel the course and orientation of the spinal nerves change (Figs. 4, 5, 6A). The dimension of the vertebral arch changes also in a cranio-caudal direction: the horizontal part of the arch increases with a simultaneous decrease of the vertical part respectively. An increasing amount of the pars interarticularis (isthmus) extends therefore laterally and covers the medial aspect of the LIPC, which renders the surgical approach more laborious in the lower lumbar spine (Fig. 6B).

In summary the LIPC is more narrow at its entry, delineated rostrally by the pedicle and dorsally by the pars interarticularis of the superior vertebra (isthmus). The exit is much larger and is covered by the facet

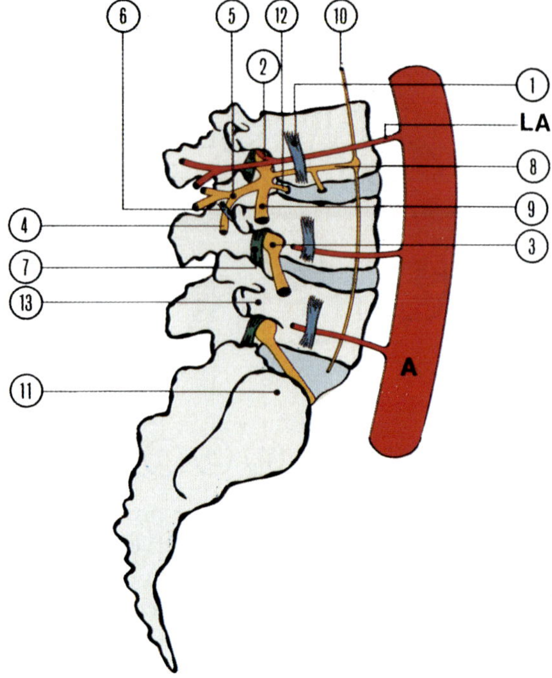

Fig. 4. Lateral view of the lumbar spine. The lumbar artery LA arises from the aorta *A* at L1-L4. Fibrotendinous arcade *1* of psoas muscle, radicular artery *2*, DRG *3*, medial branch *4* of the dorsal ramus *5*, mamillo-accessory ligament *6*, lateral shelf of the yellow ligament *7*. The ramus communicans *8* connects the ventral ramus *9* with the sympathetic chain *10*. The sinuvertebral nerve *12* is a recurrent branch of the ventral ramus which innervates the posterior longitudinal ligament, the intervertebral disc, the adjacent vessels and the anterior dura of the thecal sac. Note the progressively greater contact between the ventral ramus and the lateral aspect of the disc from L3 to L5. The L5 ventral ramus, which wraps around the lateral surface of the L5-S1 disc, is related to the disc medially, to the sacral ala laterally *11* and postero-inferiorly, and to the L5 TP *13* superiorly

joint, i.e. the superior facet of the inferior vertebra. The nervous structures cross the LIPC in its cranial part and the dorsal root ganglion is in contact with the upper pedicle immediately ventral to the isthmus. These elements are the keys to the feasability of the extraforaminal approach to ELLDH.

Indication for Operative Treatment

Indications and contraindications for surgical treatment of ELLDH are the same as for classical disc herniations. The operation is undertaken if signs and symptoms of nerve root compression fail to improve or increase during a conservative treatment course, and if a disc herniation has been

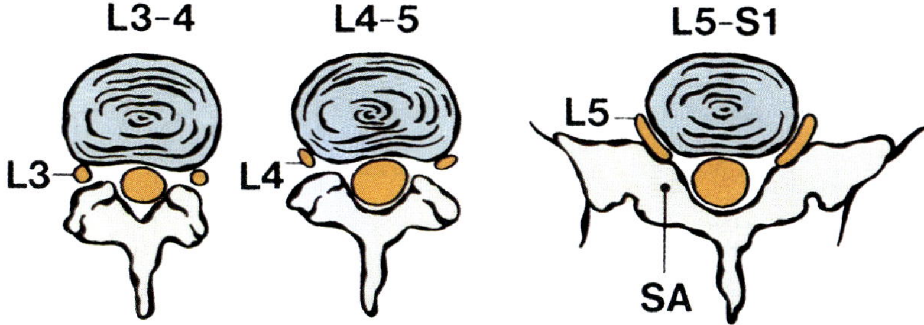

Fig. 5. The changing relationships and courses of the L3, L4 and L5 ventral rami in the axial plane at the level of the intervertebral disc space are demonstrated. Sacral ala *SA*

radiologically demonstrated in a location appropriate to explain the clinical manifestations. We require at least 7 days of strict bed-rest followed by progressive mobilisation with physiotherapy during one month. In the presence of a significant, recent and progressive motor deficit, the operation is scheduled earlier. Symptoms and signs of compression of the cauda equina are an indication for emergency surgical decompression, however an ELLDH cannot be responsible for this clinical presentation. The mere presence of an ELLDH on neuroradiological imaging is not an indication per se. Numerous patients with significant extraforaminal disc herniation on CT will become asymptomatic with conservative treatment [2, 38], probably because of the lesser bony conflict in the far lateral compartment.

The degree of associated degenerative disease has to be taken into account especially in elderly people. Femoral neuropathies in the same age group as a result of non-compressive causes such as diabetes or combined factors have to be excluded.

Preoperative Evaluation

Plain lateral and anteroposterior X-rays are requested. In cases of typical sciatica or femoral type pain syndrome, these X-rays need not to be recent, and they can be replaced by a frontal and lateral scout view on CT scan. In anticipation of disc surgery, the images will be particularly screened for any abnormality of segmentation, forward or lateral slipping, with or without spondylolysis or scoliosis and other types of degenerative pathology. The height of the iliac crests are of special interest in cases with ELLDH at L5-S1 level.

CT scan is requested in patients with a typical history and clinical signs and symptoms of disc disease with compression of one or two nerve roots. To define the origin of a monoradicular syndrome, 3 to 4 mm slices have to be made over at least two consecutive segments. The superior disc has to

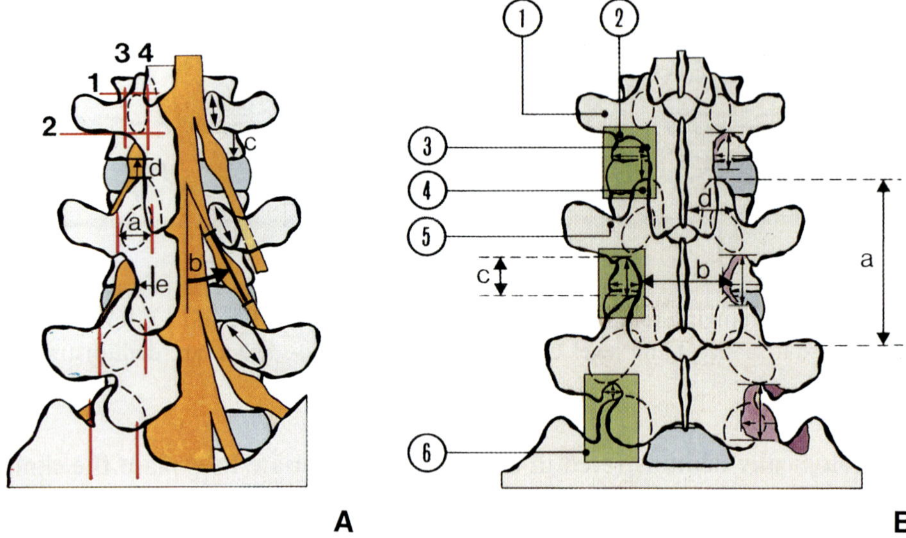

Fig. 6. (A) Lateral interpedicular compartment, pedicle and nerve alterations. The approximate locations of the borders of the pedicle: superior *1* a line drawn perpendicular to the midpoint of the vertical dimension of the facet joint; inferior *2* a line drawn parallel with the inferior aspect of the TP; lateral *3* a line along the lateral aspect of the superior articular process; medial *4* a line drawn perpendicular to midpoint of the transverse dimension of the facet joint. *a* Effective horizontal width of pedicle, *b* angle of the "foraminal" segment of the nerve, *c* distance from the base of TP to the caudal endplate, *d* distance from the superior aspect of the disc space to the superior aspect of the facet joint, *e* amount of isthmus extending lateral to the medial border of LIPC. The changes in the orientation of the long axis of the pedicle are seen on the right. (B) Operative exposure (green boxes) and osseous changes in posterior elements. The osseous landmarks are: the medial aspect of the cranial TP *1*, with its accessory process *2*, the lateral aspect of the isthmus *3* and the supero-lateral portion of the caudal facet joint *4*. For the uncommon infero-lateral ELLDH, the superior aspect of the caudal TP *5* is exposed. The supero-medial aspect of the sacral ala *6* is routinely exposed for L5-S1 ELLDH. Maximal vertical *a* and minimal horizontal dimensions of the posterior arch. Level dependent bone removal (violet)

be included in the scanning because it could carry a classical disc herniation, and the inferior disc could be the origin of an ELLDH. CT scan has therefore to cover the whole length of the spinal segments, in order to detect fragments that have migrated away from the disc, and to cover the entire LIPC where ELLDH most often are located underneath the pedicle.

In most cases CT scan will demonstrate the ELLDH (Fig. 7). The fat in the LIPC is replaced by material of a density of about 80 Hounsfield units which occupies the intervertebral foramen and/or the adjacent extrafor-

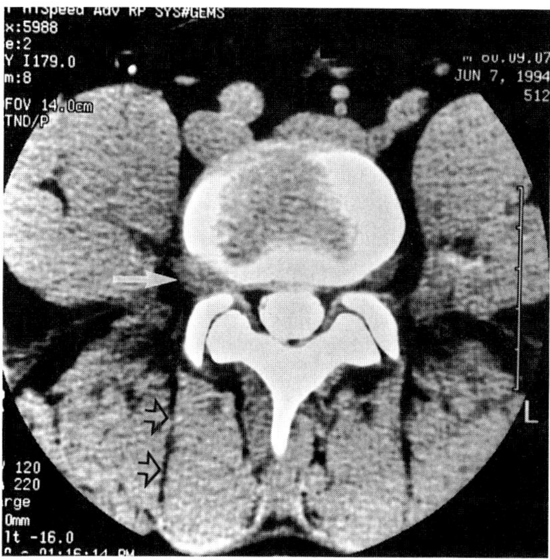

Fig. 7. Computed tomography after myelography showing a right sided extreme lateral lumbar disc herniation at the level L4-L5 (arrow). Slice thickness: 3 mm). The black arrowheads indicate the fibroadipose separation between the multifidus and the longissimus muscles which corresponds with the approximate route for the transmuscular approach

aminal area. The dorsal root ganglion can usually no longer be identified, because the whole area is covered by the disc material. Occasionally it is difficult to distinguish between a small foraminal disc fragment and a large dorsal root ganglion. Unfortunately the comparison of densities is not reliable as sequestrated disc fragments often have a lower attenuation value than intact discs. Several hints may be useful. In our experience an ELLDH has always been visible on at least two consecutive 3 mm slices, most often on three or four slices. The material is usually in contact with the next lower disc, and the latter presents an irregular bulge into the LIPC in contact with the upper pedicle. In exceptional cases, frontal and sagittal reconstructions are necessary to clarify the situation. Ultimately, the clinical presentation will determine whether a surgical exploration is indicated for a doubtful radiological finding. The most common differential diagnoses on CT scan are: connective tissue proliferation around a facet joint in cases with severe degenerative changes and conjoined nerve roots [14]. The latter are usually an incidental, clinically silent finding, requiring no surgical intervention, but occasionally myelography will be necessary to clarify the diagnosis. Less often other differential diagnoses will have to be considered, including benign and malignant tumors, granuloma, synovial and ganglion cysts, nerve root sheath cysts and diverticula, abscesses and parasitic diseases. Enlargement of the intervertebral canal, bone erosion or

destruction, infiltration of the surrounding muscles and enhancement after
i.v. contrast infusion on CT scan should raise doubts about the diagnosis
of ELLDH.

Magnetic resonance imaging (MRI) as the most recent neuroradiological imaging technique reaches actually the same accuracy rate for lumbar
disc disease. Optimal imaging parameters with MRI depend largely on the
clinical problem, the availability and the performance of the machine.
There is always a compromise between numerous factors, including spatial
and contrast resolution, signal-to-noise ratio, slice thickness, field/plane of
view and total examination time.

A typical MRI examination protocol for lumbar disc disease includes
the use of surface-receiving coils, starting with a relatively T1-weighted
sagittal image sequence using the spin echo technique and 5 mm slices. This
is followed by a T1-weighted series of axial images with a single echo and
5 mm slices. Optimal demonstration of anatomical details is given by the
echo with a short TE (< 50 ms) on the sagittal and axial images. Cortical
bone will appear as a black outline of signal void around the cancellous
bone structures which emit an intermediate signal, similar to muscle.
Annulus fibrosus, posterior ligament, dura, CSF and nerve roots are relatively hypointense and do not contrast with cortical bone or osteophytic
spurs, whereas the yellow ligament appears slightly brighter. Fat emits a
very strong signal and is invaluable for a perfect outline of the content of
the spinal canal, LIPC, and paravertebral area. The nucleus pulposus emits
an intermediate signal.

To obtain a T2-weighting in order to increase the signal of CSF and
produce a myelographic image, it is necessary to use a long TR (2.0 s) and
late echo sampling (TE > 60 ms). The standard spin echo sequences are
time consuming and not routinely performed. They have been replaced
by turbo-spin-echo sequences giving almost similar contrast in a shorter
acquisition time or by gradient-echo sequences.

T2-weighting will also increase the signal from the nucleus to a degree
which depends greatly upon its hydration. The distinction between nucleus
and annulus tends to disappear with age. Disc herniation will best be
outlined on T1-weighted images (Fig. 8), whereas disc degeneration and
compression of the dural sac are visible on T2-weighted images.

For ELLDH it is important to examine sagittal screening pictures, not
only in the median plane but also far laterally at the level of the LIPC and
beyond (Fig. 9). Axial images are essential, as they are more useful to
define precisely the lateral position of the herniation with respect to the
intervertebral foramen. Although MRI theoretically provides more information than CT scan, there are pitfalls. The absence of a signal from
cortical bone deprives the surgeon of critical information which is immediately apparent on CT scan. The possible compression of nerve roots by

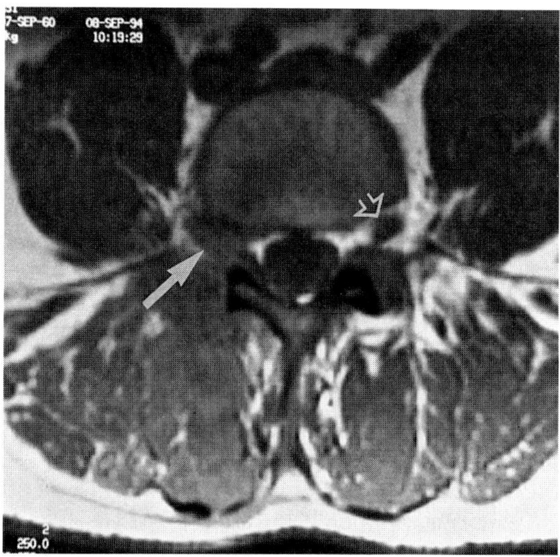

Fig. 8. Transverse T1 weighted spin-echo sequence showing the same extreme lateral lumbar disc herniation as in Fig. 7 (arrow). The left L4 dorsal root ganglion is well seen just underneath the pedicle, surrounded by extraforaminal fat (arrowhead)

osteophytes is also less apparent. Taking into account only practically relevant factors, including image quality, ease of unambiguous interpretation, examination time, availability and expenses, we still consider CT scan as the standard examination for lumbar disc disease.

Myelography is no longer indicated as a primary investigation for typical sciatic or femoral pain syndromes.

According to our findings, the myelography will be strictly normal in approximately one-fourth of cases with ELLDH [14]. The same proportion of examinations will show some associated pathology such as lumbar canal stenosis which will interfere with the radiological evaluation of the region of interest. In at least half of the patients with ELLDH, there will be a uniform abnormality of the superior nerve root sheath which is slightly shortened and enlarged at the level of the pedicle (Fig. 10). This typical manifestation of an ELLDH of the next lower disc can easily be misinterpreted as a lateral recess stenosis or a downward herniation from the upper disc space. A CT scan after myelography will clarify the situation.

Surgical Technique

Selection of Approach

There are two possible approaches to reach the LIPC from the outside: the paramuscular and transmuscular approaches (Fig. 1). The anatomical

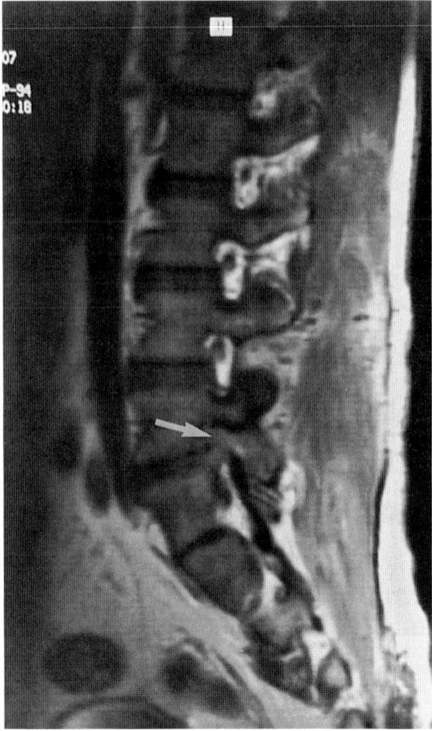

Fig. 9. Sagittal T1 weighted spin-echo sequences of the same patient with L4-L5
ELLDH as in Figs. 7 and 8. The L4 intervertebral canal (arrow) is occluded by
tissue of intermediate signal representing the extraforaminal disc herniation
originating from the intervertebral space L4-L5

landmarks are easier to identify in a paramuscular approach and it is
therefore recommended for surgeons less familiar with this technique. We
usually use a paramuscular approach in obese patients, except for L5-S1
ELLDH, and in cases with paramedian and extreme lateral lumbar disc
herniations on the same level and side. This approach allows simultaneously an extreme lateral and classical paramedian access with preservation
of the pars interarticularis. The skin incision has to be longer in order to
have enough space for retraction of the paravertebral muscles beyond the
facet joint.

All other cases with pure foraminal or extraforaminal herniations are
subjected to the transmuscular approach with the advantage of a shorter
skin incision and less tissue retraction.

Positioning

The position is identical to that for classical hemilaminotomy. Our standard laminectomy frame consists of a solid arcuate support for the chest,

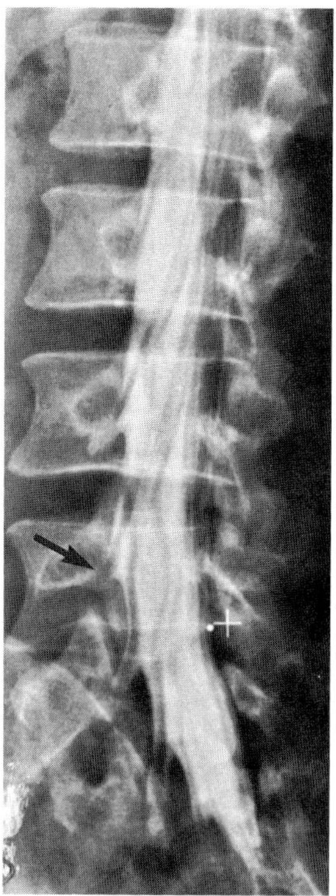

Fig. 10. Myelographic demonstration of the same right sided L4-L5 ELLDH. Note the shortening and enlargement of the L4 nerve root sleeve (arrow) beneath the pedicle of L4

the patient being otherwise positioned on the knees preventing excessive compression of the abdomen.

Prophylaxis of Infection

On the day of operation the patient takes a shower with chlorhexidine. The skin of the operative site is shaved and cleaned with a mixture of alcohol and ether. It is then rubbed for 10 minutes with an iodine liquid surgical soap. Cefazoline 1 g i.v. is administered as a single dose before the skin incision.

Operative Technique of Transmuscular Approach

First the lumbar spinous processes are identified by palpation. A lateral x-ray is taken with a spinal needle placed opposite to the superior spinous process of the concerned segment thus marking the midpoint of the the skin incision. A 5–7 cm longitudinal skin incision is made approximately

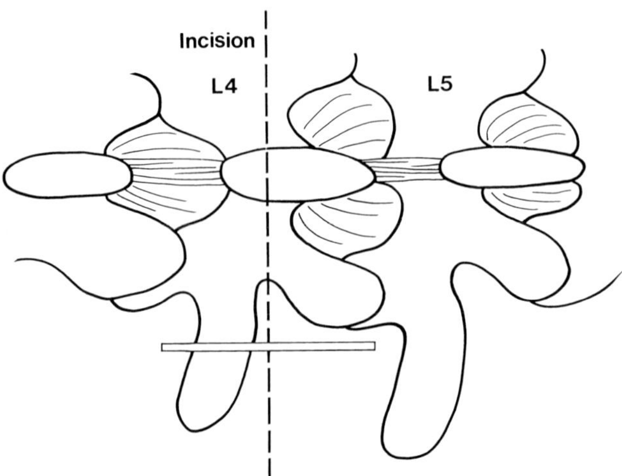

Fig. 11. Skin incision for left L4-L5 ELLDH

5 cm from the midline (Fig. 11). To provide an oblique view, the incision is 1–1.5 cm lateral to the facet joint. Thus its distance from the midline, which can be estimated from the CT scan, increases caudally until the distance becomes limited by the iliac crest at the L5-S1 level. The skin, subcutaneous tissue and posterior layer of the thoracolumbar fascia are incised revealing, through a thin adipose layer, the erector spinae aponeurosis (ESA). The space between the ESA and the erector spinae muscles is dissected with scissors medially and laterally over 3 mm in order to look for a longitudinal separation between the multifidus and the longissimus muscles. A fibrous separation usually identifies its location. If there is no distinct plane the muscle itself is split straight downward using fingers and scissors. The finger tip has to identify the base of the two adjacent transveres processes and the lateral aspect of the facet joint. The plane is enlarged until the osseous landmarks are identified: the medial aspect of the cranial transverse process and the lateral aspect of the isthmus. As soon as these structures are reached, a temporary retractor is installed and a spinal needle is placed in the corner between the base of the lower transverse process and the supero-lateral portion of the caudal facet joint. A lateral X-ray is taken; the needle tip lies exactly opposite the underlying disc. This verification is done in every case to confirm the right level. If one aims too far medially the laminar edges can be confused for the TP's of the intertransverse space.

In the depth of the operative field one can now see a medial and lateral muscle bulk and, protruding from underneath the medial muscles, the extremity of the facet joint and its white capsule. The lateral aspect of the facet joint and the base of the superior transverse process are now cleaned

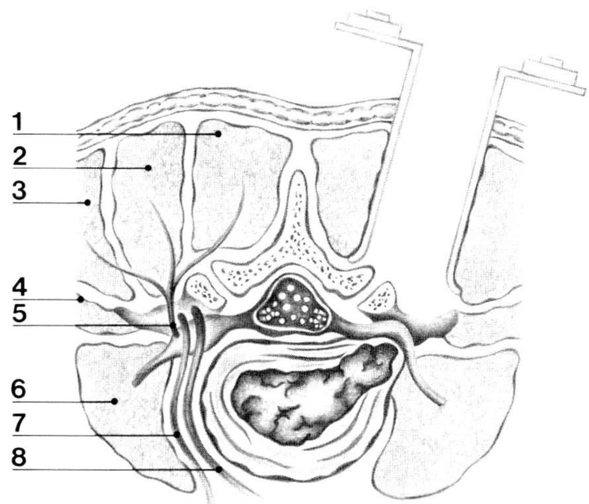

Fig. 12. Cross section at midlumbar level. Self retraining retractor. The medial blade is positioned over the facet joint, the lateral blade at the level of the transverse process. The medial blade is slightly shorter than the lateral blade. This forces the retractor in a moderately oblique direction. *1* multifidus muscle, *2* longissimus muscle, *3* iliocostalis muscle, *4* quadratus lumborum muscle, *5* ramus dorsalis of spinal nerve, *6* psoas muscle, *7* segmental lumbar artery, *8* segmental lumbar vein

from muscular attachments with scissors and periosteal elevator. The latter is useful for elevating the muscles overlying the facet joint and creating for a space for medial retraction. The definitive selfretaining retractor is now inserted (Fig. 12). We use a Caspar type retractor with parallel changeable blades and sharp tips designed for the anterior approach to the cervical spine. The shorter medial blade is placed over the dorsal aspect of the facet joint beneath the partially undermined multifidus. The slighty longer lateral blade is placed in the depth at the level of the transverse processes, somewhere between the longissimus muscle and the intertransverse ligament. If the blades have almost the same length, the step between the transverse process and the dorsum of the facet joint will force the retractor into an optimal oblique position towards the midline.

The operating microscope is now brought into position. If part of the multifidus muscle still obscures the operative view, that portion should be resected. At this stage, the base of the superior transverse process and the lateral apect of the facet joint are further exposed by cutting and removing the attachments of small muscles and ligaments. Bleeding from bone is stopped with bone wax. The accessory process is identified lying just cranial and lateral to the operative target, the isthmus. This structure has to be completely cleaned of all soft tissue to prepare for drilling. It is best to

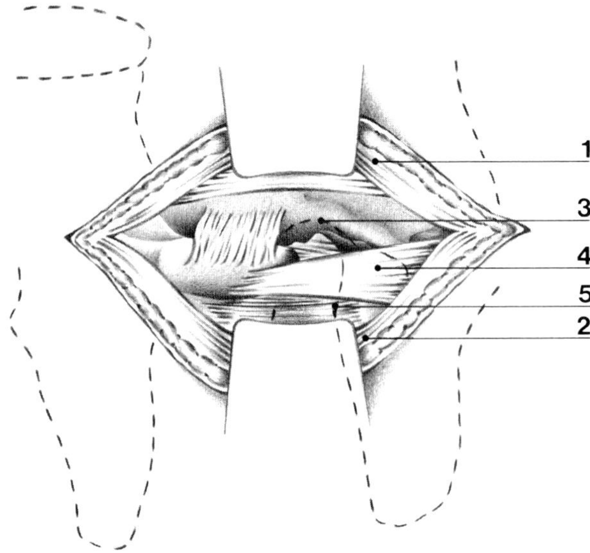

Fig. 13. View after initial placement of the retractor. The medial blade holds the bulk of the multifidus muscle *1* and the lateral blade the bulk of the longissimus muscle *2*. Deeper fibres are still attached to the bony and articular structures. The dotted line delimits the isthmic area *3* which has to be cleared of all soft tissue. Intertransversarius medialis muscle *4*, accessory process *5*

make an arcuate incision around the isthmus starting from the accessory process, cutting down to the bone and delimiting the soft tissue to be removed (Fig. 13). The facet joint capsule itself is preserved as much as possible. The angle between the base of the inferior transverse process and the facet joint is not further dissected. The medial intertransverse muscle is often detached during exposure. Any dissection in the lateral intertransverse space lateral to the lumbar artery and anterior to the horizontal leaf of the ITL (Figs. 1, 3) should be avoided because of the risk of causing troublesome bleeding and nerve injury. Unless CT scan indicates the rare instance of a herniation towards the front of the inferior TP, exposure of the spinal nerve in this area will not be needed. This prevents damage to the main trunk of the dorsal branch of the spinal nerve. In no case should one use punches to tear off soft tissues because the dorsal branch may be caught and avulsed together with part of the spinal nerve or dorsal root ganglion. The use of monopolar cautery in the intertransverse region should also be avoided [50].

A high speed pneumatic or electrical drill is used to remove the lateral part of the isthmus (Fig. 14). Drilling starts at the isthmus and is continued in an arcuate fashion. The amount of bone removal varies widely depending upon degenerative disease: Minimal or no drilling is required in younger

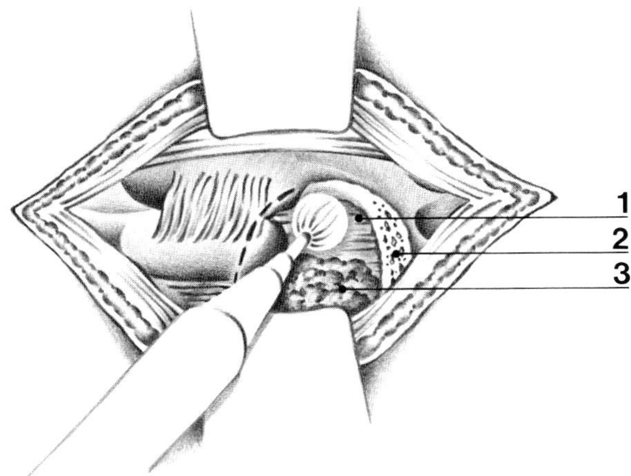

Fig. 14. Drilling of the lateral part of the isthmus and exposure of the ligamentum flavum *1*. Cranially, the drilling reaches the spongiosa of the pedicle *2*. Removal of the latero-superior part of the facet joint down to the area of the crossed line is not routinely performed and is only required to reach the spinal nerve. Extraforaminal fat *3*

people at the level L3-L4 or above; it is more extensive at lower levels, particularly in the presence of a hypertrophic facet joint. Drilling is continued in a medial and superior direction until the extremity of the yellow ligament and the spongiosa of the inferior aspect of the pedicle are reached. There is no landmark of the medial border of LIPC. When drilling, one has to remember that the dorsal root ganglion lies immediately inferior to the cranial pedicle covered by the yellow ligament. The lateral extension of the ligamentum flavum is now removed with a scalpel or microscissors. A variable quantity of foraminal fat is seen, indicating the proximity of the dorsal root ganglion. Resection of the thin layer of adipose tissue invariably discloses the dorsal aspect of the ganglion which appears surprisingly large, owing to the limited exposure and the optical magnification. Frequently, the ganglion will be pushed backwards into the opening by the underlying disc herniation. The pedicle which is just above can be seen or palpated with a hook. The ganglion serves as a new landmark and the next step includes exposure of the medial aspect of the ganglion and its junction with the spinal nerve. This usually means more removal of bone from the isthmus and the cranial part of the facet joint (Fig. 15). The ganglion is kept under visual control to drill or punch supplementary bone. In order to expose the medial aspect of the spinal nerve, the craniolateral part of the facet joint will have to be removed in most cases. The joint capsule at this level should be resected sharply before drilling bone in order to minimize distant tearing of the capsule. This enlargement allows

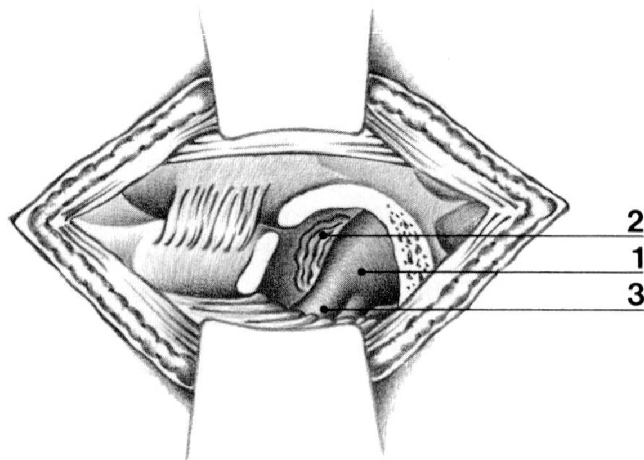

Fig. 15. Exposure of the dorsal root ganglion *1* after resection of the ligamentum flavum and of the extraforaminal fat. The junction with the spinal nerve is visible. A free fragment of herniated disc material is protruding from underneath the ganglion *2*. Spinal nerve *3*

exploration in the depth medial to the spinal nerve. The disc occupies the most caudal part of the opening (Fig. 15). It will therefore be approached obliquely from cranial to prevent extensive sacrifice of the facet joint. Visual inspection and exploration with probes will reveal a bulge extending upwards from the disc. Partially free fragments of herniated disc are most often apparent. As a rule these fragments have migrated upwards and lateral underneath the ganglion or between the pedicle and the spinal nerve. If the visible part of the disc is not ruptured, it is incised with a scalpel together with the overlying posterior longitudinal ligament. During this procedure, the ganglion is pushed laterally with the microsurgical sucker. A nerve root retractor is rarely used. Manipulation of the dorsal root ganglion should be kept to a minimum as it is highly sensitive to mechanical stimulation [5, 21]. The disc itself is now entered with small straight and curved rongeurs and nucleus pulposus tissue is removed as far as possible (Fig. 16). Larger instruments can usually not be used from this lateral approach. No attempt is made to empty completely the disc space. Rongeurs should be used cautiously as the distance to the antero-laterally related vessels is reduced compared to the interlaminar discectomy.

At the end of the operation an exploration with the hook is again performed underneath the ganglion towards the pedicle which should be clearly felt. Often a residual free fragment can be extracted from this location. Lateral dissection along the distal part of the ganglion and the spinal nerve is avoided due to the risk of injuring the radicular artery and the dorsal ramus (Figs. 2, 4). The dorsal ramus is usually not seen, espe-

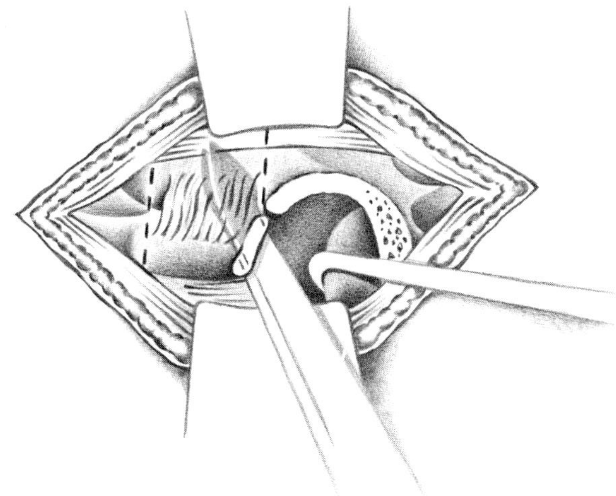

Fig. 16. Removal of the nucleus pulposus. The rongeur reaches the disc under the facet joint from above and lateral. The position of the disc is indicated by dotted lines. The blunt hook explores underneath the ganglion for sequestrated disc fragments

cially in the foraminal type of herniation, as it originates within or adjacent to the distal half of the LIPC.

The operative field is now flooded with saline and observed for any residual haemorrhage. A suction drain is rarely left in place. The aponeurosis of the erector and the thoracolumbar fascia are sutured in one layer with absorbable stiches. The skin and subcutaneous layer are closed separately.

The patient is permitted to ambulate the following day and is usually discharged home 4 days later.

Operative Technique of Paramuscular Approach

The only difference of this approach compared to the former discribed is in its initial part.

The skin incision, 6–8 cm long, is performed 4 cm lateral to the midline at the height of the superior spinous process. The thoracolumbar fascia and the aponeurosis of the erector spinae muscle are sectioned 4 cm from the midline. Dissection underneath the aponeurosis is performed to reach back to the midline. The erector spinae muscles are detached from the spinous processes and retracted far lateral beyond the lateral aspect of the facet joint to localize the base of the adjacent transverse process. Lifting up the muscle mass with a raspiratory permits detachment of the multifidus muscle by cutting with scissors. This will help to minimize damage to the facet joint capsule.

A self-retaining hemilaminectomy retractor is then introduced. The lateral retractor blade is introduced to reach the level of the transverse processes. Vigorous progressive retraction is necessary in order to visualize the isthmus and to prevent a fracture of the spinous process, where the medial blade is positioned. After radiological identification of the isthmus the operation is continued in a manner identical with the transmuscular approach.

Ten Steps of the Transmuscular Approach

1 paramedian skin incision, *2* section of thoracolumbar fascia and aponeurosis of erector spinae, *3* muscle splitting between multifidus and longissimus, *4* identification of the transverse process and facet joint, *5* lateral X-ray, *6* exposure and drilling of the lateral part of isthmus and lower third of the pedicle, *7* resection of yellow ligament, *8* exposure of the dorsal root ganglion and spinal nerve by further bone resection of facet joint, *9* incision and extraction of the disc tissue and possible free disc fragments, *10* final exploration and closure.

Discussion

The ELLDH form a specific category of disc disease. This subgroup is clearly defined by the location of a herniated disc in the lateral interpedicular compartment (LIPC) described previously [44]. ELLDH cannot however be detected on the basis of a clinical examination because there exist no specific clinical characteristics to distinguish them from classical paramedian disc herniation [38]. It is therefore, rather, an anatomical differentiation visualized by neuroradiological methods [3, 13, 18, 23, 30, 31, 40]. This difference is however very important for spinal surgeons, because of its impact on the surgical approach and on spinal stability. We consider that all ELLDH needing surgical treatment should be approached from the lateral side of the isthmus to preserve a maximum of osseous and articular structures.

The craniocaudal changes in the osseous and nervous structures have their influence on the pathophysiology. The upper lumbar nerves (L1-L3) run at an acute angle from the vertical in their brief "intraforaminal" course and are entirely posterior to the lateral aspect of the disc space in their "extraforaminal" course (Figs. 4, 5). In contrast, the L5 nerve root has an oblique, long "intraforaminal" course and in its "extraforaminal" course is intimately related to the lateral aspect of the L5-S1 disc space. Therefore, a purely lateral disc herniation in the upper lumbar spine will be too far anterior to compress the nerve while the same herniation can result in significant compression at the caudal levels (Fig. 5). This anatomical finding supports the clinical impression that herniations which are primarily lateral to the intervertebral disc space more frequently require surgery in the lower than in the upper lumbar spine.

Concerning the technical part of the transmuscular or paramuscular approaches we want to emphasise a few important practical details.

The initial difficulty is getting the right level. It is therefore important to remember that the skin incision must be at least half a segment higher than would be appropriate for a classical interlaminar approach at the same level. Digital palpation after muscle splitting can be misleading especially if one is reaching too superficially and too medially; the laminae can be confused with the transverse processes and the first sacral foramen can be misinterpreted as the narrow L5-S1 intertransverse space. We therefore recommend a perioperative X-ray with a marker at the lateral border of the target isthmus.

The dissection should never be carried ventral to the intertransverse membrane or the level of the transverse process as it can endanger branches of the segmental lumbar arteries and accompanying veins and may lead to bleeding. Even the spinal nerve from the next higher segment can be damaged. Blind monopolar coagulation in this area is therefore also contraindicated. Dissection should be started in the immediate region of the isthmus, starting from the accessory process at the base of the superior transverse process and directed medially. Further lateral exploration should only take place once the dorsal root ganglion has been identified. Deep exploration along the lateral aspect of the ganglion should also be avoided, in order to prevent possible avulsion of the radicular artery at its penetration into the ganglion; ischaemia of the nerve root or the conus medullaris can be the cause of a neurological deficit.

Other minor or major difficulties and complications are not peculiar to the extraforaminal approach and have not been encountered in our practice.

Outcome

The final outcome after discectomy by a far lateral approach for ELLDH is encouraging. Our first analysis of the postoperative results in 62 cases showed an excellent result in 66% of the patients without any residual symptoms. 27.5% of the patients noted a clear improvement with some residual symptoms of back pain. There were 5% without any notable improvement and 1.5% were aggravated [15]. The follow up period ranged from one to three years. Regarding daily activity, we noted that 91% of all operated patients returned to their preoperative activity level. We have operated on more than 250 patients with ELLDH by either the transmuscular or paramuscular approach. The recent unpublished data seem to confirm the initial positive results.

In summary, the use of the lateral approach for ELLDH is a safe and efficient procedure in experienced hands using the microsurgical technique. The major advantage is the minimal surgical approach to preserve a maximum of bony and ligamentous structures, achieving excellent long term results.

Acknowledgement

The authors are grateful to CEMCAV-CHUV responsible for the illustration.

References

1. Abdullah AF, Ditto EW, Byrd EB, Williams R (1974) Extreme lateral lumbar disc herniations: clinical syndrome and special problems of diagnosis. J Neurosurg 41: 229–234
2. Abdullah AF, Wolber PGH, Warfield JR, Gunadi IK (1988) Surgical management of extreme lateral lumbar disc herniations: Review of 138 cases. Neurosurgery 22: 648–653
3. Angtuaco EJC, Holder JC, Boop WC, Binet EF (1984) Computed tomographic discographie in the evaluation of extreme lateral disc herniation. Neurosurgery 14: 350–352
4. Behrsin JF, Briggs CA (1988) Ligaments of the lumbar spine: a review. Surg Radiol Anat 10: 211–219
5. Bogduk N, Twomey LT (1987) Clinical anatomy of the spine. Churchill Livingstone, Edinburgh
6. Bonneville JF, Runge M, Cattin F *et al* (1989) Extraforaminal lumbar disc herniations: CT demonstration of Sharpey's fibers avulsion. Neuroradiology 31: 71–74
7. Bose K, Balasubramaniam P (1984) Nerve root canals of the lumbar spine. Spine: 16–18
8. Crock HV (1981) Normal and pathologic anatomy of the lumbar spine nerve root canals. J Bone Joint Surg 63B: 487–490
9. Dommisse GF (1974) The lood supply of the spinal cord. J Bone Joint Surg 56B: 225–235
10. Ebeling U, Reichenberg W, Reulen HJ (1986) Results of microsurgical lumbar discectomy. Review of 485 patients. Acta Neurochir (Wien) 81: 45–52
11. Ebeling U, Mattle H, Reulen HJ (1990) Extreme lateral lumbar intervertebral disc displacement. Incidence, symptoms and therapy. Nervenarzt 61: 208–212
12. Epstein NE, Epstein JA, Carras R, Hyman RA, Murth Vishnubakhat S (1986) Far lateral lumbar disc herniation: diagnosis and surgical management. Neuroorthopedics 1: 37–44
13. Epstein NE, Epstein JA, Carras R *et al* (1990) Far lateral lumbar disc herniations and associated structural abnormalities. An evaluation in 60 patients of

the comparative value of CT, MRI and myelo-CT in diagnosis and management. Spine 15: 534–539

14. Fankhauser H, de Tribolet N (1987) Extreme lateral lumbar disc herniation. Br J Neurosurg 1: 111–129
15. Fankhauser H, Messikommer A, Robert JP (1994) Ergebnisse der externen Foraminotomie bei extraforaminaler lumbaler Diskushernie. In: Aktuelle Probleme in Chirurgie und Orthopädie, Vol 44: Die Intra- und extraforaminale Diskushernie. Huber, Bern, pp 109–113
16. Fankhauser H, de Tribolet N (1991) Extraforaminal approach for extreme lateral lumbar disc herniation. In: Torrens MJ, Dickson RA (eds) Operative spinal surgery. Churchill Livingstone, Edinburgh, pp 145–160
17. Gado M, Patel J, Hodges FJ (1983) Lateral disc herniation into the lumbar intervertebral foramen: Differential diagnosis. AJNR 4: 598–600
18. Goderski JC, Erickson DL, Seljeskog EL (1984) Extreme lateral disc herniation: diagnosis by computed tomographic scanning. Neurosurgery 14: 549–552
19. Hause M, Kunogi J, Kikuchi S (1989) Classification by position of dorsal root ganglia in the lumbosacral region. Spine 14: 1261–1264
20. Hollinshead WH (1969) anatomy for surgeons; Vol 3: The Back and lower limbs. Harper and Row, New York, pp 172–206
21. Hood RS (1990) surgical approach to far lateral disc herniation. Perspect Neurol Surg 1: 49–55
22. Jackson RP, Glah JJ (1987) Foraminal and extraforaminal disc herniation: Diagnoses and treatment. Spine 12: 577–585
23. Kornberg M (1987) Extreme lateral lumbar disc herniations. clinical syndrome and computed tomographie recognition. Spine 12: 586–589
24. Kurobane Y, Takahashi T, Tajima T et al (1986) Extraforaminal disc herniation. Spine 11: 260–268
25. Macnab I (1971) Negative disc exploration. J Bone Joint Surg 53A: 891–903
26. Macnab I, Dall D (1971) The blood supply of the lumbar spine and its application to the technique of intertransverse lumbar fusion. J Bone Joint Surg 53B: 628–638
27. Maroon JC, Kopitnik TA, Schulhof LA et al (1990) Diagnosis and microsurgical approach to far lateral disc herniation in the lumbar spine. J Neurosurg 72: 378–382
28. Mc Culloch JA (1990) Microsurgical approach to the foraminal herniated nucleus pulposus. In: Williams RW, Mc Culloch JA, Young PH (eds) Microsurgery of the lumbar spine. Aspen, Rockville, ML, pp 187–198
29. Motateanu M, Fankhauser H, Mansouri B et al (1986) La hernie discale lombaire extrêmement latérale. A propos d'une série de 25 cas. Neurochirurgie 32: 74–80
30. Nelson MJ, Gold LH (1983) CT evaluation of intervertebral foraminal lesions with normal or non-diagnostic myelograms. Report of ten cases. Comp Radiol 7: 155–160
31. Novetsky GJ, Berlin L, Epstein AJ, Lobo N, Miller SH (1982) The extraforaminal herniated disc: Detection by computed tomography. AJNR 3: 653–655

32. Osborne AG, Hood RS, Sherry RG (1988) CT/MR spectrum of far lateral and anterior lumbosacral disc herniations. AJNR 9: 775–778
33. Osborne DR, Heinz ER, Bullard D, Friedman A (1984) Role of computed tomography in the radiological evaluation of painful radiculopathy after negative myelography: Foraminal neural entrapment. Neurosurgery 14: 147–153
34. Osgood CP, Dujorny M, Faille R, Abassy M (1975) Microsurgical ganglionectomy for chronic pain syndromes. J Neurosurg 45: 113–115
35. Patrick BS (1975) Extreme lateral ruptures of lumbar intervertebral discs. Surg Neurol 3: 301–304
36. Pedersen HE, Blunck CFJ, Gardner E (1956) The anatomy of lumbosacral posterior rami and menigeal branches of spinal nerves (sinu-vertebral nerves). J Bone Joint Surg 38A: 377–391
37. Pfaundler S, Ebeling U, Reulen HJ (1989) Pedicle origin and intervertebral compartment in the lumbar and upper sacral spine. Acta Neurochir (Wien) 97: 158–165
38. Porchet F, Fankhauser H, de Tribolet N (1994) Extreme lateral lumbar disc herniation: clinical presentation in 178 patents. Acta Neurochir (Wien) 127: 203–209
39. Postacchini F, Montanaro A (1979) Extreme lateral herniations of lumbar discs. Clin Orthop Rel Res 138: 222–227
40. Rauschning W (1987) Normal and pathologic anatomy of the lumbar root canals. Spine 12: 1008–1019
41. Recoules D, Baron JJ, Gayet A, Pouchat JM (1984) La hernie discale lombaire du canal de conjugaison. A propos de 37 hernies opérées. Neurochirurgie 30: 301–307
42. Recoules-Arche D (1985) La chirurgie de la hernie discale du canal de conjugaison. Neurochirurgie 31: 61–64
43. Reulen HJ, Pfaundler S, Ebeling U (1987) The lateral approach to the "extracanalicular" lumbar disc herniation: A technical note. Acta Neurochir (Wien) 84: 64–67
44. Schlesinger SM, Fankhauser H, de Tribolet N (1992) Microsurgical anatomy and operative technique for extreme lateral lumbar disc herniations. Acta Neurochir (Wien) 118: 117–129
45. Siebner HR, Faulhauer K (1990) Frequency and specific surgical management of far lateral lumbar disc herniations. Acta Neurochir (Wien) 105: 124–131
46. Williams RW (1978) microlumbar discectomy. Spine 3: 175–181
47. Williams AL, Haugthon VM, Daniels DL, Thornton RS (1982) CT recognition of lateral lumbar disk herniation. AJR 139: 345–47
48. Wiltse LL (1973) The paraspinal sacrospinalis-splitting approach to the lumbar spine. Clin Orthop 91: 48–57
49. Wiltse LL, Bateman JG, Hutchinson RH (1968) The paraspinal sacrospinalis-splitting approach to the lumbar spine. J Bone Joint Surg 50A: 919
50. Zindrick MR, Wiltse LL, Rauschning W (1987) Disc herniations lateral to the intervertebral foramen. In: White AH, Ray CD (eds) Lumbar spine surgery. Techniques and complications. Mosby, St Louis, pp 195–207

Subject Index

Springer Neurosurgery

Advances and Technical
Standards in Neurosurgery

Volume 22

Edited by L. Symon (Editor-in-Chief), L. Calliauw,
F. Cohadon, J. Lobo Antunes, F. Loew, H. Nornes, E. Pásztor,
J. D. Pickard, A. J. Strong, M. G. Yaşargil

1995. 149 partly coloured figures. XV, 381 pages.
Cloth DM 328,–, öS 2295,–
ISBN 3-211-82634-3

Contents:
Advances: K. Thapar, K. Kovacs, E. R. Laws:
The Classification and Molecular Biology
of Pituitary Adenomas.
J. P. Chirossel, G. Vanneuville, J. G. Passagia, J. Chazal,
Ch. Coillard, J. J. Favre, J. M. Garcier, J. Tonetti, M. Guillot:
Biomechanics and Classification
of Traumatic Lesions of the Spine.
U. Ebeling, H.-J. Reulen: Space-Occupying Lesions
of the Sensori-Motor Region.
Technical Standards: J. P. Houtteville: The Surgery
of Cavernomas Both Supra-Tentorial and Infra-Tentorial.
A. Bricolo, S. Turazzi: Surgery for Gliomas
and Other Mass Lesions of the Brainstem.
M. Samii, C. Matthies: Hearing Preservation in Acoustic
Tumour Surgery.

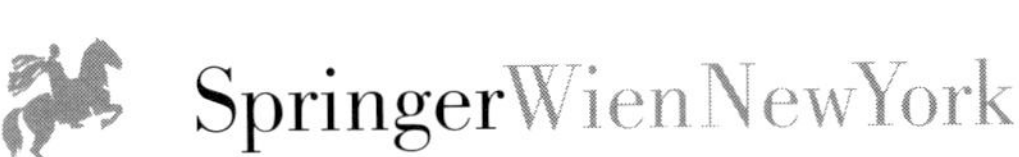

Springer Wien New York

P.O.Box 89, A-1201 Wien • New York, NY 10010, 175 Fifth Avenue
Heidelberger Platz 3, D-14197 Berlin • Tokyo 113, 3-13, Hongo 3-chome, Bunkyo-ku

SpringerNeurosurgery

Advances and Technical
Standards in Neurosurgery

Volume 21

Edited by L. Symon (Editor-in-Chief), L. Calliauw,
F. Cohadon, J. Lobo Antunes, F. Loew, H. Nornes, E. Pásztor,
J. D. Pickard, A. J. Strong, M. G. Yaşargil

1994. 69 partly coloured figures. XIII, 286 pages.
Cloth DM 251,–, öS 1756,–
ISBN 3-211-82482-0

Contents:
Advances: G. J. Pilkington, P. L. Lantos: Biological Markers
for Tumours of the Brain.
C. Daumas-Duport: Histoprognosis of Gliomas.
F. Cohadon: Brain Protection.
Technical Standards: S. F. Ciricillo, M. L. Rosenblum:
AIDS and the Neurosurgeon – an Update.
M. Choux, G. Lena, L. Genitori, M. Foroutan: The Surgery
of Occult Spinal Dysraphism.
P. Cosyns, J. Caemaert, W. Haaijman, C. van Veelen,
J. Gybels, J. van Manen, J. Ceha: Functional Stereotactic
Neurosurgery for Psychiatric Disorders: an Experience
in Belgium and The Netherlands.

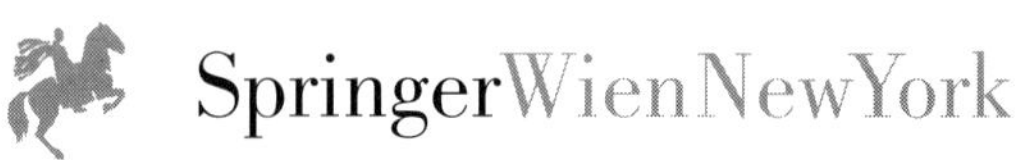

SpringerWienNewYork

P.O.Box 89, A-1201 Wien • New York, NY 10010, 175 Fifth Avenue
Heidelberger Platz 3, D-14197 Berlin • Tokyo 113, 3-13, Hongo 3-chome, Bunkyo-ku